A Practical Guide to

Human Cancer Genetics

Third edition

The third edition of this very successful book provides a comprehensive and practical guide to the diagnosis and management of inherited disorders conferring susceptibility to cancer. Issues discussed include risk assessment, genetic counselling, predictive testing and organisation of a cancer genetics service. A full reference list gives access to background literature.

With completely up-to-date molecular information, screening guidelines and management advice, this new edition will provide geneticists and clinicians in all disciplines with an invaluable resource for screening, managing and advising patients.

Shirley V. Hodgson is Professor of Cancer Genetics at St Georges Hospital, London (SW Thames Regional Genetics Service). Previously she had directed the Family Cancer Clinic at St Mark's Hospital, and the Cancer Genetics Service at Guy's Hospital.

William D. Foulkes is Associate Professor of Medicine, Human Genetics and Oncology, and Director of the Program in Cancer Genetics, McGill University, Montreal, Quebec, Canada. He directs clinical cancer genetics services at the McGill University Health Centre and at the Sir M.B. Davis-Jewish General Hospital, Montreal.

Charis Eng is Chairman and Director of the Cleveland Clinic Genomic Medicine Institute and Professor and Vice Chairman of the Department of Genetics at Case Western Reserve University, Cleveland, Ohio, USA. She is a Doris Duke Distinguished Clinical Scientist and is also Senior Editor of Cancer Research.

Eamonn R. Maher is Professor of Medical Genetics and Head of Section of Medical and Molecular Genetics at the University of Birmingham School of Medicine's Institute of Biomedical Research and Honorary Consultant in Medical Genetics at West Midlands Region Genetics Service, Birmingham, UK. He is also Editor-in-Chief of the *Journal of Medical Genetics*.

A Practical Guide to

Human Cancer Genetics

Third edition

Shirley Hodgson

William Foulkes

Charis Eng

Eamonn Maher

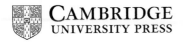

CAMBRIDGE
UNIVERSITY PRESS

CAMBRIDGE UNIVERSITY PRESS
Cambridge, New York, Melbourne, Madrid, Cape Town, Singapore, São Paulo

Cambridge University Press
The Edinburgh Building, Cambridge CB2 2RU, UK

Published in the United States of America by Cambridge University Press, New York

www.cambridge.org
Information on this title: www.cambridge.org/9780521685634

First published 2007

Printed in the United Kingdom at the University Press, Cambridge

A catalogue record for this publication is available from the British Library

ISBN-13 978-0-521-68563-4 paperback
ISBN-10 0-521-68563-X paperback

Contents

We dedicate this book to our families and to Suzanna

Preface

There continue to be rapid developments in our understanding of inherited cancer susceptibility and the importance of this for the translation of this knowledge into clinical practice. There appear to be differences in the pathways of carcinogenesis in individuals with differing inherited cancer susceptibility syndromes, which can lead to improved strategies for surveillance and management. Gene expression studies have revolutionised our understanding of many aspects of this. An example is that carriers of germline mutations in *BRCA1* have breast cancers which have particular pathological characteristics which in turn can indicate an increased chance that a woman carries a *BRCA1* mutation, and the fact that specific types of DNA damage repair is deficient in *BRCA1* mutation carriers has led to the suggestion that cancers in such women may be more sensitive to treatment with cisplatin and PARP inhibitors. The discovery of *MYH* (MUTYH)-associated polyposis has highlighted the presence of autosomal recessive inheritance patterns for conditions originally thought to be predominantly autosomal dominant conditions.

The development of sensitive counselling practices for predictive testing for cancer predisposing conditions, taking into account the psychosocial, insurance and ethical issues has been continued as part of ongoing collaboration between different genetic centres and professionals. The inclusion of nurses and genetic counsellors in the development of cancer genetics services is essential, and training is taking this into account. This edition of the book has taken into account the new developments in our understanding of many aspects of cancer genetics, from molecular pathways and new gene discoveries to the translation of this knowledge into the development of a rapidly increasing service, now forming almost half of the workload of clinical genetics services. The text has been substantially revised and rewritten, and we now have two other authors from the USA and Canada to enhance the international perspective of the book. Cancer genetics is now appreciated by an increasing number of different specialists as our understanding of clinical cancer susceptibility is becoming appreciated in many different specialities. We believe that the popularity of previous editions of this book will be improved upon and this edition will be of increasing importance for clinicians, laboratory scientists and healthcare professionals who are faced with the ever-enlarging demand for knowledge of familial cancer risks.

Acknowledgements

The authors are grateful to Dr Julia Newton-Bishop for her contribution to the section on skin cancers, and to Dr Marc Tischkowitz for his help with the section on Fanconi anaemia. They would also like to thank Professor Gareth Evans, Professor Diana Eccles, Professor Doug Easton and Dr Ros Eeles for contributing tables, Professor C. Mathew and Professor Gill Birch for comments, and Professor Patrick Morrison for illustrations.

Part one

Cancer genetic counselling

Genetic counselling in a familial cancer clinic

Demand for cancer risk assessment based upon the estimation of the genetic component of cancer risk to a given individual is increasing rapidly. This is both because of increased public awareness of the genetic aspects of cancer susceptibility and as a result of requests from clinicians for evaluation of their patients so that appropriate surveillance protocols can be developed. Risk prediction in common cancers is based upon careful assessment of family history of cancer and cancer-related syndromes, and a personal history and examination (where appropriate). The genetic risk assessment requires confirmation of the diagnosis in affected relatives whenever possible. Close links with oncologists and clinicians involved in organising surveillance are essential. Joint or multidisciplinary clinics may be appropriate in this context and, ideally, a cancer family clinic network should be developed throughout each region, province or state. Education for primary care physicians should be provided, with guidelines for appropriate referrals.

Genetic counsellors and trained genetic nurses may be increasingly employed in specialised familial cancer clinics in cancer units and primary care, with the remit of assessing empiric cancer risks on the basis of personal and family histories, and to arrange surveillance protocols (audited centrally, if possible) for individuals at moderately increased risk, reassure those at low risk, and refer those at high risk of a genetic cancer susceptibility to the Regional Genetics Centre for further evaluation, advice and management. In most countries, training in genetic counselling involves completing a 2-year Masters in Genetic Counselling, followed by Board Certification and membership of a national association (in the USA, the National Association of Genetic Counselors, and in Canada, the Canadian Association of Genetic Counsellors).

Unfortunately, in the USA and elsewhere, the demand for trained genetic counsellors exceeds the supply, and currently, it may be impractical to deploy such trained individuals in primary care or even oncology clinics. As a result, the identification of potential genetic risk for cancer is dependent on the busy primary care physician or other caregiver or in certain institutions, based on uniform questionnaires. Once a patient or family with potential genetic risk is identified, they are referred to either "high-risk clinics" or preferably clinical cancer genetics programmes, often housed in Comprehensive Cancer Centres or in broad multi-disciplinary institutes or centres of human genetics.

Most risk estimates for cancer development are empiric, based on the likelihood of a genetic contribution in the individual, and this risk estimate is increased if the individual has several affected relations on the same side to the family with the same or related cancers, multiple or early onset cancers, and if the proband has clinical features of a cancer-predisposing condition or has previously had cancer or a cancer precursor lesion (Table 1.1) (Hampel et al., 2004; Garber and Offit, 2005). Computer programs for the assessment of risk and the provision of referral guidelines have been developed and can be adapted for use in primary care or even potentially by the families themselves. Various methods of assessing the risk of an inherited *BRCA1/2* mutation being present in a family have been developed, one of the most well known being BRCAPRO, that uses a Bayesian probabilistic model (Berry et al., 2002). Several non-computer based models, such as LAMBDA (which is currently restricted to the Ashkenazim) (Apicella et al., 2003) and the Evans model (Evans et al., 2004), may outperform BRCAPRO, particularly in families with other cancers such as pancreas, prostate and peritoneal. Other programs can also predict the risk of

Table 1.1. *Family history of cancer (example guidelines for referrals)*

There are a number of questions that can help when trying to assess an individual's risk. Ask about:

(a) Age of onset in the family member
(b) Site of primary tumour
(c) Number of affected members in the family
(d) Multiple primary tumours

Possible indications for referrals

Personal history

- Early onset of cancer (e.g. breast cancer diagnosed <40 years, colorectal cancer diagnosed <45 years, etc.)
- Multiple primary cancers

Family history

- Three close relatives (same side of family) with cancer of the same or syndromically related type (e.g. breast and ovarian or colorectal and uterine)
- Two close relatives (same side of family) with cancer, or the same or related type, with at least one affected under 50 years
- One first-degree relative (mother or sister) with early onset cancer (e.g. breast cancer) diagnosed <40 years, or <45 years if colorectal cancer
- One first-degree relative with multiple primary cancers
- Two or more relatives with uncommon cancers (e.g. sarcomas, gliomas, pancreatic cancer, glioma haemangioblastomas, etc.)

breast cancer accurately, taking into account unmeasured polygenic factors (Antoniou et al., 2004). In this appropriately named BOADICEA model, the predicted mutation probabilities and cancer risks in individuals with a family history of breast and/or ovarian cancer can differ markedly from those predicted by other models. When available as a computer package, this model is likely to become commonly used in the clinic setting.

How should risk be communicated? Risk can be given as a risk of developing cancer per year, or before a certain age, or as an overall life-time risk relative to the population risk. It is appropriate to compare this risk with the background population risk (relative risk).

Screening and preventative options should be discussed, with consideration of the possibility of false-positive and false-negative results of tests and the anxiety these could cause. It should be made clear that no surveillance programme is totally reliable and it should be emphasised that the individual being screened should never ignore abnormal symptoms between screening procedures. The current state of knowledge about the efficacy of screening should be fully explained. The individual's perception of his or her cancer risk should be assessed, as should its possible effects on the individual's health–behaviour.

Predictive testing is only possible in a small proportion of families in which the germline cancer-predisposition mutation can be defined in an affected relative. Family history indicators of a high probability of finding such a mutation are given in the relevant chapters. Such guidelines are not inflexible and depend on continuing studies to determine the prevalence of mutations in different family history types.

To identify a pathogenic germline mutation in a family, it is usual to start testing with blood (or tissue) from an affected relative, following informed consent for testing for a genetic cancer susceptibility. This requires an initial approach from the individual being counselled, and some family and confidentiality problems can arise over this. It is essential that the affected relative understands the nature of the tests being performed, the possible emotional impact of a positive (or a negative) result, and its relevance in terms of insurance and employment. In many cases, such a test will not reveal a pathogenic mutation, and in a few cases a sequence change may be detected in a cancer-predisposing gene, whose significance may not be clear, necessitating further tests to clarify this (e.g. does the mutation segregate with the disease in the family?). In such cases it is important to have a rapport with the tested individual, with a clear plan for the communication of results. When a pathogenic mutation is detected in a family in which the significance of inheriting such a mutation is understood, and when the affected individuals agree to the release of their results to the family, predictive testing can be offered to at-risk individuals in that family.

Such testing optimally requires two pre-test counselling interviews at which issues such as the emotional, family, insurance and employment implications of any result can be discussed prior to testing, and the mode of inheritance and penetrance of the mutation can be explained.

Often, it is advisable to have an interval of up to 3 months between these sessions, along the lines of predictive testing for Huntingdon disease. The results should be given as soon as possible after they are available to the person tested, with a confidant (unless some prior arrangement to deliver the results to a third party has been made). Such a protocol may be varied with relevance to the condition tested for and the attitude and knowledge of the individual undertaking the test. Individuals with a low-risk result may also require post-test support because they can suffer from "survivor guilt". High-risk individuals should be offered psychological support and a clear protocol for surveillance and possible preventive action.

Insurance issues are still being debated. Currently in the UK, for policies under £500 000 for mortgages on a residence, the family history of the person whose life is insured is taken into account, but the results of genetic tests are not. There is currently a moratorium for requesting genetic test results in the UK until 2011. In the USA, despite fear and much debate, to our knowledge, no individual has been discriminated against by health insurance companies or third party payors because of visiting a cancer family clinic or because of a gene test result to date. There are US federal and often state laws protecting against discrimination by group health insurance. In a group health insurance, such protection prevents individuals from being dropped or individual premiums from being raised. Often however individuals who are self-insured can be open to such theoretical discrimination by third party health insurers.

It should not be forgotten that individuals who have had cancer may be psychologically affected by the news that they have an inherited cancer susceptibility, particularly as it may indicate that they have an increased risk for metachronous cancers, and that they could be "responsible" for handing on the susceptibility to their children – a potential cause of profound guilt feelings. A positive result also has management implications, such as the option of bilateral prophylactic mastectomy when treating unilateral breast cancer in a *BRCA1* or *BRCA2* mutation carrier.

Patient support groups are well established for familial cancer conditions such as retinoblastoma, but broader-based support groups are being developed, for breast and ovarian cancer susceptibility particularly, initiated both from the starting point of those originally concerned with support for cancer sufferers, and from genetic interest groups concerned with promoting the welfare of families with a broad spectrum of genetic disorders. "Carrier clinics" specifically for carriers of mutations in *BRCA1* and *BRCA2* are being set up, so that specific management issues can be addressed, and patient support groups are arising from these. For example, a charity, the Hereditary Breast and Ovarian Cancer Foundation (http://www.hboc.ca/) is devoted entirely to women at increased genetic risk of breast and ovarian cancer.

Since it is generally true that early diagnosis of cancer improves outcome, it would seem appropriate to identify individuals at increased cancer risk, and offer them surveillance and/or prophylactic measures to reduce their risk of cancer, or provide the earliest possible stage at diagnosis. However, the development of such a system requires robust audit of outcomes, both in terms of cancer morbidity and mortality, and of psychological effects. Clearly a threshold level of risk at which to offer screening needs to be established in the light of outcome assessment. Screening methods must be carefully evaluated and long-term survival audited.

A further question is whether families should be ascertained actively or whether this should be reactive. The Calman–Hine model (Department of Health, 1995; 1999) proposed that individuals at population or only slightly increased risk should be managed in the primary care setting, those estimated to have a moderately increased risk, for which some surveillance may be appropriate, should ideally be managed in cancer units and primary care, and only those at high risk referred to genetics centres for specialised genetic counselling and predictive testing as appropriate. This has been developed in the Kenilworth model, and promoted as the optimal way of managing genetic cancer susceptibility from the population to tertiary care (NHS Cancer Plan, 2000; Hodgson et al., 2000). Certain difficulties have been encountered in trying to establish this model of care. Clearly there is a need to put in place clinics in primary and secondary care where family history taking and risk estimation can be undertaken, and education/guidelines provided to non-genetics professionals to help triage families at this service level. There is some reluctance in primary care to become too involved in this because of the time required to evaluate family histories. As a result, in the USA, CD-ROM's or other computerised systems, such as GRAIDS, that aid in triage are being advocated (Westman et al., 2000; Sweet et al., 2002).

Specialist cancer genetics nurse-led clinics can be set up for groups of general practices or in district hospitals to undertake such evaluation, in collaboration with the local genetics centre. Nurses in these clinics are trained in pedigree taking and risk assessment, and can "triage" patients into those who can be reassured, those who can be referred for surveillance because of a moderately increased risk, and those who should be referred to the genetics centre. Close links are maintained with the genetics centre with regular discussion of difficult families or problems with risk assessment. Such health care delivery developments are being piloted in the UK under the Department of Health White Paper Initiative on Genetics, in collaboration with Macmillan Cancer Relief. Telephone clinics are being assessed as part of these assessments. Computerised systems are needed to maintain pedigree data, ensure the smooth running of appropriate surveillance programmes, and document screening outcomes in relation to risk. These could be maintained in secondary and primary care but monitored in the genetics centre, if secure data transfer is made available. Audit of surveillance strategies in individuals at moderately increased risk is vital in order to assess the efficacy (specificity, sensitivity and cost–effectiveness) of such strategies in the long term. The genetics centre provides specialist genetic counselling for families in which it is likely that some individuals carry a mutation conferring a strong genetic susceptibility to specific cancers. Predictive testing can be offered to individuals from families in which a mutation is identified and screening and prophylactic measures offered only to those testing positive for the mutation. This also saves costs in screening for those at low risk. Multidisciplinary clinics for carriers of *BRCA1* and *BRCA2* carriers are helpful for managing these individuals and their families.

The delivery of a comprehensive service of this type requires a good deal of co-ordination and audit, which is best organised centrally. The genetics centre should be responsible for providing education and continuing support for nurses and genetic counsellors working in primary and secondary care, and for providing educational study-days, literature and referral guidelines for non-genetics professionals. Courses aimed at educating health professionals to be able to run "family history clinics" are required in the development of such a service. Such nurse-led clinics could utilise computer packages, which additionally could provide printed risk information for the patients and for maintaining practice and hospital patient notes.

Part two

Genetics of human cancers by site of origin

2

Central nervous system

Primary central nervous system (CNS) neoplasms affect about 1 per 10 000 of the population. Although the incidence of brain tumours increases with advancing age, intracranial neoplasms are the most common cause of solid cancer in children. The distribution and histological type of brain tumour differ in children and in adults. In children, brain tumours most often arise in the posterior fossa, and the most frequent tumour types are medulloblastoma, spongioblastoma (including cerebellar astrocytoma and optic nerve glioma) and ependymomas. In adults, most tumours are supratentorial, and meningiomas and gliomas are the most frequent type. Familial brain tumours may occur as part of a rare specific inherited cancer syndrome (Table 2.1). Epidemiological studies have suggested that there is a small increased risk of cerebral neoplasms among relatives of brain tumour patients compared to controls: Choi et al. (1970), Gold et al., 1994 found a ninefold increase in the incidence of brain tumour among relatives of patients with glioma compared to controls, whereas Burch et al. (1987) found a (statistically insignificant) sixfold increase among relatives of brain tumour patients. Nevertheless, the absolute risk to relatives is small, 0.6 per cent in the study by Choi et al. (1970). Miller (1971) found a ninefold increase in the expected number of sib pairs among children with brain tumours,

Table 2.1. *Genetic disorders associated with tumours of the CNS.*
Details of individual conditions are given in Part Three

Neurofibromatosis type 1
Neurofibromatosis type 2
von Hippel–Lindau disease
Li–Fraumeni syndrome
Familial adenomatous polyposis
Turcot syndrome (including homozygous mismatch gene mutations)
Tuberose sclerosis
Gorlin syndrome
Ataxia telangiectasia
Werner syndrome
Blue rubber bleb naevus syndrome

and a similar excess of families in which one child died of brain tumour and another of cancer of bone or muscle. Soft tissue sarcomas and brain tumours occur as part of the Li–Fraumeni syndrome. Mahaley et al. (1989) found a family history of cancer in 16–19 per cent of patients with brain tumours (similar to the expected incidence), but that the incidence was 30–33 per cent in patients with glioblastoma multiforme, malignant lymphoma and neuroblastoma. A family history of neurofibromatosis was obtained in 1.6 per cent of cases. The genetic implications of specific CNS tumours are described below.

Vestibular schwannoma (acoustic neuroma)

This tumour accounts for around 8 per cent of all intracranial tumours and has an incidence of 13/million per year (Tos and Thomsen, 1984). Although sometimes called acoustic neuromas, these are Schwann cell tumours. They usually arise from the vestibular nerve, but they can develop on the fifth cranial nerve, and less often on the ninth and tenth nerves. Within the spinal canal, they usually arise on the dorsal spinal root. Familial and bilateral vestibular schwannoma are features of neurofibromatosis type 2 (NF2). About 4 per cent of vestibular schwannoma are bilateral and all patients with bilateral tumours have NF2 (see Part Three). Sporadic vestibular schwannoma is typically seen in the fifth and sixth decades of life, which is about 20 years later than in patients with NF2. The clinical features and diagnostic criteria for NF2 are discussed in Part Three. Although vestibular schwannoma in NF2 is usually bilateral, it can be unilateral. Multiple extracranial schwannomas (cutaneous and spinal) may be inherited as a dominant trait and is allelic with NF2 (Evans et al., 1997). Those mosaic for an *NF2* gene mutation may present with milder- and later-onset disease (see p. 239). Although vestibular schwannoma in NF2 is usually bilateral, it can be unilateral. Multiple extracranial schwannomas (cutaneous and spinal) without vestibular schwannomas may be inherited as a dominant trait (Evans et al., 1997a). Although both sporadic and NF2-associated vestibular schwannoma show somatic *NF2* tumour gene mutations and allele loss and extracranial schwannomas from familial schwannomatosis cases may have NF2 inactivation, linkage studies have mapped familial schwannomatosis to chromosome 22 but have excluded linkage to *NF2* (Menon et al., 1990a; Irving et al., 1994; MacCollin et al., 2003).

Choroid plexus tumour

Choroid plexus neoplasms are rare (0.5 per cent of all brain tumours), and are most frequent in infancy. The majority of choroid plexus tumours are benign papillomas, but up to 30 per cent are classified as carcinomas.

Childhood choroid plexus tumours in sibling pairs have been reported in three families. In the most recent report, the parents were consanguineous and autosomal recessive inheritance was suggested (Zwetsloot et al., 1991). Tumours of the choroid plexus have been reported in the X-linked disorder Aicardi syndrome (Robinow et al., 1986) and in a girl with hypomelanosis of Ito and a constitutional (X;17)(q13;p13) translocation (Steichen-Gersdorf et al., 1993). Choroid plexus carcinoma has been described in families with Li–Fraumeni syndrome (Garber et al., 1990; Yuasa et al., 1993). Two further kindred in which the index patient had choroid plexus tumour and relatives had additional early-onset neoplasms have been described (see Garber et al., 1990). The associated tumours in the first family were cerebral glioma (two siblings), lung cancer (mother) and optic glioma (niece); in the second family, one sibling had ventricular ependymoma and another neuroblastoma. A germline p53 mutation was also identified in a woman with early-onset osteosarcoma and choroids plexus papilloma (Rutherford et al., 2002). Choroid plexus angiomas were reported in two out of four patients with Perlman syndrome reported by Henneveld et al. (1999).

Ependymoma

These glial cell tumours of the brain and spinal cord occur both sporadically and in association with cancer susceptibility syndromes. In children, the tumour usually presents as a posterior fossa mass. Ependymoma may be a feature of NF2 (see Part three) and has been reported as part of Turcot syndrome (Torres et al., 1997). Familial ependymoma consistent with autosomal dominant inheritance with incomplete penetrance has been described (Gilchrist and Savard, 1989; Nijssen et al., 1994). In both cases the tumours showed mosaicism for complete or chromosome 22 monosomy, and malignant ependymoma has been reported in association with a constitutional t(1;22)(p22;q11.2) which did not interrupt the *NF2* gene. Furthermore, Yokota et al. (2003) reported a family with two cases of spinal ependymoma which demonstrated 22q allele loss.

Gliomas (including astrocytoma and glioblastoma)

Astrocytoma and glioblastoma account for about 4 per cent of brain tumours in childhood and 17 per cent in adults. Genetic conditions associated with a predisposition to glioma include neurofibromatosis type 1 (NF1), NF2, Li–Fraumeni syndrome, tuberose sclerosis, Gorlin syndrome, Turcot syndrome and Maffucci syndrome (see Part three). The precise tumour type in some cases can be correlated with specific disorders, for example in tuberose sclerosis a benign astrocytic tumour (subependymal nodule) is typically seen, although giant cell astrocytoma can occur. However, in NF1 and Turcot syndrome, both astrocytoma and glioblastoma multiforme may be seen. Kibirige et al. (1989) found that of 282 children with astrocytoma, 21 had neurofibromatosis and 4 had tuberose sclerosis, and there was evidence that a similar proportion might have had Li–Fraumeni syndrome.

Familial glioma not associated with the inherited syndromes described above occurs, but is uncommon, and has been reviewed in detail by Vieregge et al. (1987). Of 39 reports, most (60 per cent) were of affected siblings, and one quarter was of affected twins or of individuals with affected relatives in two generations. There were three pairs of monozygotic twins with glioma. In most affected sibling cases, the onset in the second sibling was usually within 5 years of that of the first sibling. A high incidence of cerebral glioma was found in an isolated inbred community by Armstrong and Hanson (1969) and Thuwe et al. (1979). Glioblastoma multiforme is rare in children, but Duhaime et al. (1989) reported an affected sib pair aged 2 and 5 years with simultaneous onset of symptoms. Thus, although familial glioma not associated with a specific genetic syndrome does occur, it is infrequent.

Van Meyel et al. (1994) investigated 16 kindreds with familial glioma for evidence for germline mutations in exons 5–9 of the *TP53* gene and exon 24 of the *NF1* gene. No mutations were identified. A study from the Mayo Clinic of 15 brain cancer patients who had a family history of brain tumours found that one had a germline *TP53* mutation, and another had a germline hemizygous deletion of the *CDKN2A/ARF* region (see below). No germline mutations were seen in *PTEN* or *CDK4* (Tachibana et al., 2000).

One clear, but very rare association that has emerged is the joint familial occurrence of various types of brain tumours (including glioma) and melanoma (Kaufman et al., 1993; Azizi et al., 1995; Bahuau et al., 1997), subsequently found to be due in part to hemizygous deletions of a region of chromosome 9p21 that includes the open reading frames of both *CDKN2A* (p16) and *ARF* (p14) (Bahuau et al., 1998; Tachibana et al., 2000). Interestingly, p14 appears to be critical, as there is one report of a nervous system tumour–melanoma family segregating a deletion that does not disrupt *CDKN2A* structure (Randerson-Moor et al., 2001). The situation is complicated, because p14[ARF] is formed from the products of exon 1β and exon 2 of *CDKN2A*, whereas p16 is formed from exon 1α and exon 2 of *CDKN2A*; nevertheless, the reading frames are different and have no amino acid homology, although both are cell cycle regulators. In brain tumour–melanoma kindreds, deletions studies of this region may be warranted if clinical testing for *CDKN2A* mutations has been undertaken, and is negative.

Haemangioblastoma

These vascular tumours occur most frequently in the cerebellum followed by the spinal cord, brain stem and, least frequently, supratentorially. Approximately 30 per cent of all cerebellar haemangioblastomas occur as part of von Hippel–Lindau (VHL) disease (see Part three). All patients with multiple CNS haemangioblastomas have VHL disease. Hemangioblastoma is a benign tumour but may recur if surgical removal is not complete. In such cases the possibility of a new primary (and hence a diagnosis of VHL disease) should also be considered. The risk of VHL disease is highest in younger patients: the mean ages at diagnosis of cerebellar haemangioblastoma in this disease and in non-familial cases are 29 and 48 years, respectively. All patients with apparently sporadic haemangioblastomas should be screened for subclinical evidence of VHL disease. In addition, *VHL* mutation analysis is helpful, particularly in patients aged <50 years. Germline VHL gene mutations were detected in 4 per cent of apparently sporadic haemangioblastoma cases without clinical or radiological evidence of VHL disease (Hes et al., 2000). In view of the possibility of false negative mutation analysis results (e.g. if mosaic), younger patients (<40 years) may be kept under review in case evidence of VHL disease develops later.

Statistical analysis of the age at onset of cerebellar haemangioblastoma in VHL disease and sporadic cases is compatible with a retinoblastoma-like model of tumorigenesis (Maher et al., 1990a). Both VHL disease-associated and sporadic cerebellar and spinal haemangioblastomas show chromosome 3p allele loss and somatic *VHL* gene mutations.

Haemangioma

Familial cavernous haemangiomas of the brain may be inherited as a dominant trait with incomplete penetrance. In familial cases, cavernous haemangiomas are often multiple but may be asymptomatic and only detected by magnetic resonance imaging (MRI) scanning. A locus for familial cavernous haemangiomas (*CCM1*) was mapped to chromosome 7q in families of Mexican-American descent but there is evidence of locus heterogeneity (Gunel et al., 1996; Polymeropoulos et al., 1997). Subsequently, germline mutations in *KRIT1* were identified (Laberge-le Couteulx et al., 1999). In a molecular genetic survey of 121 cerebral cavernous haemangioma probands with familial and/or multiple lesions, Cave-Riant et al. (2002) found germline *KRIT1* mutations in 43 per cent. Two further familial cerebral cavernous haemangioma loci have been mapped: *CCM2* at 7p and *CCM3* at 3q (Craig et al., 1998), and these are estimated to account for about 20 and 40 per cent of families, respectively. Characterisation of the *CCM2* gene was reported by Liquori et al. (2003).

Meningeal haemangioma and facial naevus flammeus constitute the Sturge–Weber syndrome, and cerebral vascular lesions occur in Rendu–Osler–Weber syndrome. Although the Sturge–Weber syndrome is sometimes designated the fourth phakomatosis, there is no evidence of a genetic basis and there is no predisposition to neoplasia. Cutaneous and CNS haemangiomas and arteriovascular malformations can be dominantly inherited with variable expression and incomplete penetrance (Brown and Shields, 1985; Leblanc et al., 1996).

Medulloblastoma

This tumour accounts for about 25 per cent of all brain tumours in children and has an incidence of approximately 1/100 000 per year. Medulloblastoma occurs predominantly in the first two decades of life, with a peak incidence between 3 and 5 years of age. Familial medulloblastoma appears to be uncommon, but has been reported in twins and siblings (Hung et al., 1990). Familial non-syndromic medulloblastoma occurs rarely (von Koch et al., 2002). Genetic disorders associated with medulloblastoma include Gorlin syndrome, familial adenomatous polyposis, blue rubber bleb naevus syndrome and ataxia telangiectasia (see part three). Gorlin syndrome is caused by germline mutations in the *PTCH* gene which encodes the sonic hedgehog receptor (see p. 196). In addition, germline and somatic mutations in another of the sonic hedgehog pathways, *SUFU* (encoding the human suppressor of fused), may be found in a subset of children with medulloblastoma (Taylor et al., 2002). Medulloblastoma may also occur in patients with homozygous *BRCA2* mutations (Fanconi Anaemia Type D1, see p. 195) (Offit et al., 2003; Hirsch et al., 2004).

Meningioma

The most common benign brain tumour, meningioma, accounts for about 15 per cent of all primary brain tumours. The frequency of meningioma increases with advancing age and it is more common in women. Multiple or familial meningioma is associated with (i) NF2, (ii) pure familial meningioma and (iii) constitutional chromosome 22 rearrangements. Meningioma also occurs with increased frequency in Werner syndrome and Gorlin syndrome (see Part three).

Multiple meningioma is frequent and occurs in approximately 35 per cent of patients with NF2 (see Part three). Expression of NF2 is variable, so a careful search for evidence of NF2 and a detailed family history should be performed in all patients with multiple or familial meningioma, or with a young age at onset. Although many reports of familial meningioma may be variants of NF2, dominantly inherited meningioma with no evidence of NF2 does occur. However, signs of NF2 should be assiduously sought in all cases of familial meningioma as these may not be obvious. For example, Delleman et al. (1978) reported a family in which four members in two generations had meningiomas with no evidence of neurofibromatosis, but another relative had multiple meningiomas and bilateral vestibular schwannomas. Rearrangements of chromosome 22 have been associated with meningioma: multiple tumours developed in the third decade in a mentally retarded patient with a ring chromosome 22 (breakpoints p12 and q13.3) (Arinami et al., 1986), and familial meningiomas associated with a Robertsonian chromosome 14;22 translocation have also been described (Bolger et al., 1985). In addition, Pulst et al. (1993) reported exclusion of linkage to the NF2 kindred with familial meningioma.

Nerve root tumours

The commonest nerve root tumour is the benign schwannoma or neurolemmoma, and the most frequent site is the eighth cranial nerve (see Vestibular schwannoma, page 12, Part Two). Multiple schwannomas occur in NF2 (see part three). Although familial extracranial schwannomatosis has been considered to be allelic with NF2 (Evans et al., 1997a), MacCollin et al. (2003) excluded NF2 as a susceptibility locus for familial schwannomatosis. Schwannomas occur in the Carney complex (see part three), most commonly in the upper gastrointestinal tract and sympathetic nerve chains.

Neuroblastoma

This tumour of postganglionic sympathetic neurons is the most common solid tumour in children. Most cases are sporadic; familial cases (in which predisposition to neuroblastoma is inherited as an autosomal dominant trait) account for less than 1 per cent of the total. However, in a statistical analysis of the age at onset of neuroblastoma, Knudson and Strong (1972) estimated that 22 per cent of neuroblastomas could result from a germinal mutation and follow a "single-hit" mutation model, as in inherited retinoblastoma (Knudson, 1971). The mean age at diagnosis of familial cases is 9 months (60 per cent at less than 1 year) compared to 30 months (25 per cent at less than 1 year) in non-familial cases (Kushner et al., 1986), and familial tumours are frequently multiple (Robertson et al., 1991). Despite these data, no neuroblastoma susceptibility gene has been identified, despite numerous suggestive leads (see below), suggesting that the classical "two-hit" model does not apply to neuroblastoma. Nevertheless, neuroblastoma is occasionally seen in disorders associated with abnormal neural crest differentiation such as NF1 and Hirschsprung disease, and in overgrowth disorders such as Beckwith–Wiedemann syndrome and hemihypertrophy. However, the risk of neuroblastoma in siblings or offspring of most patients with neuroblastoma is less than 6 per cent (Kushner et al., 1986).

Cytogenetic and molecular genetic studies have implicated inactivation of a tumour suppressor gene on chromosome 1p and oncogene activation in the pathogenesis of neuroblastoma (Brodeur and Fong, 1989; Brodeur, 1990). Approximately 80 per cent of neuroblastoma cell lines show chromosome 1p terminal deletions, and molecular studies suggest the critical region for allele loss is chromosome band 1p36 (Brodeur and Fong, 1989). Cytogenetic studies of neuroblastoma reveal double minute bodies or chromosomally integrated, homogeneously staining regions in 90 per cent of cell lines and 30 per cent of primary tumours. These cytogenetic findings were predicted to result from gene amplification and subsequently it was shown that an oncogene related to the viral oncogene V-*MYC* and designated N-*MYC* was amplified in neuroblastoma. Both chromosome 1p deletions and N-*MYC* amplification are found more frequently in advanced disease and both are associated with a poorer prognosis irrespective of tumour stage (Brodeur and Fong, 1989; Rubie et al., 1997). Brodeur (1990) has suggested that neuroblastoma patients can be divided into three groups, those with: (i) hyperdiploid or near-triploid tumour karyotype, which is usually seen in children aged less than 1 year with localised disease and a good prognosis; (ii) near-diploid or near-tetraploid tumour karyotype, usually seen in older children with more advanced slowly progressive disease which is frequently fatal and (iii) near-diploid or tetraploid karyotype with chromosome 1p deletions or N-*MYC* amplification, usually seen in older children with advanced, rapidly progressive disease.

Linkage to chromosome 1p36 markers has been excluded in familial neuroblastoma and although there are reports of an association between neuroblastoma and Hirschsprung disease, there is no evidence of *RET* mutations causing familial neuroblastoma (Hofstra et al., 1996; Maris et al., 1996). More recently, linkage to chromosome 16p12–13 has been reported using seven families with at least two cases of neuroblastoma (Maris et al., 2002). The linked region, when including loss of heterozygosity data, is 14.5 cM. Others have not replicated these findings (Perri et al., 2002).

In familial neuroblastoma, screening by urinary catecholamine estimations should commence at birth and continue until the age of 6 years. Population screening of infants for neuroblastoma by urine screening was initially advocated, but it was already well established that occasionally, neuroblastoma can regress spontaneously, reducing the likelihood that screening would reduce mortality. It has been suggested that there are two subsets of neuroblastoma and that screening may preferentially detect those patients with a more favourable prognosis who would not have gone on to develop more aggressive tumours.

Woods et al. (1996) found that screening for neuroblastoma by urinary assay of homovanillic acid and vanillymandelic acid at 3 weeks and 6 months increased the incidence of neuroblastoma in infants without decreasing the frequency of unfavourable advanced-stage disease in older children. This was confirmed by the final results of the Quebec screening programme, which showed that there was no significant reduction in mortality due to neuroblastoma among screened Quebec children compared with any other control group (Woods et al., 2002).

Pineal tumour

A proportion of children with bilateral retinoblastoma will develop a pineal tumour (the so-called trilateral retinoblastoma). Familial pinealblastoma occurs rarely (Peyster et al., 1986). Extragonadal germ cell tumours may arise in the pineal gland and be associated with Klinefelter syndrome or 46XY gonadal dysgenesis.

Primitive neuroectodermal tumours

Cerebral primitive neuroectodermal tumours (PNET) can occur predominantly in childhood and arise most frequently in the posterior fossa, but can occur anywhere in the brain. Medulloblastoma is the most common form of PNET (see above), but CNS malignant rhabdoid tumours are another subset. Germline mutations in *P53*, *PTCH* (Gorlin syndrome) and *APC* may be associated with susceptibility to centeal PNETs. In contrast to the peripheral type, such as Ewing sarcoma, t(11;22)(q24;q12) is uncommon in the central type.

Taylor et al. (2000) reported a kindred with two affected relatives with a posterior fossa brain tumour in infancy (cerebellar malignant rhabdoid tumour) and posterior fossa choroids plexus carcinoma and a germline *SMARCB1* (*hSNF5*) splice-site mutation. Inheritance was autosomal dominant inheritance with incomplete penetrance and mice heterozygous for an *SNF5* deletion developed T-cell lymphomas and rhabdoid tumours (Roberts et al., 2002). In addition, a neonate with a malignant rhabdoid tumour of the kidney and a brain PNET was found to have a de novo *SMARCB1* germline deletion (Kusafuka et al., 2004).

Supratentorial PNETs are very rare tumours, but appear to be particularly associated with homozygous *PMS2* mutations (De Vos et al., 2004). Other features of recessively inherited *PMS2* mutations are café-au-lait lesions and susceptibility to haematological malignancies. A family history of colorectal cancer is often absent. Biallelic mutations in *BRCA2* causing Fanconi anaemia subtype D1 (see p. 195) predispose to solid tumours including medulloblastoma (Offit et al., 2003; Hirsch et al., 2004).

3

Eye

The ocular tumours discussed in this section include retinoblastoma, haemangioblastoma, optic nerve glioma, meningioma and melanoma. Ocular rhabdomyosarcoma is discussed with rhabdomyosarcoma of other sites on pages 136 and 137. Genetic disorders associated with significant ocular manifestations (neoplastic and non-neoplastic) include neurofibromatosis type 1 (NF1), neurofibromatosis type 2 (NF2), von Hippel–Lindau (VHL) disease, tuberose sclerosis and familial adenomatous polyposis (see Part Three).

Retinoblastoma

Retinoblastoma is the commonest malignant ocular tumour of childhood and affects 1 per 20 000 children. The tumour is derived from primitive retinal cells (retinoblasts) and usually presents in early childhood (90 per cent before the age of 5 years). Less than 10 per cent of children with retinoblastoma have a positive family history (where inheritance is autosomal dominant), but new mutations are frequent and approximately 40 per cent of retinoblastoma patients have a genetic predisposition. Retinoblastoma holds a unique place in human cancer genetics as the paradigm of the tumour suppressor gene.

Retinoblastoma typically presents as leukocoria (white eye, cat's eye reflex) or strabismus. It is bilateral in about 30 per cent of cases, and these children have a younger age at diagnosis (mean 8 months) than those with unilateral tumour (mean 25 months). Bilateral or multifocal tumours occur in patients with germline mutations of the retinoblastoma (*RB1*) gene, but about 15 per cent of children with a single tumour will have a germline mutation. The 40 per cent of all children with retinoblastoma who carry a germline retinoblastoma gene mutation are at risk for secondary tumours, especially osteosarcoma and soft tissue sarcomas (see below). This predisposition is exacerbated in those who receive radiotherapy. A few individuals (less than 2 per cent) with germline retinoblastoma gene mutations may develop a retinoma. These benign retinal lesions appear as focal translucencies with cottage-cheese-like calcification and underlying choroidal and retinal pigment epithelial disturbance. A retinoma is thought to result when a second *RB1* mutation occurs in a retinoblast which is almost differentiated. About 2 per cent of all patients with retinoblastoma also have an

Table 3.1. *Risk of retinoblastoma in relatives of a child with retinoblastoma and no family history*

Retinoblastoma in proband	Relationship to proband	Risk of carrying *RB* mutation[1] (%)	Risk of developing retinoblastoma tumour[1] (%)	Risk of developing retinoblastoma tumour[2] (%)
Bilateral	Offspring	50	45	44
Bilateral	Sibling or dizygotic twin	5	2.7	2
Bilateral	Offspring of unaffected sibling	0.5	0.27	
Bilateral	First cousin	0.05	0.027	
Bilateral	Monozygotic twin	100	90	
Unilateral	Offspring	7.5	5.7	1
Unilateral	Sibling or dizygotic twin	0.8	0.4	1
Unilateral	Offspring of unaffected sibling	0.08	0.04	
Unilateral	First cousin	0.008	0.004	
Unilateral	Monozygotic twin	10	5.4	

[1] The calculated risks from Musarella and Gallie (1987) take into account the retinoblastoma mutation rate and assume that 90 per cent of individuals with a germline mutation will develop a tumour and 15 per cent of patients with unilateral retinoblastoma have a germline mutation.
[2] The risks from Draper et al. (1992) for siblings relate to the first child, when there are further unaffected siblings the risk will be lower.

intracranial lesion, usually in the pineal. The association of pineal tumour and retinoblastoma is often termed trilateral retinoblastoma and occurs in patients with germline retinoblastoma mutations. The retinoblastoma mutation is non-penetrant in approximately 10 per cent of obligate carriers. Although there is no detectable paternal age effect on new mutations for retinoblastoma, most new hereditary mutations develop in paternal germ cells (Zhu et al., 1989). An excess of males among patients with bilateral sporadic disease has been noted, and Naumova and Sapienza (1994) suggested the involvement of genomic imprinting effects.

About 60 per cent of retinoblastomas result from somatic (acquired) mutations inactivating both alleles of the retinoblastoma gene. Such patients develop single tumours and there is no risk to their offspring. However, 15 per cent of patients with single tumours will have a germline mutation. Risk estimates for the relatives of isolated cases of retinoblastoma are given in Table 3.1. The later estimates of

Draper et al. (1992) are lower in some cases than earlier estimates. Genetic counselling for the relatives of patients with isolated unilateral retinoblastoma is complicated by the possibility of mosaicism of a germline *RB1* mutation (Lohmann et al., 1997).

Individuals with genetic retinoblastoma (germline mutation) are at increased risk for second tumours, but children with non-genetic tumours are not. The risk of second primary neoplasms reflects a genetic predisposition to non-retinoblastoma tumours and the effects of treatment (e.g. radiation). Draper et al. (1986) estimated that the cumulative probability of a second primary neoplasm in genetic retino-blastoma patients at 18 years after diagnosis is 8.4 per cent for all tumours and 6 per cent for osteosarcoma. The risks for osteosarcoma outside and within the radiation fields were 2.2 per cent and 3.7 per cent respectively, and thus patients with genetic retinoblastoma may be more sensitive to radiation-induced oncogen-esis. The most common site of osteosarcoma outside the radiation field is in the femur, and genetic retinoblastoma patients are at a 200– 500-fold increased risk of this complication. Soft tissue sarcomas also occur with increased frequency in patients with genetic retinoblastoma. Studies of non-ocular cancer in relatives of retinoblastoma patients have demonstrated that retinoblastoma mutation carriers are at increased risk of a variety of other cancers (overall relative risk 11.6) includ-ing cancer of the lung (relative risk 15), malignant melanoma and bladder cancer (Sanders et al., 1988). Moll et al. (1996) estimated cumulative incidences of second primary tumours in hereditary retinoblastoma of 4 per cent and 18 per cent at ages 10 and 35 years respectively. Eng et al. (1993) reported a cumulative probability of death from a second primary neoplasm of 26 per cent at 40 years after bilateral retinoblastoma. The most common second primary tumours were bone and con-nective tissue neoplasms and malignant melanoma. Eng et al. (1993) also demon-strated that radiotherapy increased the risk of a second primary tumour and suggested that all patients with inherited retinoblastoma should receive lifelong surveillance for second primary tumours. In a follow up study of UK hereditary retinoblastoma cases, Fletcher et al. (2004) found a cumulative cancer incidence and mortality of 69 and 48 per cent respectively. In contrast to patients treated by radiotherapy, sarcomas accounted for only a minority of tumours and there was an increased mortality for lung cancer (standardised mortality ratio (SMR) = 7), bladder cancer (SMR = 26) and all other epithelial cancers combined (SMR = 3.3).

The retinoblastoma gene was initially assigned to chromosome 13 band q14 by reports of children with retinoblastoma and interstitial deletions of chromo-some 13. About 3 per cent of children with retinoblastoma will have a cytogenet-ically visible chromosome 13 deletion or translocation. Retinoblastoma cases with constitutional chromosome deletion may have associated mental retardation and most have reduced serum levels of esterase D (the gene for which maps close to the retinoblastoma gene). Genetic linkage studies confirmed the mapping of retinoblastoma to 13q14 and subsequently a candidate gene was isolated by Friend et al. (1986). This gene (*RB1*) spans 200 kb, is associated with a 4.7 kb RNA transcript which encodes a 110 kDa nuclear phosphoprotein with DNA-binding activity. The retinoblastoma gene was predicted to function as a tumour suppressor gene and confirmatory evidence for this hypothesis was the demonstration that introducing the *RB1* gene (via a retrovirus vector) suppressed the tumorigenicity of retinoblastoma and osteosarcoma cell lines (Huang et al., 1988).

The cloning of the retinoblastoma gene has enabled the presymptomatic identification of individuals with germline mutations by a variety of techniques. A series of intragenic restriction fragment length polymorphisms (RFLPs) has been described, and these RFLPs are informative in about 95 per cent of families and usually allow accurate presymptomatic diagnosis of at-risk relatives in families with two or more affected members (Wiggs et al., 1988). However, linkage analysis is not helpful in families with only a single affected individual. Mutation detection rates of 80 per cent or more were reported by Lohmann et al. (1996) and Houdayer et al. (2004) using a variety of molecular genetic techniques. Germline deletions are not infrequent and an appropriate deletion scanning approach (e.g. Multiplex Ligation-dependent Probe Amplification (MLPA) etc.) should be performed as part of the mutation detection strategy. *RB1* mutations are heterogeneous, and generally no clear genotype–phenotype associations have been described except that promoter mutations and some intragenic mutations with residual protein activity may display reduced penetrance (Kratzke et al., 1994; Cowell et al., 1996). The identification of a germline mutation in a unilateral sporadic case distinguishes those individuals with simplex retinoblastoma and a new germline mutation from non-hereditary cases. When a germline mutation is identified, other relatives can be tested. When histopathological material (formalin fixed paraffin embedded) from a deceased patient is available, mutation analysis can be undertaken on the tumour tissue, and further investigations undertaken to determine if a characterised mutation is somatic or germline.

In the absence of molecular genetic diagnosis, the parents and siblings of all children with retinoblastoma should undergo thorough ophthalmological assessment. Offspring and siblings of retinoblastoma patients should be followed up from birth, with complete retinal examination: examination should be performed at birth and monthly until 3 months of age without anaesthesia, then under general anaesthetic every 3 months until the age of 2 years, then every 4 months until the age of 3 years. Thereafter, examinations without general anaesthesia are performed every 6 months until the age of 5 years, and then every 12 months until the age of 11 years (although the frequency and duration of screening can be modified according to the results of DNA analysis). Parents of children with apparently sporadic retinoblastoma must be examined to exclude a regressed tumour or retinoma because this would identify the child as having a germline *RB1* gene mutation. Children with retinoblastoma will require careful follow-up to detect new tumours or recurrence. New tumours occurred in 11 per cent of children studied by Salmonsen et al. (1979). Traditionally, all children with retinoblastoma are followed up with regular retinal examinations under general anaesthesia. However, the application of DNA techniques to identify *RB1* gene mutations in tumours and constitutional DNA enables follow-up to be restricted to those shown to have germline *RB1* mutations. This not only enhances management of at-risk relatives, but is also a cost-effective strategy (Noorani et al., 1996). Survivors of bilateral retinoblastoma (and unilateral retinoblastoma in those with germline retinoblastoma gene mutations) are at high risk of osteosarcoma in adolescence, and of the occurrence of other cancers (see above).

Retinal astrocytic hamartoma

This benign, non-progressive tumour is most commonly seen in patients with tuberose sclerosis, and occurs in about 50 per cent of patients with this disorder. Retinal astrocytomas not associated with tuberose sclerosis differ from those in tuberose sclerosis in that a proportion appear to be true neoplasms and may invade locally (Arnold et al., 1985).

Optic glioma

Although rare, glioma is the commonest optic nerve tumour in childhood. Optic glioma is associated with NF1 (see Part Three) in a third of cases, and Lewis et al. (1984) reported that 10–15 per cent of patients with NF1 develop an optic glioma (which may be bilateral), although Huson et al. (1988) found only two out of 135 patients had a symptomatic glioma. McGaughran et al. (1999) estimated an actuarial risk of optic glioma in NF1 patients of 3.7 per cent at age 10 years and 6.2 per cent at age 25 years. All patients with optic glioma, and their families, should be assessed for evidence of NF1. Histological appearance is of a low-grade (pilocytic) astrocytoma, spontaneous regression may occur, and many consider these tumours to be congenital hamartomas rather than acquired neoplasms (Riccardi and Eichner, 1986). Optic gliomas usually originate in the optic nerves or chiasm. Presentation is usually with visual impairment, and painless proptosis occurs with optic nerve gliomas. Most NF1-associated optic gliomas are orbital. Computerised tomography (CT) or magnetic resonance image (MRI) scanning will demonstrate optic glioma and differentiate from optic nerve meningioma. The natural history of optic glioma is not well defined. Most are non-progressive, and conservative management is usually preferred, treatment (surgery or radiotherapy) of optic nerve glioma is indicated for progressive visual loss associated with proptosis. Treatment of chiasmal lesions is more difficult, but again most are non-progressive and conservative management is pursued.

Ocular choristoma

Ocular choristomas are congenital lesions, which are deposits of normal tissue in an abnormal location, and are the most common epibulbar and orbital tumours in children, with an incidence of about 1 per 5000 (Mansour et al., 1989). Dermoid and epidermoid cysts are both included in this group. Ocular choristomas may be associated with Goldenhar syndrome (hemifacial microsomia) or epidermal naevus syndrome. In the latter disorder, choristomas are frequently bilateral and extensive. Goldenhar syndrome is usually sporadic, but in rare cases can be familial. Familial choristoma with dominant inheritance not associated with Goldenhar syndrome occurs rarely (Mansour et al., 1989).

Cavernous haemangioma

This rare ocular tumour should be distinguished from retinal haemangioblastoma (capillary haemangioma). Mean age at diagnosis is 23 years, and less than 10 per cent are bilateral. Cavernous haemangioma is usually non-progressive and serious complications are uncommon. Retinal or optic disc cavernous haemangiomas are associated with cutaneous vascular lesions in about 28 per cent of patients, and in some patients with intracranial cavernous haemangioma (Lewis et al., 1975). A triad of ocular, central nervous system and cutaneous cavernous haemangiomas can be dominantly inherited with variable expression and incomplete penetrance (Brown and Shields, 1985). Thus the finding of retinal cavernous or choroidal haemangioma is an indication to search for features of systemic or familial disease (Sarraf et al., 2000). Germline *KRIT1* (*CCM1*) mutation (see p. 15) has been reported in association with retinal and cerebral cavernous haemangiomas (Laberge-le Couteulx et al., 2002).

Haemangioblastoma

Retinal haemangioblastoma (angioma) is the most common presentation of VHL disease (Maher et al., 1990b). The exact proportion of patients with retinal haemangioblastoma who have this disease is unclear. The most frequent estimate is 40 per cent but Neumann and Wiestler (1991) detected evidence of the disease in

Table 3.2. *Estimated probability of underlying VHL disease in a patient with a solitary ocular angioma after careful ophthalmic screening*

Other negative information	Probability by age group (years)			
	<20	21–40	41–60	>60
None	0.30	0.30	0.30	0.30
DNA	0.11	0.11	0.11	0.11
Systemic screening	0.27	0.13	0.06	0.02
Parent history	0.19	0.13	0.09	0.09
Parent history + systemic screening	0.17	0.05	0.02	0.01
DNA + parent history	0.06	0.04	0.03	0.03
DNA + systemic screening	0.10	0.04	0.02	0.01
DNA + systemic screening + parent history	0.06	0.01	0.00	0.00

Source: From Webster et al. (2000).

86 per cent of their patients with retinal angiomatosis. All patients with retinal angioma should be investigated for subclinical manifestations of VHL disease (see Part Three). All patients with multiple retinal angiomas have VHL disease, but in atypical cases, expert ophthalmological review is helpful to confirm that the lesions are haemangioblastomas and are not a vascular lesion (e.g. Coat disease) that is not associated with VHL disease. Webster et al. (1998) investigated 17 cases with VHL-like solitary ocular angioma and no evidence of other complications of this disease in themselves or in family members. All 17 cases were negative for germline *VHL* mutations. The mean age of presentation was 30.9 years (median 27.5, range 3–52). The estimated prevalence of non-VHL ocular angioma was 9.0×10^{-6} (95 per cent confidence interval (CI) = $3.3–19 \times 10^{-6}$). The estimated risk of there being underlying VHL disease in a patient with a solitary ocular angioma was 30 per cent; this risk decreased with negative DNA and clinical screening and also with increasing age (Table 3.2). Webster et al. (1999) concluded that sporadic ocular angioma can occur in the absence of VHL disease. The tumours are similar in anatomical location, and cases are similar in age of presentation and degree of visual morbidity compared to those with the disease.

Melanoma

Uveal melanoma is the most common primary intraocular malignancy in adults, with an incidence 6/million per year (lifetime risk 1 in 2500) (Canning and Hungerford, 1988). Familial cases are uncommon and account for about

0.6 per cent of all patients (Singh et al., 1996). Canning and Hungerford (1988) reviewed 14 kindreds with familial ocular melanoma. The mean age at diagnosis is significantly younger in familial than in sporadic cases (42 and 56 years respectively) and inheritance can be autosomal dominant with incomplete penetrance. Intraocular melanoma may be associated with familial atypical mole-melanoma syndrome (p. 142), ocular melanocytosis and NF1 (see Part Three) (Singh et al., 1995). The molecular basis for uveal melanoma susceptibility has not been defined, although *CDKN2A* and *BRCA2* have been excluded as susceptibility genes (Hearle et al., 2003).

Meningioma

Optic nerve meningioma is an uncommon tumour that may present at any age but predominantly occurs in middle-aged women. Most tumours are unilateral, but a small proportion of patients have bilateral involvement. Optic nerve sheath meningioma may complicate NF2 (see Part Three), when it is usually unilateral but can be bilateral (Cunliffe et al., 1991).

4

Cardiorespiratory system and thorax

Head and neck cancer

General

Squamous carcinomas of the head and neck (a grouping which includes tongue and mouth, nasopharynx and larynx) are associated with cigarette smoking and alcohol ingestion (although the risk factors for different sites may differ). In addition, specific head and neck cancers may be associated with familial cancer syndromes such as hereditary non-polyposis colon cancer syndrome and Li–Fraumeni syndrome (larynx) and Fanconi anaemia (oral cancer). Foulkes et al. (1996) reported a relative risk of 3.7 for developing head and neck cancer in first-degree relatives of an affected case, but the relative risk was almost 8 if the index case had multiple primaries. Spitz et al. (1994) reported an association between mutagen susceptibility (bleomycin-induced chromosome breakage) and multiple primary head and neck cancers, and while new data from the Spitz group (Wu et al., 2002) and others (Cloos et al., 2000) have confirmed or extended these findings, some researchers have questioned the significance of these observations (Szekely et al., 2003), and the bleomycin sensitivity assay is not used clinically. Interestingly, IGF-1 levels also predict the risk of second primary head and neck cancers, and such an assay could be clinically useful (Wu et al., 2004).

Specific sites

Nasopharynx

Cancers of the nasopharynx account for 0.1 per cent of all cancers, and differ from tumours in other parts of the pharynx by not being associated with tobacco or alcohol. There is a high incidence (lifetime risk 1.6 per cent) of nasopharyngeal carcinoma among the southern Chinese (100-fold higher than that of European populations), and both environmental (high dietary intake of salted fish and, particularly, Epstein–Barr virus, EBV) and genetic factors (association with HLA A2, Bw46 and B17 haplotypes) have been implicated. Lu et al. (1990) have supported the presence of a susceptibility gene(s) linked to the HLA region in southern Chinese. Their results are consistent with a recessive gene which produces a 20-fold increase in relative risk in homozygotes and would be responsible for approximately two-thirds of cases in the southern Chinese (Easton and Peto, 1990). Using meta-analysis, Burt et al. (1996) also demonstrated a significant association with HLA types in non-Chinese populations. This work has been followed up by more detailed studies, indicating that the extended haplotype HLA-A*3303-B*5801/2-DRB1*0301-DQB1*0201/2-DPB1*0401, specific to the south Chinese ethnic group, is associated with a significant 2.6-fold increased risk for nasopharyngeal carcinoma (Hildesheim et al., 2002). There is no associated risk for non-Chinese populations.

Molecular and cytogenetic studies of nasopharyngeal carcinoma have shown consistent deletions of the short arm of chromosome 3 (Huang et al., 1991). Recently, linkage to chromosome 3p21 has been reported in familial nasopharyngeal carcinoma ascertained in Hunan province, China (Xiong et al., 2004). Another group has reported linkage to chromosome 4 in familial nasopharyngeal carcinoma in Guangdong province (Feng et al., 2002), which is situated immediately south of Hunan (South China), so there is strong evidence for genetic heterogeneity and a major environmental factor, EBV infection. Notably, there is little evidence for risk of other cancers in families affected by nasopharyngeal carcinoma (Jia et al., 2004).

Larynx
Cancers of the larynx account for 1 per cent of all cancers, and are associated with tobacco smoking and alcohol. Carcinoma of the larynx has been reported in families with HNPCC, *BRCA2* mutations and in Muir–Torre and Li–Fraumeni syndromes (see part three). Allelic variants in the glutathione-S-transferase family of genes have been associated with laryngeal cancer susceptibility (Trizna et al., 1995) and meta-analyses of squamous cell carcinoma of the head and neck (including larynx cancer) have shown a very modest (~20 per cent) but statistically significant increased risk for these cancers in individuals null for *GSTM1*. Results for *GSTT1* were borderline or null (Hashibe et al., 2003; Ye et al., 2004). Bleomycin sensitivity has also been reported as a risk factor for head and neck cancer, as discussed above. Most recently, in an adjusted analysis, the AA genotype in the alcohol dehydrogenase 3 gene (*ADH3*), resulting in homozygosity for valine at position 349 was associated with an increased risk for upper aerodigestive tract cancer, particularly among those with low consumption of alcohol or tobacco (Nishimoto et al., 2004).

Tumours of the thymus

Thymomas are rare tumours of the thymic epithelium that usually occur in adults (average age at onset of 48 years) and are usually sporadic. About 65 per cent are benign, but when they occur in children they are more likely to be malignant. Familial occurrence is rare, but a sibship has been described in which two of three siblings died of thymoma (Matani and Dristas, 1973). Malignant epithelial tumours of the thymus (thymic carcinoma and thymoma) have also been described once in two members of a sibship (Wick et al., 1982).

Other tumours that may involve the thymus are carcinoids, germ cell tumours, neurogenic tumours, thymolipomas and Hodgkin disease. About one-third of thymic carcinoids are associated with multiple endocrine neoplasia type 1 (MEN 1), and Teh et al. (1997) have suggested that adult MEN 1 patients (aged more than 25 years) should be screened for this tumour. A recent prospective study of 85 patients with MEN 1 followed over a mean of 8 years found that with intensive screening, seven patients (8 per cent) developed thymic carcinoids (Gibril et al., 2003). Of relevance for risk assessment, MEN 1 patients with and without carcinoids did not differ except for the preponderance of males and the presence of another foregut carcinoid (usually gastric). The tumours were hormonally inactive. Despite appropriate surgery, the tumour recurred in all patients who were followed up for more than 12 months. Magnetic resonance imaging appeared to be the best way of detecting bony metastases. This poor prognosis has also been seen in other series, and some authors consider that adjuvant chemotherapy should be offered (Tiffet et al., 2003).

Tumours of the lung

Lung (bronchial) cancer accounts for 19 per cent of all cancers and 29 per cent of cancer deaths in the UK. The two most common histological types of lung cancer (small cell and squamous) are known to be strongly related to cigarette smoking. It is estimated that 90 per cent of lung cancer in males and 80 per cent in females is attributable to cigarette smoking. Adenocarcinoma (moderately associated with smoking) and alveolar cell carcinoma (not associated with smoking) account for 10 per cent of all lung cancer. In addition to smoking, other environmental agents such as asbestos and radiation have been associated with lung cancer.

Familial clustering of lung cancer occurs, but as relatives of lung cancer patients are more likely than average to be smokers or passive smokers, careful studies are required to distinguish the effects of shared environment (e.g. asbestos exposure) and lifestyle (e.g. smoking) from that of genetic predisposition. Although studies of the familial incidence of smoking-related lung cancer should be interpreted cautiously, there is evidence for an increased risk of lung cancer among relatives of affected patients. Tokuhata and Lilienfeld (1963) and Ooi et al. (1986) found a threefold increased lung cancer incidence in both smoking and non-smoking relatives of lung cancer patients. Sellers et al. (1990)

performed segregation analysis which allowed for variable age at onset and smoking history in affected patients. They concluded that familial clustering of lung cancer was consistent with Mendelian codominant inheritance of a rare autosomal gene with variable age at onset. It was estimated that at age 50 years, 69 per cent of lung cancer resulted from genetic factors acting in combination with smoking, but that at age 70 years, 72 per cent of lung cancer could be attributed to environmental factors alone. In a subsequent analysis, Sellers et al. (1994) provided further evidence that Mendelian factors may influence the occurrence of smoking-related cancers in the relatives of lung cancer probands. In an attempt to distinguish genetic susceptibility effects from environmental carcinogen exposure, Schwartz et al. (1996) analysed the family histories of non-smokers with lung cancer. They found a 7.2-fold increased risk of lung cancer in the first-degree relatives of non-smokers who developed lung cancer aged 40–59 years. Risk of lung cancer was also increased in the offspring of non-smoking cases. These findings suggest that a subset of relatives of early-onset, non-smoking lung cancer cases is at increased genetic risk (Spitz et al., 2003). An epidemiological study from Sweden showed standard incidence rates (SIR) for lung cancer in offspring of cases of 1.87 for adenocarcinoma and 1.86 for squamous cell carcinomas. The population attributable fraction was 2.77 per cent for familial lung cancer (Li and Hemminki 2003).

The rare alveolar cell carcinoma is not smoking related, and familial clustering has been reported: Paul et al. (1987) reported three brothers with alveolar cell carcinoma who shared HLA-A28, and Joishy (1977) reported simultaneous onset of alveolar cell carcinoma in identical twins. Adenocarcinoma of the lung (which is also not strongly smoking related) has been reported to occur in Li–Fraumeni syndrome (see part three) and, in transgenic mice with *p53* mutations. Compared with the general population, hereditary retinoblastoma survivors have a higher mortality from lung cancer standardised mortality ratio = 7.0 (Fletcher et al., 2004).

As only 5–10 per cent of all smokers develop lung cancer, there has been considerable interest in identifying genetic factors that might predispose to lung cancer by increasing susceptibility to environmental carcinogens. Genetic polymorphisms in the activation or detoxification of carcinogens (such as those in tobacco smoke) could be associated with interindividual susceptibilities to lung cancer. There have been numerous association studies between lung cancer risks and polymorphisms in candidate genes such as those encoding cytochrome P450 enzymes (e.g. *CYP2E1*, *CYP1A1*, *CYP2D6*), *N*-acetyltransferase (*NAT2*) and glutathione-*S*-transferases (e.g. *GSTM1* and *GSTT1*).

DNA damage repair defects have also been implicated (Spitz et al., 2003). Polymorphic variants in the *OGG1* gene (a base excision repair gene involved in the repair of oxidative damage of DNA damage) may alter the susceptibility of smokers to lung cancer (Le Marchand et al., 2002).

Although significant associations have been reported, these have not always replicated (see Hirvonen, 1995). These inconsistencies may reflect differences in study design and interethnic differences in polymorphism frequencies. Further molecular investigations should facilitate the identification of genetic susceptibility factors and may lead to methods to identify individuals most at risk from exposure to environmental carcinogens. While this might be advantageous in modifying occupational exposure, screening smokers to identify the minority at highest risk of developing lung cancer is likely to be impractical because it would have no effect on other smoking-related disorders such as coronary atherosclerosis.

Patients with MEN 1 have been identified with leiomyomas of the lung (McKeeby et al., 2001). Neuroendocrine tumours of the lung may show LOH at 11q and at 3p to a lesser extent, indicating possible involvement of the *MEN1* and/or *FHIT* (Ullmann et al., 2002).

Pleural synovial sarcomas have been described, showing a characteristic X:18 translocation (Carbone et al., 2002).

Cardiac tumours

Primary cardiac tumours are rare, being found in less than 0.1 per cent of autopsies. The most common tumour is myxoma, which accounts for up to 50 per cent of the total. Most myxomas are sporadic and occur in the over-50 years age group. However, familial myxoma has been described and may occur as a dominant trait. Familial myxomas are more frequently multiple and have an earlier age at diagnosis (20–40 years) than in sporadic cases. Cardiac myxomas occur in the autosomal dominantly inherited Carney complex (NAME syndrome; see part three) which is characterised by the occurrence of cardiac myxoma, spotty pigmentation and cutaneous myxomas, pituitary and adrenocortical tumours (Carney, 1995). Cardiac myxoma is the most serious complication of Carney complex and all individuals at risk for familial cardiac myxoma should be screened regularly by echocardiography.

Cardiac rhabdomyomas are rare and most affected patients have tuberose sclerosis (see part three). These are usually asymptomatic, are most frequent in infants, and often involute with age.

Cardiac fibromas are a feature of Gorlin syndrome (see part three), although they occur in only a small proportion (approximately 3 per cent) of patients with this disorder (Gorlin, 1987; 1995).

5

Endocrine system

Thyroid tumours

The incidence of primary epithelial cancer of the thyroid is 0.7 per 100 000 in males and 1.9 per 100 000 in females in the UK. Overall, the annual incidence of thyroid cancer is between 0.9 and 5.2 per 100 000 people, with a ratio of women to men of 2–3:1. Thyroid cancer is the most rapidly rising incident cancer in women and the second most rapidly rising incident cancer in men in the USA. Whether the papillary or follicular histology is favoured is dependent on the amount of dietary iodine in a particular region. Papillary carcinoma (PTC) accounts for more than 50 per cent of cases in the UK and USA, the next most common type of thyroid cancer being follicular carcinoma (FTC). Less frequent types are medullary (MTC), anaplastic (undifferentiated), Hurthle cell and squamous cell carcinomas. Other non-epithelial malignancies that may be observed in the thyroid include lymphomas and sarcomas, but these are rare.

PTC of the thyroid

Genetic susceptibility to PTC can be seen in familial adenomatous polyposis syndrome (FAP), Cowden syndrome (CS), possibly Carney complex (CNC) and in a familial site-specific syndrome. These syndromes are described in detail in the next section. Thyroid cancers can be detected in 5–25 per cent of FAP patients. It should be noted that there is preliminary evidence that what is commonly referred to as "PTC" in FAP is not identical to classic PTC. FAP-related thyroid cancer is of a distinct cribiform subtype (Harach et al., 1994). In contrast to classic PTC, FAP-related thyroid cancers do not show the typical fir tree branching papillary pattern, and psammoma bodies are rare or non-existent. This distinct architecture seen in *APC*-related thyroid carcinomas is very unusual in sporadic PTC (Harach et al., 1994). CS-related thyroid carcinomas are only rarely PTC (Harach et al., 1999). While thyroid tumours, for example, PTC, have been reported in CNC, it is currently unclear if PTC are true component cancers of CNC.

Several putative loci, but no genes, have been identified for non-syndromic familial PTC and are summarised in Table 5.1.

Sporadic PTC are characterised by somatic translocations between one of several genes and the intracellular domain of *RET* (at intron 11) termed

Table 5.1. *Familial PTC (reviewed in (Eng, 2000a))*

Syndrome	Chromosomal location	Comments
PTC with cell oxyphilia	*TCO*, 19p13.2	Oncocytic PTC
PTC without oxyphilia	19p13.2	
Multinodular goitre (MNG)	*MNG1*, 14q31	MNG and PTC
	MNG2, Xp22	MNG only
PTC and renal tumours	1q21	PTC, thyroid nodular disease, papillary renal cell carcinoma
PTC and clear cell renal cancer	t(3;8)(p14.2;q24.1)	
FNMTC	*NMTC1*, 2q21	Follicular variant of PTC

RET/PTCn. The precise frequency is unknown but could range from 10–60 per cent. Typically, the 5′ translocation partner encodes a protein which can force dimerisation of the kinase domain of RET, for example, leucine zippers (Santoro et al., 1990; Lanzi et al., 1992; Sozzi et al., 1992; Bongarzone et al., 1993; 1994). It would appear that PTC tumours without *RET/PTC* translocations harbour a relatively high frequency of somatic gain-of-function *BRAF* mutations (Kimura et al., 2003; Soares et al., 2003). As somatic *BRAF* mutations and the presence of the *RET/PTC* translocation or *RAS* mutations are mutually exclusive, it is suggested that activation of the RAS-RAF-MAP kinase pathway is important in PTC development but that two insults to this pathway are not necessary.

FTC of the thyroid

FTC is a proven component cancer in CS and Werner syndrome. In CS, FTC is the major component of thyroid cancer (Harach et al., 1999). However, rarely, PTC and the follicular variant of PTC are also observed (Marsh et al., 1998). In Werner syndrome, thyroid carcinoma, mainly FTC, is more commonly observed in Japanese patients than those from elsewhere. Both syndromes are discussed in detail in the next section.

The molecular aetiology of sporadic FTC remains unknown. A publication reporting a high frequency (50 per cent) of somatic *PAX8/PPARG* translocations in FTC initially suggested that this was the initiating event (Kroll et al., 2000). Subsequently, the frequency of this *PAX8/PPARG* translocation, which inactivates *PPARG* by a dominant negative mechanism, was found to be much less (10 per cent) in sporadic FTC (Aldred et al., 2003b). Instead, loss-of-function by a haploinsufficient mechanism, seems to occur more frequently and play some role in FTC development (Aldred et al., 2003b). Microarray expression strategies have been used to attempt to elucidate the molecular pathogenesis of sporadic FTC (Aldred et al., 2003b).

MTC of the thyroid

MTC, which is a carcinoma of the parafollicular C-cells, is a proven component cancer of multiple endocrine neoplasia type 2 (MEN 2), caused by germline mutations in the *RET* proto-oncogene. This syndrome is detailed in the next section. While C-cell hyperplasia was believed to be pathognomonic for MEN 2, once *RET* was identified as the MEN 2 susceptibility gene, it was discovered that this association no longer holds true and indeed, C-cell hyperplasia can be found in truly sporadic MTC (Eng et al., 1995b; Marsh et al., 1996b).

The aetiology of sporadic MTC is also not well known. Amongst all presentations of MTC, clinical epidemiologic studies have shown that 25 per cent can be attributable to MEN 2. Occult germline mutations in the *RET* proto-oncogene can be found in 5–15 per cent of apparently sporadic MTC, that is, without obvious syndromic features or family history (Blaugrund et al., 1994; Eng et al., 1995c; Wohlik et al., 1996; Schuffenecker et al., 1997). Due to these accumulating data, the general recommendations are to offer *RET* mutation analysis to all presentations of MTC irregardless of age, presence of syndromic features or family history.

Somatic *RET* mutations have been reported to occur in 10–80 per cent of sporadic MTC (Eng et al., 1994b; 1995c; Hofstra et al., 1994; Marsh et al., 1996a). The great majority of somatic *RET* mutations are M918T. Of note, somatic mutations have been found to occur in patches or subpopulations even within a single tumour (Eng et al., 1996b; 1998). Up to 80 per cent of sporadic MTC harbour at least one subpopulation with somatic M918T mutation (Eng et al., 1996a). It remains controversial whether somatic M918T in the primary tumour portends a poor prognosis. Unfortunately, because some studies have used mixed primary and metastatic tumours (e.g. Schilling et al., 2001), and because of the presence of subpopulations and the varied mutation detection technologies employed, whether M918T status is associated with prognosis remains unknown. Nonetheless, one well-designed study did not show a difference in clinical outcome with or without somatic M918T (Marsh et al., 1996b). In general, MEN 2-associated MTC do not carry somatic intragenic *RET* mutation as a second genetic event (Eng et al., 1995b). However, there are rare instances of somatic M918T occurring in MEN 2-associated MTC (Marsh et al., 1996a). It is also believed that duplication of the mutated *RET* allele in MEN 2A-associated MTC may contribute to carcinogenesis (Koch et al., 2001).

Benign neoplasias of the thyroid

Benign thyroid neoplasias such as follicular adenomas, multinodular goitres and hamartomas are components of CS (see below). Due to the risk of recurrence and the risk of thyroid cancer in CS patients or in those with a proven germline *PTEN* mutation, a total thyroidectomy should be performed if surgery is being considered for these benign thyroid lesions.

Parathyroid tumours

Parathyroid neoplasias are very common, however, familial hyperparathyroidism occurs at a frequency of about 0.14 per 100 000 and for the most part, occurs as part of the multiple endocrine neoplasia syndromes (MEN; see p. 220 and 222), with chief cell hyperplasia as the usual histologic change. The genetic differential diagnosis of parathyroid hyperplasia or parathyroid adenoma includes MEN 1, caused by germline *MEN1* mutations; MEN 2, caused by germline *RET* mutations; and hyperparathyroidism jaw tumour syndrome (HPT-JT), caused by germline mutations in *HRPT2*. Familial site-specific hyperparathyroidism can be caused by germline *MEN1* mutations as well as due to HPT-JT (Teh et al., 1998; Kassem et al., 2000). Germline mutations in the calcium-sensing receptor gene have been identified in benign familial hypocalciuric hypercalcaemia and, in homozygous form, cause neonatal severe hyperparathyroidism with parathyroid hyperplasia (Pollak et al., 1993). While parathyroid disease is very common in MEN 1 and often the first component neoplasia to manifest, hyperparathyroidism in MEN 2 occurs in 15–30 per cent of MEN 2A cases and likely manifests relatively later in life (Schuffenecker et al., 1998). Germline *RET* C634R is particularly associated with the development of hyperparathyroidism in MEN 2A (Mulligan et al., 1994; Eng et al., 1996a).

Parathyroid carcinoma is extremely rare but it is believed to be a component neoplasia of HPT-JT (Carpten et al., 2002). It is unclear, however, whether parathyroid carcinoma is a true component cancer of MEN 1 as well.

Somatic loss of heterozygosity (LOH) of markers on 11q13 as well as somatic *MEN1* mutations have been described in parathyroid hyperplasias (Friedman et al., 1992). Somatic mutations in *HRPT2* occur with a relatively high frequency in sporadic parathyroid carcinomas (Howell et al., 2003; Shattuck et al., 2003). Surprisingly, occult germline mutations in *HRPT2* were found in 3 of the 15 apparently sporadic patients with parathyroid carcinoma (Shattuck et al., 2003).

Those at risk for parathyroid hyperplasia and/or adenoma should undergo routine clinical surveillance. Management for parathyroid disease for MEN 2 is discussed in that section below.

Pituitary tumours

Tumours of the pituitary gland rarely complicate genetic conditions other than MEN 1 (see section below). The most common pituitary tumour in MEN 1 is prolactinoma (Burgess et al., 1996b), but there are several reports in the literature of familial pituitary adenomas without clinical evidence of MEN 1. Mostly, these are examples of familial acromegaly (Bergman et al., 2000; Gadelha et al., 2000; Tamura et al., 2002) and rarely of prolactinoma (Berezin and Karazik, 1995). Molecular genetic investigations have been used to argue for and against the hypothesis that familial acromegaly is allelic with *MEN1* (Bergman et al., 2000; Gadelha et al., 2000; Tamura et al., 2002). Pituitary adenoma may develop in CNC (see section below) and chromophobe adenomas may possibly have an increased frequency in Maffucci syndrome (see section below) (Schnall and Genuth, 1976).

Both somatic tumour suppressor gene inactivation and oncogene activation have been implicated in the pathogenesis of pituitary tumours. Chromosome 11 allele loss (the *MEN1* gene maps to chromosome 11q13) is the most frequent event in sporadic pituitary adenomas, and chromosome 13 allele loss is also frequent. Accordingly, there exist somatic *MEN1* mutations in sporadic pituitary adenomas (Zhuang et al., 1997). Some growth-hormone-secreting pituitary tumours have been found to contain somatic mutations which inhibit the GTPase activity of a G-protein alpha chain and convert it to a putative oncogene *gsp* (Lyons et al., 1990). This results in activation of adenyl cyclase and bypasses the need for trophic-hormone-mediated activation. Similar mutations have been found in McCune–Albright syndrome (see below).

Adrenal gland tumours

Tumours of the adrenal glands arise from either the medulla or the cortex. Adrenal medullary tumours include neuroblastomas (p. 17), embryonal tumours and phaeochromocytomas.

Phaeochromocytoma

Phaeochromocytomas are derivatives of the neural crest and arise from adrenal chromaffin cells. Extra-adrenal (chromaffin) paragangliomas may be referred to as extra-adrenal phaeochromocytomas. Medical textbooks have traditionally suggested that approximately 10 per cent of phaeochromocytomas are heritable, 10 per cent are extra-adrenal, and 10 per cent are malignant. However, the frequency of heritable phaeochromocytoma has been underestimated and in one population-based study, 25 per cent of unrelated, apparently sporadic presentations of phaeochromocytomas, without syndromic features or family history, were found to harbour germline mutations in one of four genes, *VHL, RET, SDHD* or *SDHB* (Neumann et al., 2002). Due to this and related findings, all presentations of phaeochromocytomas, irregardless of age, syndromic features or family history, should be considered for mutation analysis in the setting of cancer genetic consultation which includes genetic counselling. The genetic differential diagnosis of phaeochromocytoma includes MEN 2 caused by germline mutations in the *RET* gene, von Hippel–Lindau (VHL) disease caused by *VHL* mutations, the phaeochromocytoma–paraganglioma syndrome caused by germline mutations in the *SDHB, SDHC* and *SDHD* gene and very rarely, NF 1 (Maher and Eng, 2002; Eng et al., 2003) (see below and section to follow). Familial site-specific phaeochromocytomas are mainly attributable to germline mutations in *VHL, SDHD*, or *SDHB* (Woodward et al., 1997; Astuti et al., 2001a). Such families with phaeochromocytomas as well as chemodectomas or glomus tumours are almost always due to germline mutations in *SDHB, SDHC* or *SDHD* (Maher and Eng, 2002).

In general, like virtually all inherited neoplasias, the mean age at diagnosis for heritable phaeochromocytoma is lower, and there will be a higher incidence of bilateral tumours and multi-focal disease when compared to sporadic phaeochromocytoma. Nonetheless, these clinical features, the clinical hallmarks of heredity, are syndrome-dependent (and hence, dependent on susceptibility gene involved). For example, in the population-based study on non-syndromic phaeochromocytomas, while the mean age at presentation in individuals without germline mutations (sporadic) was 44 years, the mean age was 36 years for those shown to carry a *RET* mutation (MEN 2), 18.3 years for VHL and approximately 27 years for those found to have germline *SDHD/SDHB* mutations (Neumann et al., 2002). NF 1-related phaeochromocytomas are usually diagnosed relatively older, around 40 years. Further, of those found to carry germline mutations, about one-third presented with multi-focal disease compared to two-thirds with a solitary lesion (Neumann et al., 2002).

There has been scant information regarding somatic mutations in sporadic phaeochromocytoma except for relatively low frequencies of somatic *VHL* mutations, somatic *RET* mutations and somatic *SDHD* mutations (Eng et al., 1995a; Gimm et al., 2000; Astuti et al., 2001). Interestingly, differential distributions of frequencies of LOH at 1p, 3p and 22q exist between VHL-related phaeochromocytomas and those of sporadic tumours (Bender et al., 2000). In VHL-related phaeochromocytomas, almost all showed LOH of markers around *VHL* at 3p with LOH of markers at 1p and 22q being 15 and 21 per cent respectively. In contrast, sporadic tumours showed LOH at 3p in only 21 per cent of samples but relatively high frequencies of 1p and 22q marker LOH (Bender et al., 2000). In MEN 2-related phaeochromocytoma, it is believed that

Table 5.2. *Sample surveillance protocol for SDH mutation carrier (see also text)*

Proven *SDHB* mutation carrier
1. Annual 24 h urine for catecholamines and vanyllylmandelic acid measurements from age 5 years.
2. Annual abdominal MRI scans from age 7 years (abdominal and thoracic every 3 years).
3. MRI neck age 20 years and every 3 years thereafter.

Proven *SDHD* mutation carrier (paternally transmitted)
1. Annual 24 h urine for catecholamines and vanyllylmandelic acid measurements from age 5 years.
2. Two yearly abdominal MRI scans from age 7 years (abdominal and thoracic every 5 years).
3. MRI neck age 20 years and every 1–2 years thereafter.

amplification of the mutant *RET* allele could contribute to carcinogenesis in an unknown proportion of tumours (Huang et al., 2000).

Individuals at risk for phaeochromocytoma should be offered annual surveillance. The precise measures for clinical surveillance are dependent on the specific syndrome at-risk for and the institution. In general, annual physical examination paying particular attention to the retinal examination and blood pressure measurements, especially with orthostatic manoeuvres, and a 24-hour urinary catecholamines and vanyllylmandelic acid measurements are performed. Some centres advocate serum catecholamine, vanyllylmandelic acid and chromogranin-A measurements as well. Further investigation may include MIBG and computerised tomography (CT) or magnetic resonance imaging (MRI) scans and selective venous sampling as appropriate. Recently, positron emission tomography (PET) scanning is performed for surveillance in certain centres. Full details of screening protocols in VHL disease, NF1 and MEN 2 are described in part three and a sample screening protocol for *SDHB* and *SDHD* gene carriers is suggested in Table 5.2.

Adrenocortical adenoma and carcinoma

Adrenocortical tumours are rare (incidence approximately 0.2 per 100 000 per year) and may be benign or malignant. The most frequent presentation is with Cushing syndrome with or without associated virilisation, sometimes with primary aldosteronism; oestrogen-producing tumours are rare. Adrenocortical carcinomas are proven component cancers in Li–Fraumeni syndrome caused by germline *TP53* mutations (see below for complete discussion of this syndrome). Indeed, early onset (under the age of 4 years) or bilateral disease carries a high likelihood of germline *TP53* mutation (Malkin et al., 1990; Eng et al., 1997). In a series of 14 patients with adrenocortical carcinoma unselected for family history,

11 (82 per cent) carried a germline *TP53* mutation. Interestingly, the same two mutations (at codons 152 and 158) were present in 9 of the 11 mutation-positive cases. In another series of 36 cases of childhood adrenocortical carcinoma in southern Brazil, 35 carried an identical R337H mutation (Ribeiro et al., 2001). Some believe that adrenocortical carcinomas can be found at increased frequencies in Beckwith–Wiedemann syndrome (Wiedemann, 1983).

A macroscopically and histologically distinctive type of adrenocortical hyperplasia called primary pigmented nodular adrenocortical disease (PPNAD) is a component neoplasia of CNC (NAME syndrome), and is discussed below. PPNAD can be clinically diagnosed by its paradoxical response to dexamethasone challenge (Stratakis et al., 1999). Benign adrenocortical lesions, usually non-functional, are reported in MEN 1 patients, some believe as frequently as 20–40 per cent. Adrenocortical nodular hyperplasia and rarely adenoma may be seen in McCune–Albright syndrome (see below). Hypercortisolism is often associated with macronodular hyperplasia of the adrenal cortex.

Glomus tumours (non-chromaffin paraganglioma)

Glomus tumours are benign tumours of the head and neck region derived from neural crest and are situated predominantly at the carotid bifurcation and jugular foramen. Glomus tumours, sometimes referred to as chemodectomas, are the most common type of paraganglioma in the head and neck region. They are non-chromaffin paragangliomas, that is, they do not secrete but instead are sensing organs. Glomus tumours have an incidence of approximately 1 in 30 000 and are usually sporadic and unilateral. However, about a third of multiple cases are familial, with an autosomal dominant inheritance pattern. Bilateral disease is significantly more frequent in familial (32–38 per cent of cases) than in non-familial (4–8 per cent) cases (Grufferman et al., 1980; Parry et al., 1982). Six per cent of patients with familial chemodectomas develop second primary tumours, predominantly other paragangliomas. The inheritance of some instances of familial glomus tumours show maternal imprinting: descendants of affected females who inherit the gene do not develop glomus tumours, but heterozygote descendants of affected males do (van der Mey et al., 1989). Two loci for familial glomus tumours in Dutch kindred have been mapped to the long arm of chromosome 11: PGL1 at 11q23.1 and PGL2 at 11q13 (Heutink et al., 1992; 1994; Mariman et al., 1995). Germline mutations in *SDHD* on 11q23.1 (PGL1) was described in families with glomus tumours with and without thoracic/adrenal paragangliomas (Baysal et al., 2000). In mutation-positive families, maternal imprinting was demonstrated. Perhaps because of maternal imprinting, occult germline *SDHD* mutations are evident in a relatively high frequency of apparently sporadic adrenal phaeochromocytoma or paraganglioma patients (Gimm et al., 2000). Subsequently, germline mutations in *SDHB* (PGL4) in individuals and families with paraganglioma and/or phaeochromocytomas were described (Astuti et al., 2001a). Interestingly, only two families with paragangliomas have been described with germline *SDHC* (PGL3) mutations (Niemann and Muller, 2000). The gene on 11q13 underlying PGL2 has yet to be identified and only a single Dutch family is linked to this locus. Paragangliomas may occur in CNC (p. 176).

Pancreatic endocrine tumours

Non-endocrine pancreatic tumours are described on page 52.

Pancreatic endocrine tumours (islet cell adenomas such as gastrinoma, insulinoma, glucagonoma, VIPoma, somatostatinoma) may occur in up to 1.5 per cent of autopsies but are mostly asymptomatic. Pancreatic endocrine tumours are a feature of MEN 1 and VHL disease (see part three).

6

Gastrointestinal system

Tumours of the gastrointestinal system are among the most common tumours in humans, and although environmental influences have been clearly implicated, heredity is recognised as being of major importance in their aetiology.

Oesophageal tumours

The incidence of squamous cell carcinoma of the oesophagus shows marked geographical variation, with a high frequency in the Caspian littoral of Iran, certain parts of the interior of China and the Transkei region of South Africa, and a low incidence in European and North American whites. Oropharyngeal tumours are also commoner in areas with a high incidence of oesophageal cancer. These findings are thought to be the result of differences in exposure to ingested carcinogens rather than of major genetic factors, although the at-risk individuals who develop this cancer in these high-risk areas are predominantly of Mongol or Turkic origin. The incidence of oesophageal cancer in the UK is 6 per 100 000, and it is commoner in males. Almost all (98 per cent) of oesophageal cancers are squamous carcinomas.

Early studies suggested that genetic factors do not play a major role in most cases of oesophageal cancer as there did not appear to be an increased risk to relatives of index cases (Mosbech and Videbaek, 1955), and recent studies in the United States have been in agreement (Dhillon et al., 2001). However other studies, particularly those in high-incidence regions such as China, have come to the conclusion that the familial occurrence of oesophageal cancer probably does have a Mendelian basis, with both autosomal dominant (Zhang et al., 2000) and recessive (Carter et al., 1992) models favoured. A genome-wide search indicated that chromosome 13 could harbour such a gene, but sequence analysis of known candidate genes, such as *BRCA2*, have been inconclusive (Hu et al., 2002; N. Hu, 2004). Interestingly, gene expression studies indicate that true differences exist between familial and non-familial oesophageal cancer, suggesting that there are susceptibility genes to be found (Su et al., 2003).

The autosomal dominant condition of late onset tylosis, with hyperkeratosis of the palms and soles from late childhood or adolescence (palmoplantar keratoderma), is associated with a high incidence of oesophageal carcinoma in affected individuals (Harper, 1973; p. 163). Tylosis with onset in infancy does not appear to be associated with any increased risk of oesophageal cancer. Thickening of the skin of the pressure areas of the soles of the feet is seen, and oral leucokeratosis and follicular hyperkeratosis occur. The incidence of oesophageal cancer in gene carriers (heterozygotes) reaches 95 per cent by the age of 63 years, and the mean age at onset of the cancer is 45 years (Shine and Allison, 1966). Prophylactic oesophagectomy with interposition of a segment of colon has been suggested for affected individuals. The gene for this condition has been mapped to chromosome 17q, but distal to the keratin gene cluster on 17q (Hennies et al., 1995; Kelsell et al., 1996). Gene identification has proved to be difficult (Risk et al., 2002; Langan et al., 2004).

There is an increased risk of oesophageal cancer in Fanconi anaemia (Alter, 1996; see p. 195), and possibly also in epidermolysis bullosa (p. 153), dyskeratosis congenita (p. 152) and congenital abnormalities of the oesophagus, such as strictures. The risk of oesophageal cancer is increased in coeliac disease (p. 178) and is more common in the adult-onset form, but is probably uncommon when coeliac disease is diagnosed and treated in childhood or infancy. There is an increased risk of oesophageal cancer in achalasia. This condition is not usually genetic, but its familial occurrence has been described occasionally (Frieling et al., 1988). Nevertheless it may occur rarely as part of a genetic condition (autosomal recessive), characterised by achalasia, alacrimia and sensorimotor polyneuropathy, and known as Allgrove syndrome (Kasirga et al., 1996).

There is also an increased risk of adenocarcinoma of the oesophagus (possibly 10 per cent) in Barrett oesophagus, in which columnar rather than squamous epithelium is found with chronic ulcerative oesophagitis. Although this is usually sporadic, some familial cases have been described, and 70 families have recently been reported (Drovdlic et al., 2003). Importantly, there was no excess of extra-oesophageal cancers in these families. In unselected individuals with Barrett oesophagus, it is among older males that most familial cases are encountered (Chak et al., 2002).

In tylosis, annual oesophagoscopy is recommended unless prophylactic oesophagectomy has been performed and, because of the high risk of cancer in this disorder, immediate oesophagectomy is advisable if dysplasia is detected. However, in other conditions in which the risk of carcinoma is less, the appropriate course of action if an abnormality is found may not be so clear, and results from an observational study of individuals undergoing surveillance for Barrett oesophagus found that there was no impact on overall mortality (MacDonald et al., 2000). Nevertheless, those with a family history are likely to be screened by endoscopy, even if they do not have long-segment disease. Screening for oesophageal cancer by endoscopy with multiple biopsies to detect dysplasia is performed in some high-risk areas in China (Spigelman and Phillips, 1991).

Salivary gland tumours

Tumours at this site occur with a frequency of about 1 per 100 000 population. They are commoner in Spanish, Eskimo, Indian and Cantonese Chinese populations, but do not appear to have a strong genetic basis. Familial occurrence of mixed salivary tumours has been reported infrequently (Klausner and Handler, 1994), and it is difficult to know whether the familial incidence is determined by hereditary or environmental factors. However, similarities in the epidemiology of nasopharyngeal carcinoma and salivary gland tumours suggest that they may have a similar aetiology, perhaps involving Epstein–Barr virus (EBV) infection (Ponz de Leon, 1994). Several Greenland Inuit families have been described with two or more siblings affected, and there was an increased risk of other cancers in these sibships (Merrick et al., 1986). Other studies from Greenland show that a significant fraction of all cases occurring among Greenland Inuit cluster in families (Albeck et al., 1993). Cancer incidence in this part of the world differs from that seen in more temperate climates: compared to the Caucasian population in Denmark (1973–1995), high standardised incidence ratios (SIRs) were found for cancers of the salivary gland and nasopharynx (EBV-related cancers), oesophagus, stomach (probably related to a dried fish diet) and cervix (HPV-related). Low SIRs were seen for testis, bladder, prostate, breast and hematologic cancers (Friborg et al., 2003).

A proportion of salivary gland adenomas may be shown to have abnormalities of chromosomes 7, 8, 9, 15, 18, 19, 21, 22 and Y. Translocations involving chromosome 8 with a breakpoint at 8q12 are frequently observed, often also involving chromosome 3 or 12 (Mark and Dahlenfors, 1986; Sahlin and Stenman, 1995). This is thought to result in promoter swapping between the genes for a zinc finger protein and beta catenin (Kas et al., 1997).

Submicroscopic deletions on chromosome 3p may be detected in pleiomorphic adenomas of the salivary glands with t(3:8)(p21;q12), as demonstrated by loss of heterozygosity at loci from this region (Sahlin et al., 1994).

Rare families with familial neuroendocrine carcinoma of the salivary glands and deafness and enamel hyperplasia (siblings) are described (Michaels et al., 1999).

MALT lymphomas may occur in the lymphoid tissue of the salivary glands, often associated with a translocation T (14:18 (q.32;q.21) (Streubel et al., 2003). MALT lymphomas may develop in benign lesions developing from long-standing Sjogren's syndrome. There has been a case report of a 3-year old child with a plexiform neurofibroma involving the submandibular salivary gland that mimicked an intra-glandular tumour (Bourgeois et al., 2001). There was a family history of neurofibromatosis.

Gastric tumours

Benign tumours of the stomach are uncommon. Polyploid adenomas occur in less than 1 per cent of the population, and may occur in association with intestinal metaplasia. They predispose to carcinoma. Gastric polyps occur in familial adenomatous polyposis (in up to two-thirds of patients, but with a lower potential for malignant transformation than the colonic adenomas, see p. 167), in Peutz–Jeghers syndrome and in Cowden syndrome. Gastric polyposis (with malignant potential) limited to the stomach has been described in three generations of a family (dos Santos and de Magalhes, 1980).

Hyperplastic gastric polyps are five times as common as gastric polyps, and have a much lower risk of malignancy. They are found with increased frequency in pernicious anaemia and in familial adenomatous polyposis (Debinski et al., 1995) and the Peutz–Jeghers syndrome (Ushio et al., 1976; Williams et al., 1982). Carcinoids, lymphomas, sarcomas and leiomyosarcomas may also arise in the stomach; a family with primary B-cell gastric lymphoma in a father and his two daughters has been described (Hayoz et al., 1993).

Gastric carcinoma

The incidence of gastric cancer (which is adenocarcinoma in 97 per cent of cases) shows marked geographical variation, being 88 per 100 000 males in Japan, and 22 and 11 per 100 000 in the UK and USA respectively. Women have about half the male incidence. There is a twofold to threefold excess risk of gastric cancer in the first-degree relatives of affected patients, particularly in cases diagnosed under the age of 50 years (Lehtol, 1978). Two major histological variants of gastric cancer are recognised; diffuse and intestinal type gastric cancer. The latter is preceded by chronic gastritis, atrophy and metaplasia. However, the diffuse histological type does not have recognised precursor changes (Correa and Shiao, 1994). An association between blood group A and gastric cancer (particularly the diffuse type) has long been recognised. This could in part be due to the association of this blood group with pernicious anaemia, which itself carries a higher than expected risk of gastric cancer (McConnell, 1966). The risk of gastric cancer in relatives of index cases appears to be much more pronounced when the histological type in the index case is diffuse (seven times the risk in matched controls) rather than of the intestinal type (1.5 times higher than in control families) (Macklin, 1960), but only a small proportion of diffuse gastric cancers occur in families with an autosomal dominant gastric cancer susceptibility.

The diffuse type of gastric carcinoma demonstrates a nearly equal sex ratio (compared with a male preponderance in the intestinal type), a younger patient age distribution, and little change with geographical migration, relative to the intestinal type. Chronic atrophic gastritis is found with increased frequency in relatives of index cases with pernicious anaemia and gastric adenocarcinomas but, specifically, it has been demonstrated to be more frequent in the relatives of index cases with diffuse spreading carcinoma than in controls; this has not been seen with other gastric cancer types (Kekki et al., 1987). Evidence suggests there may be an association between chronic *Helicobacter pylori* infection and intestinal-type chronic gastritis and cancer susceptibility: an increased frequency of infection with this organism has been reported in stomach cancer patients (Scott et al., 1990). Chronic gastritis may have a hereditary component, but the nature of this and its relationship to *Helicobacter* infection have not been clearly elucidated (Kekki et al., 1987). Ménétrièr's disease is also associated with an increased risk (10 per cent) of gastric cancer – possibly because atrophic gastritis occurs in this aetiologically obscure disease.

There are many reports of families in which there is a strikingly high incidence of gastric cancer, following an autosomal dominant pattern of inheritance (Triantafillidis et al., 1993). Napoleon Bonaparte came from such a family (Creagen and Fraumeni, 1973). Gastric carcinoma occurs as a component of hereditary non-polyposis colorectal cancer (HNPCC; see p. 200; Ohue et al., 1996; Cristofaro et al., 1987; Chuev et al., 1996; Lynch et al., 1990a). An increased incidence of stomach cancer has also been noted in the close relatives of women with the medullary or tubular histological types of breast cancer. Some of these families may have Li–Fraumeni syndrome (Burki et al., 1987) and gastric carcinoma has also been described in some families with *p53* mutations (Varley et al., 1995). Lobular breast cancer may be seen in families with germline *CDH1* mutations (see below).

Adenocarcinoma of the stomach is reported in familial adenomatous polyposis (Jagelman et al., 1988), and is also reported to be more frequent in ataxia telangiectasia (Haerer et al., 1969; see p. 157) and in patients with immune deficiency. IgA deficiency is associated with an increased risk of intestinal metaplasia and of gastric cancer. The inheritance of IgA deficiency is not clear-cut and may be multifactorial (Grundbacher, 1972). Gastric cancer occurs with increased relative risk in carriers of germline *BRCA2* mutations (Breast Cancer Linkage Consortium, 1997; Jajubowska et al., 2002). Gastric carcinoma (particularly of the intestinal type) is also part of the spectrum of cancers found in HNPCC, and displays replication errors (RER) characteristic of the condition in such families. The average age at diagnosis of gastric carcinoma in HNPCC has been reported to be 56 years (Arnio et al., 1997).

The International Gastric Cancer Linkage Consortium (IGCLC) defined Hereditary Diffuse Gastric Cancer (HDGC) as (a) families with two or more cases of diffuse gastric cancer in first or second-degree relatives with one affected aged <50 years or (b) three cases of diffuse gastric cancers in first or second-degree relatives at any age (Caldas et al., 1999). HDGC is genetically heterogeneous. Germline mutations in the E-cadherin (CDH1) gene were described initially in three Maori kindreds with familial diffuse gastric cancer, but have since been reported worldwide (Gayther et al., 1998; Guilford et al., 1998; Richards et al., 1999; Brooks-Wilson et al., 2004). Overall, about 30 per cent of patients with HDGC will have a germline CDH1 mutation and this rises to about 50 per cent in younger onset cases (<50 years) with a positive family history. However isolated early onset cases of diffuse gastric cancer are unlikely to have germline CDH1 mutations (Brooks-Wilson et al., 2004). CDH1 mutation carriers are estimated to have a cumulative risk of 67 and 83 per cent in men and women respectively at age 80 years (Pharoah et al., 2001). In addition there is an increased risk of breast cancer, particularly lobular, with a cumulative risk of 39 per cent in women with germline CDH1 mutations. Gastric cancer screening in high-risk individuals (e.g. by annual gastroscopy) is problematical because of false-negative results. Hence in CDH1 mutation carriers, prophylactic gastrectomy should be considered (despite significant morbidity and mortality). Indeed multifocal early diffuse gastric cancers were detected in prophylactic gastrectomy specimens from individuals with CDH1 truncating mutations (Huntsman et al., 2001). For mutation carriers for whom prophylactic gastrectomy is not acceptable, chromoendoscopic surveillance using the methylene blue/congo red staining may facilitate early cancer diagnosis (Shaw et al., 2005).

For individuals at risk for familial gastric cancer without CDH1 mutations, endoscopy with eradication of H. pylori infection is performed as an initial step. Subsequently endoscopies may be performed 1–2 yearly, depending on the family history.

Hepatic tumours

Cancer of the liver typically occurs as hepatocellular carcinoma or intrahepatic bile duct cancer (cholangiocarcinoma) in adults and as hepatoblastoma in childhood.

Hepatoblastoma

This rare tumour usually presents below the age of 3 years, is more common in males than in females and shows no association with hepatitis B infection or cirrhosis. It may occur in the "overgrowth syndromes" which include congenital hemihypertrophy (Muller et al., 1978; p. 200), Beckwith–Wiedemann syndrome

(BWS) (p. 170), Sotos syndrome and Bannayan–Riley–Ruvalcaba syndrome. Of the overgrowth syndromes, Weaver and Marshall–Smith syndromes seem to be associated with the smallest risk of embryonal tumours (Cohen, 1989). Hepatoblastoma may occur in children with familial adenomatous polyposis (Herzog et al., 2000) (p. 184).

Congenital abnormalities are common in children with hepatoblastoma, and have been reported in up to a third of cases. The abnormalities described include hemihypertrophy, polycystic kidney disease and abnormalities of the urinogenital system, many of which occur in the overgrowth syndromes. Familial cases occasionally occur (Hartley et al., 1990).

There is no consensus regarding screening for hepatoblastoma and other embryonal tumours in BWS and other overgrowth syndromes. However, the risk of neoplasia in children with this disorder is increased if hemihypertrophy is present and children with BWS and loss of methylation at KvDMR1 appear to be at higher risk of hepatoblastoma than Wilms tumour (Cooper et al., 2005). In high-risk cases, physical examination, serum alphafetoprotein and abdominal ultrasound may be performed in the neonatal period, then every 3 months until the age of 3 years, and then every 6 months until the age of 6 years (Chitayat et al., 1990).

Hepatocellular carcinoma

Most cases of hepatocellular carcinoma occur in adults, appear to be sporadic, and are related to environmental carcinogens such as hepatitis B viral infections and aflatoxin. The marked geographical variations in the incidence of hepato-cellular carcinoma (it is frequent in Africa and Asia, reaching an incidence of 40 per 100 000 males) are thought to be caused by environmental factors. The incidence in the UK is 1–1.6 per 100 000, and it is commoner in males. Familial clustering of hepatocellular cancer has occasionally been reported (Fernandez et al., 1994; Drinkwater and Lee, 1995), and the relative risk of the cancer in the first-degree relatives of index cases with primary liver cancer has been assessed to be 2.4 (Fernandez et al., 1994). However familial clustering of hepatitis B virus is common as a consequence of perinatal transmission and this is regarded as the main cause of familial hepatocellular carcinoma in high-prevalence areas (Tai et al., 2002).

Liver cancer may occur as a complication of chronic liver disease and cirrho-sis of a variety of causes (although it is rare in biliary cirrhosis), some of which have a genetic basis (see Table 6.1). In haemochromatosis, the incidence of hepatic car-cinoma is usually only increased if cirrhosis has developed. Haemochromatosis is a common condition affecting about 1 in 300 individuals of Northern European descent. However many cases are asymptomatic and women are less severely

Table 6.1. *Genetic causes of liver cancer*

Important causes	Less commonly associated
Haemochromatosis	Galactosaemia
α_1-Antitrypsin deficiency	Hereditary fructose intolerance
Glycogen storage disease	Iron overload in thalassaemia
Type I (hepatic)	Iron overload in hereditary haemorrhagic telangiectasia
Type IV	Acute intermittent porphyria
Tyrosinaemia	Common bile duct atresia
Fanconi anaemia	Neonatal hepatitis
Wilson disease	Cystic fibrosis
	De Toni–Fanconi syndrome
	Werner syndrome
	Familial cirrhosis
	Indian childhood cirrhosis
	Neonatal giant cell hepatitis
	Neonatal haemochromatosis
	Porphyria cutanea tarda

affected than men because of menstrual blood loss (Brind and Bassendine, 1990). Hepatocellular carcinoma develops in up to one-third of cirrhotic cases, in whom the relative risk of hepatoma may be 200 (Edwards et al., 1982). Treatment by phlebotomy before cirrhosis develops appears to prevent malignancy (Niederau et al., 1985), although occasionally liver cancer has been reported in the absence of cirrhosis. The *HFE* gene is closely linked to the MHC class I gene cluster at 6p21 (Feder et al., 1996). The two common *HFE* mutations, *C282Y* and *H63D* are readily screened for. A diagnosis of haemochromatosis can be made in *C283Y* homozygotes and *C282Y/H63D* compound heterozygotes. Screening of at-risk relatives is important as early diagnosis allows treatment with prophylactic phlebotomy, and the prevention of cirrhosis from developing will reduce the risk of hepatocellular cancer (Harrison and Bacon, 2005).

Alpha-1 antitrypsin deficiency, particularly with the ZZ phenotype, predisposes to hepatocellular carcinoma (Eriksson et al., 1986). This is an autosomal recessive condition with a frequency of 1 in 2000 births. Alpha-1 antitrypsin is a serum protease inhibitor encoded by a gene on chromosome 14q31–q32. The phenotype (Pi type) is determined by isoelectric focusing of serum, and both parental alleles are expressed. PiMZ heterozygotes may also have an increased risk of hepatocellular cancer, but not those with the null–null phenotype. The commonest phenotype in the UK (PiM) is associated with normal levels of AAT, PiZ is associated with 15 per cent levels of serum AAT, and null variants are associated with no detectable levels. About 10 per cent of PiZZ individuals develop neonatal cholestatic jaundice, and 25 per cent of these develop cirrhosis. PiZ adults have a risk relative to the normal population of 7.4 for cirrhosis, and 20 for hepatocellular carcinoma (higher in males) (Brind and Bassendine, 1990; Perlmutter, 1995).

Individuals with type 1 (hepatic) glycogen storage disease, an autosomal recessive condition due to deficiency of glucose-6-phosphatase, often develop liver adenomas, and hepatoblastomas and hepatocellular carcinomas have been described (Ito et al., 1987). Glycogen storage disease type IV (due to a glycogen debrancher enzyme defect) is also associated with cirrhosis and hepatic cancer.

Hepatoma is a significant cause of death in individuals suffering from the autosomal recessive condition of hereditary tyrosinaemia (due to a defect in the fumaryl acetoacetase gene on chromosome 15q; Rootwelt et al., 1996), consequent upon the progressive liver disease with cirrhosis in this condition. About a third of affected children develop liver cancer if they survive to the age of 5 years (Fisch et al., 1978).

Other inherited disorders (e.g. galactosaemia, hereditary fructose intolerance) may result in chronic liver damage and so predispose to carcinoma of the liver. Wilson disease, an autosomal recessive copper storage disorder, can cause cirrhosis in the absence of successful therapy with chelating agents. The risk of intra-abdominal malignancy (hepatomas, cholangiocarcinomas and poorly differentiated adenocarcinomas of unknown primary) is substantial in patients followed for >10 years and surveillance by abdominal ultrasound may be indicated (Walshe et al., 2003). Iron overload can produce cirrhosis of the liver in thalassaemia, and hereditary haemorrhagic telangiectasia may occasionally predispose to liver carcinoma. The hepatic porphyrias can be associated with cirrhosis, and primary liver carcinoma (not always in the presence of cirrhosis) has been described in patients with acute intermittent porphyria (Gubler et al., 1990). Common bile duct atresia, neonatal hepatitis, cystic fibrosis and the De Toni–Fanconi syndrome are also associated with a risk of cirrhosis and potentially of liver cancer.

Hepatic carcinoma is described in Fanconi anaemia (Alter, 1996) and may sometimes be secondary to androgen therapy for the pancytopenia (Mulvihill et al., 1975). Werner syndrome may also carry an increased risk for liver cancer. Familial cases of cirrhosis without a known predisposing cause have been described, but this group is probably heterogeneous and often environmental in aetiology. Indian childhood cirrhosis, with onset between 6 and 18 months of age, has been described with familial occurrence (in about 30 per cent of cases) in India, Pakistan, Sri Lanka and Burma, but the clinical course is usually too rapid for liver cancer to have time to develop. Multifactorial inheritance has been suggested for this condition (Kumar, 1984). Neonatal giant cell hepatitis is a rare autosomal recessive disorder or group of disorders (including neonatal haemochromatosis) in which primary hepatic cancer has occasionally been described (Sandor et al., 1976).

There are occasional reports of familial hepatomas in the literature, occurring without cirrhosis, but these are rare. In one family, affected individuals also suffered from maturity onset diabetes mellitus of the young (MODY) (Foster et al., 1978), Bluteau et al. (2002) demonstrated somatic and germline mutations in *TCF1* at 12q24 in patients with hepatic adenomas. MODY type 3 is caused by heterozygous germline mutations in the *TCF1* that encodes hepatocyte nuclear factor 1 (HNF1). Thus *TCF1* inactivation, with or without MODY3, is important in the pathogenesis of hepatic adenoma. The incidence of second malignancies in individuals with hepatocellular carcinoma has been reported to be high (9 per cent), and the second primaries were of the types seen in the cancer family syndrome, suggesting the involvement of a similar genetic predisposition in these conditions (Miyanaga et al., 1989). A specific mutation in *TP53* (a GC to TA transversion at codon 249) can be frequently demonstrated in sporadic cases of hepatocellular carcinoma, and is probably related to the mutagenic action of aflatoxin B1 and possibly also the hepatitis virus (Harris, 1991; Wands and Blum, 1991).

Cholangiocarcinoma of the liver

This liver tumour develops from the epithelial cells of the bile duct and occurs more often in males than females; it is 15 times less common than hepatocellular carcinoma. It occurs in individuals about 10 years older than those with hepatocellular carcinoma, and chronic liver disease is not such an important aetiological feature. In patients with ulcerative colitis, the risk of biliary tract tumours is about ten times greater than in the general population, and may be related to the duration and severity of the colitis. This association is particularly seen in patients of certain HLA haplotypes (HLA B8). Familial aggregation of biliary tract tumours is rarely reported. Periampullary cancers are seen in familial adenomatous polyposis (p. 184), and bile duct cancers may also occur with congenital dilatation of the bile ducts, or with congenital absence of the gallbladder and cystic ducts.

Hepatic angiosarcoma

This rare tumour (occurring in the 50–70-year age group) may be associated with environmental exposure to agents such as vinyl chloride monomer, Thorotrast and inorganic arsenic in up to 25 per cent of cases (Schottenfeld and Fraumeni, 1982).

Tumours of the gallbladder

Cancer of the gallbladder is relatively rare, with an incidence of 2 per 100 000, is commoner in females, and has a peak incidence in the seventh decade. Most gall-bladder cancers (95 per cent) are adenocarcinomas, and cholelithiasis appears to be the most important predisposing factor. The frequency is very high in North American Indians, and commoner in the Japanese and in Caucasians than in negroid races. There is an increased relative risk of this cancer in the first-degree relatives of index cases–of up to 14 (Fernandez et al., 1994). Familial clustering is very rare, but two families in which several cases of this disorder occurred were described in Hispanic Indians from New Mexico, perhaps reflecting a higher genetic risk for this cancer in this racial group (Devor and Buechley, 1979). Developmental abnormalities of the pancreatobiliary ducts, including chole-dochal cysts, are associated with malignancy in situ, but these are rarely familial.

Biliary tract cancer appears to occur with increased frequency in HNPCC and may be part of the spectrum of cancers to which individuals with HNPCC are predisposed (Aarnio et al., 1995; see p. 200).

Pancreatic cancer

In recent years, the incidence of pancreatic cancer has been increasing in indus-trialised nations, and it now occurs with a frequency of 8–10 per 100 000 popu-lation and is more common in males. Pancreatic cancer accounts for about 5 per cent of all cancer deaths. Tumours of the endocrine pancreas are described on page 41.

Up to 6 per cent of individuals with pancreatic carcinoma may have a positive family history of the condition, and there is up to fivefold increased risk of this cancer in the first-degree relatives of index cases (Fernandez et al., 1994; Ghadirian et al., 2002). However, familial clustering is relatively rare, but the tumour may occur as part of the spectrum of malignancies in HNPCC (p. 200), in hereditary cutaneous malignant melanoma families, (p. 139), in fami-lies segregating BRCA1, and especially BRCA2 mutations (see below, and p. 75). It also occurs as part of Li–Fraumeni syndrome (p. 215), and it is thought to occur with increased frequency in Peutz–Jeghers syndrome (p. 241), and in ataxia telangiectasia (p. 167) (Flanders and Foulkes, 1996). The occurrence of pancreatic cancer in kindred with several cases of breast cancer is a significant predictor of a germline mutation in BRCA2 (Ozcelik et al., 1997; see below). In addition, families have been reported in which several cases of cancer of the pan-creas have occurred in a sibship, albeit with late age at onset. Although autoso-mal recessive inheritance has been suggested (Friedman and Fialklow, 1976), there is evidence of autosomal dominant inheritance in other affected families

(Ehrenthal et al., 1987; Lynch et al., 1990a; Evans et al., 1995), and dominant inheritance with incomplete penetrance would be a unifying explanation. The age at onset, histology, sex distribution and survival of familial pancreatic cancer appear to be similar to those of non-familial cases. Mutations in *CDKN2A* (encoding p16) on chromosome 9p21 are present in some families with multiple cases of cutaneous malignant melanoma, and in some families, the risk of pancreatic cancer is very high (Goldstein et al., 1995; 2004; Ghiorzo et al., 1999; Lynch et al., 2002; de Vos tot Nederveen Cappel et al., 2003). By contrast, in familial pancreas cancer, if there are no cases of melanoma, *CDKN2A* mutations are not found (Lal et al., 2000; Bartsch et al., 2002).

Mutations in the breast cancer susceptibility gene, *BRCA2*, are found in some familial pancreas cancer kindred (Murphy et al., 2002; Hahn et al., 2003), although several of the mutations were *BRCA2:6174delT*, and studies that did not include a high proportion of Ashkenazi Jews tended to have lower *BRCA2* mutation frequencies. Nevertheless, there is an excess of pancreas cancers in breast cancer families carrying *BRCA2* mutations (Cancer risks in *BRCA2* mutation carriers. The Breast Cancer Linkage Consortium 1999), and there is also a twofold increase in risk in carriers of mutations in *BRCA1* (Thompson and Easton, 2002).

The Fanconi Anaemia genes have been implicated in pancreatic cancer but the true contribution of these genes is uncertain (Rogers et al., 2004).

One family has been described with a specific form of hereditary pancreas carcinoma, where there is clear architectural distortion within the pancreas, and a high incidence of dysplasia. In some cases, preventive pancreatectomy has been carried out, and incipient, or early cancers were identified. The gene has been linked to the telomeric regions of chromosome 4q (Eberle et al., 2002), but it seems likely that this gene will account for a very small proportion of familial pancreas cancer. Pancreatic cancer is reported to occur in familial adenomatous polyposis (p. 184), although the tumours usually, actually arise from the ampulla of Vater.

There is an increased risk of adenocarcinoma of the pancreas in hereditary pancreatitis, a well described but uncommon autosomal dominant condition associated with attacks from childhood of recurrent pancreatitis in affected family members (Kattwinkel et al., 1973). The condition has been mapped to chromosome 7q and mutations in the cationic trypsinogen gene *PRSS1* have been detected in affected individuals (Whitcomb et al., 1996). A recent survey showed that among 112 families in 14 European countries (418 affected individuals), 58 (52 per cent) families carried a *R122H* mutation, 24 (21 per cent) had the *N29I* mutation and 5 (4 per cent) had the *A16V* mutation. Other mutations were very rare, but 19 per cent of all families had no identified mutations in *PRSS1* (Howes et al., 2004). Other genetic causes of chronic pancreatitis, such as *CFTR* (Sharer et al., 1998; Pezzilli et al., 2003) or *SPINK1* (Witt et al., 2001) mutations do not appear to frequent in those with pancreatic cancer (Malats et al., 2001; Pezzilli et al., 2003; Teich et al., 2003), but there could be instances where it would be worthwhile to look for specific mutations, such as ΔF508 in *CFTR* and N34S in *SPINK1* in individuals with pancreas cancer in the context of chronic pancreatitis.

Pancreatic cancer has been described in a case of Williams syndrome, possibly secondary to hypercalcaemia (Jensen et al., 1976). Pancreatoblastoma has been described in the BWS (Koh et al., 1986; see p. 170) and rarely, in familial adenomatous polyposis (Abraham et al., 2001). Overexpression of IGF2 may underlie these cancers in both conditions (Kerr et al., 2002).

Screening for pancreatic cancer is extremely difficult because minor abnormalities detected by screening may be difficult to interpret as there is no clear premalignant lesion, and there are no well-recognised protocols. However, abdominal and endoscopic ultrasonography and endoscopic retrograde cholangiopancreatography (ERCP) have been suggested as possible screening methods, although the latter is probably too invasive except for the most high-risk families, where structural abnormalities may be identified (Brentnall et al., 1999); serum CA 19.9 does not appear to be suitably sensitive, but islet amyloid polypeptide may detect early pancreatic cancer. *KRAS* mutations are common in pancreatic carcinomas and their detection in pancreatic juice may also be a helpful diagnostic marker; a combination of such indicators may be developed for use in screening for pancreatic cancer in time (Lynch et al., 1996b; Urrita and DiMagno, 1996), but as yet no clinically useful tests of this type have emerged.

Tumours of the small intestine

Benign tumours of the small gut are uncommon, the most frequent being leiomyomas and lipomas. Malignant small intestinal tumours are also rare, accounting for about 1 per cent of all intestinal neoplasms (incidence of 0.5 per 100 000 population in the UK). In order of decreasing frequency, these are adenocarcinomas, carcinoids, lymphomas and leiomyosarcomas.

Gastric, duodenal and jejunal adenomas have been reported in 8 per cent, 31 per cent and 53 per cent of patients with familial adenomatous polyposis respectively (De Pietri et al., 1995; see p. 167), and upper gastroenterological malignancy is the commonest cause of death in individuals with familial adenomatous polyposis coli who have had a colectomy (Burt et al., 1994).

Adenocarcinoma of the small bowel has been reported in families with HNPCC (p. 200), with a high-relative risk (100–300 in individuals with HNPCC) (Lynch et al., 1989b; Vasen et al., 1996), and a high proportion of small intestinal carcinomas (about 45 per cent) appear to demonstrate RER characteristic of cancers in HNPCC (Hibi et al., 1997).

Crohn's disease is associated with an increased risk of small intestinal carcinoma, usually in chronic cases (Fresko et al., 1982). Crohn's disease and ulcerative colitis are multifactorial conditions, but the familial contribution is becoming increasingly appreciated, with sibling relative risks of 30–40 for Crohns and 10–20 for ulcerative colitis, and with the identification of a susceptibility locus, NOD2/ CARD2 which is one of several susceptibility gene loci for this multifactorial condition (Mathew and Lewis, 2004).

Coeliac disease in adults is associated with an increased risk of small bowel lymphoma and, less commonly, of carcinoma (Holmes et al., 1980; see p. 178). Small bowel lymphomas may develop as a complication of immune deficiency disorders.

Pancreatoduodenal endocrine tumours may occur in multiple endocrine neoplasia type 1 and these require aggressive management (Bartsch et al., 2000).

Hamartomatous polyps occur in the small intestine in Peutz–Jegher syndrome (p. 241), and there is a significant risk of malignant degeneration in these polyps, resulting in a 2–13 per cent lifetime risk of CRC in affected individuals (Jenne et al., 1998).

Other small bowel tumours are rare but may have genetic implications, carcinoid tumours are discussed on page 58, hamartomatous polyposis of the upper gastrointestinal tract has been reported in Gorlin syndrome (p. 196), small intestinal neurofibroma may complicate NF1 (p. 230), and angiomas of the small gut occurs in hereditary haemorrhagic telangiectasia. There have been rare reports of familial polyposis of the entire gastrointestinal tract, but these may be cases of familial adenomatous polyposis (Yonemoto et al., 1969). Gastrointestinal stromal tumours (GIST), leiomyomas and leiomyosarcomas may occur, and germline C-KIT mutations have been described in individuals with familial GISTs and hyperpigmentation (Robson et al., 2004).

Upper gastrointestinal endoscopy on a regular basis is advocated for individuals with familial adenomatous polyposis (p. 184) and Peutz–Jegher syndrome (Debinski et al., 1995; p. 241).

Gastrointestinal polyposis

Disorders associated with gastrointestinal polyposis may be classified according to the histological type of the polyps (Hodgson and Murday, 1994; see Table 6.2). Adenomatous polyps occur in familial adenomatous polyposis (p. 184), Turcot syndrome (p. 250), MYH polyposis (p. 230) and in HNPCC (p. 200) and occasionally in Cowden syndrome (p. 179). Hamartomatous polyps occur in Peutz–Jegher syndrome (p. 241), juvenile polyposis, p. 211 (Hyer et al., 2000; p. 155; Zhou et al., 2001b; Erdman & Barnard, 2002), and the hereditary mixed

Table 6.2. *Conditions associated with gastrointestinal polyposis*

1. Adenomatous polyposis
FAP
MYH-associated polyposis
HNPCC
Turcot syndrome

2. Hamartomatous polyposis
Juvenile polyposis
Cowden disease
Ruvalcaba–Myhre–Smith syndrome
Peutz–Jeghers syndrome
Gorlin syndrome
McCune–Albright syndrome
Cronkhite–Canada syndrome
Tuberose sclerosis (few, rectal polyps)
Hereditary mixed polyposis syndrome

3. Inflammatory polyps
Inflammatory bowel disease
Devon polyposis

4. Ganglio/neurofibromata
Neurofibromatosis type 1
MEN 2B

5. Hyperplastic polyposis

polyposis syndrome (HMPS) (Whitelaw et al., 1997), Cowden syndrome p. 179 (Gentry et al., 1978; Eng, 2003), Ruvalcaba–Myhre syndrome (p. 169), McCune–Albright syndrome and occasionally in Gorlin syndrome. The Cronkhite–Canada syndrome, characterised by hamartomatous (juvenile) polyps throughout the whole intestine and associated with alopecia, onychodystrophy and abnormal pigmentation of adult onset, is probably not genetic (Daniel et al., 1982) but does predispose to CRC (Zugel et al., 2001).

Almost 50 per cent of cases of juvenile polyposis are due to germline mutations in *SMAD4* or *BMPR1A* which encode proteins involved in TGF beta signalling (Houlston et al., 1998; Howe et al., 2001; Sayed et al., 2002). There is a significant risk of colorectal malignancy in juvenile polyposis and Peutz–Jegher syndrome.

Hereditary mixed polyposis syndrome causes an autosomal dominant predisposition to colorectal polyps of varying histological type including sessile, hamartomatous and adenomatous polyps, and early onset CRC. The locus for the susceptibility gene has been identified as CRAC1 on chromosome 15q in Ashkenazi Jewish families but the gene has not yet been identified (Jaeger et al., 2003).

Small rectal hamartomatous polyps have recently been described in tuberose sclerosis (p. 246), but these are thought to be of no clinical significance (Gould et al., 1990). Inflammatory polyps are associated with ulcerative colitis and Crohn disease. Gastrointestinal polyps, predominantly neurofibromas, are found in NF1 (p. 230), possibly in up to 25 per cent of cases (Hochberg et al., 1974). A diffuse ganglioneuromatosis of the gastrointestinal tract is described in MEN 2B (p. 224), with hyperplasia of the ganglion cells, leading to malfunction of the bowel (Fryns and Chrzanowska, 1988). Rarely, autosomal dominant inheritance of intestinal neurofibromatosis has been described without other associated manifestations of neurofibromatosis (Heiman et al., 1988). Devon polyposis has been described in one family in which multiple inflammatory fibroid polyps were found in the upper gastrointestinal tract in members of three generations of a family from Devon, UK. There did not seem to be an increased risk of cancer in these individuals (Anthony et al., 1984).

Tumours of the colon and rectum

Malignant disease of the large bowel is one of the commonest causes of cancer death, with an incidence of 32 per 100 000 population in the UK, but a much lower incidence in parts of Africa (2.5 per 100 000 in Nigeria) and in Asia. Almost all (98 per cent) large bowel cancers are adenocarcinomas. Adenomas of the colon are thought to have the potential to develop into malignancy, and coexist in 75 per cent of cases in which more than one primary carcinoma is present in the colon; one or more adenomas are present in about a third of cases of colon carcinoma. It is thus probable that most carcinomas develop from adenomas (Morson, 1966). The incidence of solitary colonic polyps in the general population is age-related, reaching 34 per cent in the sixth decade and 75 per cent in those over the age of 75 years (Lanspa et al., 1990). It has been calculated that the risk of invasive cancer in a single polyp is approximately 0.25 per cent per year, but for larger and/or villous polyps, the risks are up to 50 times higher (Eide, 1986), indicating that screening guidelines need to be modified by the pathological findings at each colonoscopy. Inflammation is probably also a predisposing factor for bowel cancer, since ulcerative colitis and Crohn disease are associated with an increased risk of colon carcinoma (Judge et al., 2002).

Genetic factors are important in the pathogenesis of cancer, and a comprehensive family history should be part of the assessment of all patients with CRC. Early age at diagnosis in the affected relative is an important predictor of

Table 6.3. *Family history and risk of death from colon cancer: empiric risk estimates for counselling*

Affected relatives	Relative risk of CRC	Lifetime risk of CRC
General population		1 in 50
One first-degree relative	×3 (OR 1.8)	1 in 17
One first degree aged <45 years	×5 (OR 3.7)	1 in 10
One first and one second degree		1 in 12
Both parents		1 in 8.5
Two first-degree relatives	(OR 5.7)	1 in 6
Three first-degree relatives		1 in 3

Odds ratios (OR) figures from St John et al., 1993; lifetime risks from Houlston et al., 1990.

risk. Empiric risk estimates based on the number of relatives affected by (and age at diagnosis of) CRC are given in Table 6.3 and indicate that risk increases with earlier age at diagnosis and increased numbers of affected relatives. Twin studies indicate that 35 per cent of CRCs are partly due to inherited factors (Lichtenstein et al., 2000). Identification of individuals at increased genetic risk of colon cancer is important because screening can be offered to high-risk individuals, and evidence is accumulating that this is likely to be effective in reducing morbidity and mortality from CRC.

It is estimated that about 5 per cent of CRC occur in individuals with a dominantly inherited predisposition. Genetic conditions associated with colonic polyps carry an increased risk of CRC (Table 6.4). These include familial adenomatous polyposis (p. 184), Turcot syndrome (p. 250), juvenile polyposis (p. 211) and Peutz–Jeghers syndrome (p. 241). The former conditions are characterised by the development of colorectal adenomas, whereas the latter are characterised by gastrointestinal hamartomas, which are potentially premalignant although adenomas have more malignant potential. A rare familial syndrome of familial giant hyperplastic polyposis coli has been described which predisposes to CRC (Jeevaratnam et al., 1996). More recently, the importance of some types of hyperplastic polyps, particularly as precursors of right-sided microsatellite unstable colon cancers, has been stressed (Jass et al., 2002).

Germline *PTEN* mutations are also associated with hamartomatous gastrointestinal polyps but unlike the genes listed above, mutation carriers (affected with Cowden or Ruvalcaba–Myhre–Smith syndromes) do not seem to have a greatly increased risk of CRC, but there may be some risk in specific families.

Familial adenomatous polyposis is the commonest of these disorders, but accounts for fewer than 1 per cent of all cases of colon cancer. A larger proportion

Table 6.4. *Conditions characterised by colorectal polyposis*

	Gene(s)
Adenomatous polyposes	
Familial adenomatous polyposis (FAP)	*APC*
Attenuated polyposis/multiple adenomas	*APC, MYH*
Hamartomatous polyposes	
Juvenile polyposis	*BMPR1A, SMAD4*
Peutz–Jegher syndrome	*LKB1/STK11*
Hereditary mixed polyposis syndrome	*CRAC1*

of colon cancer (probably 2–3 per cent) is accounted for by HNPCC (Evans et al., 1997b; Salovaara et al., 2000), an autosomal dominant inherited predisposition to CRC, otherwise known as Lynch syndrome (p. 200), in which bowel cancers occur with high frequency at an early age (on average two decades earlier than sporadic cases). Mutations in one of several genes involved in the repair of DNA mismatch errors (*MLH1, MSH2, MSH6, PMS2* and possibly *MLH3*) have been found to cause HNPCC (both "Lynch syndrome type I" (hereditary site-specific colon cancer) and "Lynch syndrome type II" (sometimes called the "family cancer syndrome" because of the occurrence of extra-colonic cancers) (p. 201), and microsatellite instability (MSI) is seen, where multiple allelic changes are demonstrable in tumour DNA when compared to the constitutional DNA of the patient. It is evident that there is no clear distinction between the "Lynch I" and "Lynch II" syndromes; both predispose to early onset and an increased proportion of right-sided colon cancers (65 per cent versus 25 per cent in sporadic cases) with a risk of multiple primary CRC. Nevertheless, the risk of extra-colonic cancers seems to be higher in individuals with *MSH2* rather than *MLH1* mutations (Vasen et al., 2001), and *MSH6* mutations particularly predispose to endometrial cancer (Wijnen et al., 1999). These extra-colonic malignancies comprise mainly endometrial, ovarian, pancreatic, gastric and urinary tract cancers (Wijnen et al., 1999). Full details of HNPCC are given on page 200. The Muir–Torre syndrome is HNPCC associated with sebaceous adenomas and other characteristic skin lesions. HNPCC and Muir–Torre syndrome are allelic (i.e. due to mutations in the same gene) but Muir–Torre syndrome is much more often due to mutations in *MSH2* than in *MLH1* (Lucci-Cordisco et al., 2003). Germline methylation of the *MLH1* promoter, and mutations in *MLH3* and *EXO1* may account for a small proportion of CRC cases with MSI-positive tumours (Wu et al., 2001;

Liu et al., 2003; Laiho et al., 2002; Brassett et al., 1996; Suter et al., 2004), but this area remains controversial.

The term HNPCC is something of a misnomer (Umar et al., 2004a), since colonic adenomas do occur in patients with this condition. Although they are not more common than in the general population, the adenomas progress more rapidly through the adenoma–carcinoma sequence than in normal individuals (Jass, 1995a). This has implications for the frequency with which colonoscopic surveillance should be performed in these individuals. It is very rare for more than 50 polyps to develop in this condition, which distinguishes it from classical familial adenomatous polyposis in which there is a minimum of 100 colonic adenomas. There are, however, families with intermediate numbers of polyps that cannot easily be classified as HNPCC or familial adenomatous polyposis (sometimes known as attenuated familial adenomatous polyposis, AFAP or AAPC), and affected individuals in some such families may be demonstrated to have germline mutations in exons 3 or 4 of the *APC* gene (Spirio et al., 1993; Gismondi et al., 2002). Others may have MYH-associated polyposis, an autosomal recessive condition characterised by variable numbers of colonic adenomas and relatively early onset CRC, with usually 30–100 adenomas (Halford et al., 2003; see p. 230). A subgroup of HNPCC-related CRC may be distinguished by the occurrence of flat adenomas in the right hemicolon (Lynch et al., 1993), but it seems likely that this is merely another variant of HNPCC. However, serrated adenomas are common in HMPS, characterised by colonic adenomas and hamartomas and early onset CRC. This has been linked to the CRAC1 locus within an ancestral Ashkenazi haplotype between D15S1030 and D15S118 on chromosome 15 (Jaeger et al., 2003).

A polymorphism in the *APC* gene, a T-A mutation germline mutation (predicted to result in a change from isoleucine to lysine position 1307 of the protein, see familial adenomatous polyposis section, p. 184) confers an approximately twofold increase in the risk of CRC. The mechanism for this at a molecular level appears to be that the polymorphism which converts an AAATAAAA sequence to $(A)_8$, predisposes to the development of somatic mutations in the *APC* gene (Laken et al., 1997). This mutation is common (about 6 per cent) in individuals of Ashkenazi Jewish origin, but is very rare in other ethnic groups. The relative risk, or odds ratio for CRC in association with this mutation is about 1.5–1.8 (Gryfe et al., 1999), which is generally thought to be insufficient to warrant colonoscopic surveillance. The mutation is at least 2200 years old (Niell et al., 2003) and has probably become frequent in this population by genetic drift.

There is possibly a slightly increased relative risk of colon cancer in individuals with germline *BRCA1* mutations, but this is accompanied by a decrease in risk for rectal cancer, and this increased risk has not been reported in men (Thompson and Easton, 2002). Overall, the risks are probably not clinically important. In support of the absence of an effect, there is no apparent increased risk for CRC for Ashkenazi Jewish carriers of *BRCA1:185delAG* or *BRCA1:5382inC* (Ford et al., 2004; Struewing et al., 1997; Kirchhoff et al., 2004; Niell et al., 2004).

NAT2 (which alters the ability to acetylate N-acetyl transferase) and other metabolic gene variants may alter susceptibility to colonic adenomas and cancer in the general population and alter polyp density in FAP (Crabtree et al., 2002; Jass, 2004), but are unlikely to cause a sufficiently increased CRC risk to be clinically important on their own. It may be that multiple variants in different genes including *MLH1*, *MSH2*, *APC*, *AXIN1* and *CTNNB1* (beta catenin) can contribute to susceptibility to colonic adenomas and cancer (Fearnhead et al., 2004; Lammi et al., 2004).

Identification of high-risk families

Efficient screening for HNPCC requires that high-risk individuals are targeted for mutation testing. Approximately 10 per cent of patients with CRC have an affected first-degree relative, and 2 per cent have two affected first-degree relatives. However, the frequency of families that fulfill the "Amsterdam Criteria" (AC) for HNPCC is less than 5 per cent of all cases (Stephenson et al., 1991; Peel et al., 1997). Most population-based mutation analysis studies start with individuals with microsatellite unstable cancers and then look for germline mutations in these cases only: these studies have found that between 1 and 4 per cent of all CRC is due to germline mutations in either *MLH1* or *MSH2* (Peel et al., 2000; Salovaara et al., 2000). Some patients with early onset CRC with no family history still have germline mutations in the mismatch repair genes (Dunlop et al., 1997) and these may account for a substantial proportion of CRC in patients diagnosed below 35 years, but only a minority of older cases.

In families not fulfilling the Amsterdam or Bethesda criteria for HNPCC (see Table 6.2), pathological tumour analysis by immunohistochemical stains (IHC) gives a high specificity for the diagnosis of HNPCC and indicates the gene which may be mutated in the germline, although MSH2 and MSH6 staining may both be lost in tumours in people with germline mutations in MSH2. Measurement of MSI in tumours is less specific because approximately 15 per cent of all CRCs may be MSI positive, and does not indicate which gene is likely to be involved in the germline. Some cases, especially older women with MSI-high cancers, may have somatic *MLH1* inactivation. The specificity of MSI for HNPCC is increased considerably if two tumours from the same individual demonstrate MSI positivity (Frayling et al., personal communication).

It is reasonable to start looking for *MLH1* and *MSH2* mutations in cancers that show a high level of MSI-H or loss of the respective proteins by

Table 6.5. *Frequency of germline MLH1 and MSH2 mutation carriers in early onset CRC (from Mitchell et al., 2002)*

Age range (years)	Number of index cases	MLH1 mutation carriers		MSH2 mutation carriers	
		Number	%	Number	%
<30	50	7	14	7	14
<40	12	1	8.3	1	8.3
<45	38	1	2.6	2	5.3
<50	135	6	4.4	6	4.4

immunohistochemistry (IHC) in CRC sections, as this strategy is very unlikely to miss highly-penetrant germline mutations (Umar et al., 2004a). It is, however, notable that most studies demonstrating this have not included screening for genomic deletions, which may account for up to 25 per cent of all disease-causing mutations (Charbonnier et al., 2002; Wagner et al., 2003), and detection of deletions should be part of routine screening.

In terms of identifying those at risk, it should be remembered that some patients with early onset CRC without a family history of HNPCC have germline mutations in mismatch repair genes (Dunlop et al., 1997). If cases of CRC unselected for family history are studied with HNPCC mutation analysis, the mutation detection rate is dependent on the age at diagnosis of CRC in the case (Mitchell et al., 2002; see Table 6.5). Familial clustering of CRC that does not fulfill the AC for a diagnosis HNPCC is less likely to be due to germline *MLH1* or *MSH2* mutations. In early studies only about 8 per cent of families not meeting the rather stringent AC1 had detectable mutations although some may have deletions or other gene rearrangements (Wijnen et al., 1997). More recent data suggest this is an under-estimate, and detailed searches can find mutations in many more, as long as MSI-H is present in the CRC of the subject of the mutation analysis (Wagner et al., 2003), and would be considered to be very likely if MSH2 protein is absent, even if the family clustering in no way fulfils AC. In this context, looking for *BRAF* mutations (Davies et al., 2002) in the colorectal tumour may be a good step following MSI and IHC, as among MSI-H cancers that do not express MLH1, the presence of a *BRAF* mutation makes a germline *MLH1* mutation much less likely. Interestingly, loss of expression of MSH2 is rarely if ever associated with *BRAF* mutations (Wang et al., 2003a; Koinuma et al., 2004; Domingo et al., 2004).

Pathological features and molecular diagnosis

Colorectal cancers with MSI-high features characteristically have increased mucin secretion, differentiation and lymphocytic infiltrate. This is seen both in sporadic tumours and those arising in HNPCC. There is now evidence that sporadic MSI-H cancers develop in adenomas with a somatic *BRAF* mutation and DNA methylation, particularly of MLH1, whilst those in HNPCC arise in adenomas with somatic mutations in APC, beta catenin and/or K-ras. This also translates into morphological differences, HNPCC cancers showing more tumour budding (de-differentiation), and sporadic tumours being more heterogeneous and displaying mucin secretion (Jass, 2004; McGivern et al., 2004).

Over the past 15 years, molecular genetic studies of colon cancer have provided strong evidence for a multistep pathogenesis. This work started out with a simple linear model involving at least five genes (Fearon and Vogelstein, 1990). It now appears that this model is too simplistic, but it has provided a framework for many other studies.

APC mutations are thought to occur early in the process and may cause spindle aberrations via the interaction of APC with the kinetochore at mitosis through connections with the microtubules, leading to chromosome abnormalities (Powell, 2002). Originally, it was thought that the critical factor is the accumulation of mutations rather than the particular order in which they occur, but more recent work, focusing on the idea of cell-type specific "gatekeepers" suggest that there are genes which act as rate-limiting steps: it is likely that such genes are altered early in the carcinogenetic process. For example, in most CRC, biallelic *APC* mutations (or mutation plus loss of heterozygosity) occur at an early stage (Powell et al., 1992). These early alterations (such as the loss of sequences C-terminal to the beta catenin regulatory domain (Sidransky, 1997) could lead to a screening test for early CRC based on the detection of such mutations in stool: a stool test for *APC* mutations has been developed (Traverso et al., 2002). Other assays are based on multiple genes: for example, stool analysis of three gene markers (*TP53*, *BAT26* and *KRAS*) detected 71 per cent of CRC patients and 92 per cent of those whose tumours actually had an alteration in these genes (Dong et al., 2001). Despite these and other encouraging findings, commercial stool tests remain unadopted in the clinical setting.

Surveillance strategies

Screening of patients at increased risk of colon cancer is likely to prevent early death, but large-scale studies are of course difficult to conduct. In Finland, one study has found that HNPCC family members who undergo colonoscopy have a much lower CRC incidence rate, probably due to removal of adenomas. The overall death rates were 10 versus 26 subjects in the study and control groups ($P = 0.003$), 4 versus 12 in mutation-positive subjects ($P = 0.05$) (Jarvinen et al., 2000). In addition, the benefits of a genetic register for ascertaining and coordinating the screening of individuals at risk for familial adenomatous polyposis are now well recognised (Kinzler & Vogelstein, 1996; King et al., 2000).

Predictive testing for HNPCC is now available for the presymptomatic diagnosis of this condition in families in which the pathogenic mutation has been defined, so that it is becoming possible to target high-risk asymptomatic individuals for screening, as for familial adenomatous polyposis. Guidelines for screening individuals at risk for HNPCC are regular colonoscopy (every 1–2 years) from the age of 25 years, and those with a family history that includes cancers at other sites, including endometrium, should be offered screening for other cancers as appropriate (see p. 200). In addition to detecting presymptomatic colonic carcinomas, such screening allows the endoscopic detection and removal of adenomas. It is presumed (but not proven) that most cancers in patients with HNPCC arise from adenomas and that excision of the latter will prevent the development of colon cancer. Colonoscopy is the investigation of choice because of the preponderance of right-sided tumours in this condition.

In familial CRC families without evidence for HNPCC, surveillance for CRC should take into account the financial costs of screening and the possibility of adverse effects of screening by colonoscopy in particular, and balance this with the individual's estimated risk of CRC.

The risks of colonoscopy are small but significant; (Williams and Fairclough 1991) in a population-based study, serious complications were recorded in 2 per 1000 colonoscopies (Gatto et al., 2003). The 14-day death rate is around 5–10 per cent of the perforation rate (Anderson et al., 2000; Gatto et al., 2003).

Individuals who do not appear to be part of a dominant pedigree with CRC family which conforms to the revised AC for HNPCC (so-called AC2, which includes non-CRC as part of the criteria) (Vasen et al., 1999) but who are at increased genetic risk of CRC because of a family history of colon cancer, and who may fit Bethesda criteria (Umar et al., 2004a; Rodriguez-Bigas et al., 1997) may also be offered screening, although the optimal screening protocol for such individuals has not been established. Houlston et al., (1990) suggested that colonoscopy (e.g. commencing at the age of 25 years and repeated every 5 years if normal and every 3 years if adenomas are found) should be offered to individuals with an empiric risk of dying from CRC greater than 1 in 10–12. However, Dunlop (2002) performed a meta-analysis of published data on surveillance results in HNPCC, and proposed that individuals with a first-degree relative diagnosed before 45 years age, or with two affected first-degree relatives,

Table 6.6. *Example of suggested screening for colon cancer when no molecular testing is available*

1 FDR age <45 years	Colonoscopy on two occasions or 5 yearly	Begin usually at 5 years before diagnosis in relative, but not <25 years
1 FDR & 1 SDR Both age >70 years	Reassure No colonoscopy	
1 FDR & 1 SDR average age 60–70 years	Single colonoscopy	Age 55 years
Two FDR or 1 FDR & 1 SDR average age <60 years	5 yearly colonoscopy*	Age 45–75 years Refer to genetics centre if average age < 50 years
Both parents affected	Single colonoscopy	Age 55 years
Three close relatives Amsterdam criteria positive	1–2 yearly colonoscopy	Refer to genetics centre Begin age 25 years or before
Three close relatives Not Amsterdam criteria positive	5 yearly colonoscopy*	Refer to genetics centre Begin age approximately 40 years
FAP/MYH polyposis	Annual sigmoidoscopy/ colonoscopy from teenage years	Refer to genetics centre

FDR: first-degree relative; SDR: second-degree relative

Protocol adapted from the St Marks Hospital (London) screening protocol. *Three yearly colonoscopy if a few adenomas detected. Twice yearly if multiple/large adenomas. Data from St John et al. (1993) show a low detection rate of colorectal cancer below 35 years in familial colorectal cancer excluding HNPCC. In HNPCC, screening should begin at 25 years (Vasen et al., 1993). Neoplasia is unlikely to progress from normal colon to colorectal cancer (excluding HNPCC) in <5 years after a normal colonoscopy, but after adenomas have been detected, a 3 yearly interval is preferable (Winawer et al., 1993).

Other screening recommendations: Individuals with two first-degree relatives with CRC or relative diagnosed <45 years offered colonoscopy at 35 and 55 years only (Dunlop 2002).

5 yearly colonoscopy from 40 years or from 10 years < youngest diagnosis in family (Winawer et al., 2003).

5 yearly colonoscopy from 50 years or from 10 years < youngest diagnosis in family (Australian NHMRC).

should be offered two colonoscopies, one at 35 years age, or at presentation (whichever was the later), and a second at 55 years age if the first one was clear. These guidelines are published on the British Society of Gastroenterology Website http://www.bsg.org.uk/clinical_prac/ guidelines.htm. The precise screening protocol employed in individuals with a risk less than 1 in 10 and greater than 1 in 12 will depend on local facilities, patient preference and careful assessment of the risk/benefit in individual cases. Such protocols require long-term assessment and audit on a multinational basis and attempts to meet these requirements are in progress. However, an example of screening guidelines that could be used is shown in Table 6.6 derived from the Anglian Region and St Marks experience, but these are still under revision (Westergaard, 1996).

Chemoprophylaxis

There is some evidence that COX-2 inhibitors may reduce the development of colonic neoplasia in susceptible individuals, and aspirin, sulindac and non-absorbable starch are being assessed in large-scale trials such as Concerted Action Polyp Prevention (CAPP), but their clinical use is still under evaluation, particularly in view of adverse effects associated with these drugs (Zha et al., 2004).

7

Reproductive system

Breast cancer

Background: epidemiology and family history

Breast cancer is the most common cancer in women, accounting for 20 per cent of all new cases of cancer. The lifetime risk of breast cancer in the UK is one in nine females, with an incidence of <10 per 100,000 women aged <30 years, rising to 300 per 100 000 in women aged over 85 years. Similar, but slightly higher rates are seen in North America. It is rare in men (<1 per 100 000). Breast cancer incidence shows marked geographical variation: it is much less common in Asian than in Caucasian women, and less frequent in South America and Spain than in Northern Europe, North America and Australia. In India, the prevalence is lower (although rising) except amongst Parsee women. In North America, the incidence of breast cancer appears to have increased in recent years; some of this increase is due to mammographic detection of ductal carcinoma in situ leading to early diagnosis of minimally-invasive ductal carcinoma.

In 1948, Penrose and colleagues observed that breast cancer may have a hereditary basis in some families (Penrose et al., 1948). A genetic influence on breast cancer susceptibility is suggested by twin studies, as the concordance for breast cancer in identical twins (0.28) is more than twice that in dizygotic twins (0.12) (Petrakis, 1977; Bishop and Gardner, 1980). A statistically significant heritable factor of 27 per cent was observed for breast cancer (95 per cent confidence interval (CI): 4–41) in the three-country study of 44 788 pairs of twins (Lichtenstein et al., 2000). By contrast, the factor for prostate cancer was 42 per cent, so clearly these percentages do not reflect the contribution of known genes to these diseases.

There is an increased risk of breast cancer among female relatives of breast cancer patients and this increased relative risk (RR) is more pronounced when the index case has bilateral disease or early (pre-menopausal) age at onset. For patients aged 55 years or older at diagnosis, the RR of breast cancer in a first-degree female relative is about 1.8, and this increases to 3–4 when more than one first-degree relative is affected (Mettlin et al., 1990) (Figs 7.1 and 7.2).

A large study (7496 women with breast cancer and 7438 controls) of the risks of breast cancer in women in relation to their family history found that, compared

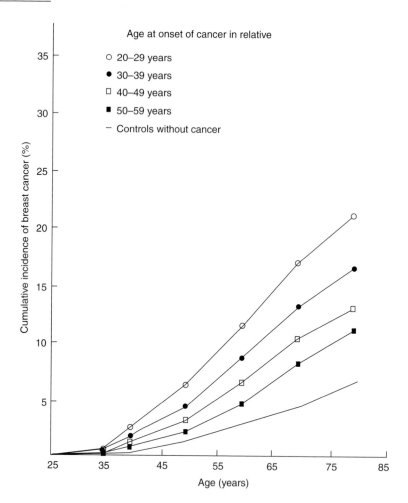

Fig. 7.1. Cumulative incidence of breast cancer in women whose first-degree relative developed breast cancer. From Claus et al. (1994).

to women with no affected relative, the risk ratio for breast cancer was 1.80 (99 per cent CI 1.69–1.91), 2.93 (99 per cent CI 2.30–3.64) and 3.90 (2.03–7.49), respectively for one, two and three or more affected first-degree relatives ($P < 0.0001$ each). Risk ratios were greatest at young ages, and with younger age at diagnosis in the relative. For women with zero, one or two or more first-degree affected relatives, the estimated cumulative risk of breast cancer up to age 50 years was 1.7, 3.7 and 8.0 per cent, respectively, corresponding to incidences up to age 80 of 7.8, 13.3 and 21.1 per cent, and death from breast cancer of 2.3, 4.2 and 7.6 per cent. There was no evidence for an autosomal recessive effect. An important finding was that other factors such as hormones and diet did not vary by family history.

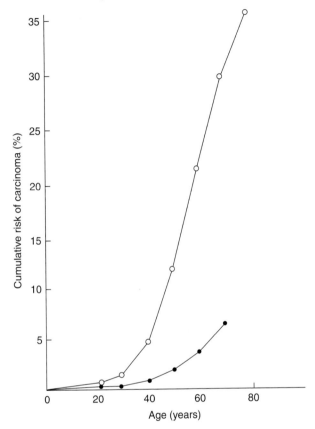

○ Two first-degree relatives diagnosed 40–49 years
   (e.g. mother and sister affected) with breast cancer

● Controls (no cancer in relative)

Fig. 7.2. Cumulative incidence of breast cancer in women with two first-degree relatives with breast cancer diagnosed aged 40–49. From Claus et al. (1994).

Among women with one affected relative, the cumulative incidence of breast cancer between ages of 20 and 80 was 12.3 per cent if the relative was over 60, but 16.1 per cent if under 40. Another key finding was that most breast cancers in women with a family history of breast cancer were likely to occur after the age of 50, even if there were two affected relatives (Collaborative Group on Hormonal Factors in Breast Cancer, 2001).

For a woman aged 30 with a mother and a sister affected with breast cancer, the cumulative risk of breast cancer to age 70 has been found to be 17.4 per cent, significantly lower than the 43 per cent risk to be expected if all such familial clusters were due to highly penetrant mutations in susceptibility genes (Peto et al., 1996), suggesting that most such familial clusters are not due to these genes. A detailed assessment of the age-specific risk of breast cancer in a woman with one or two relatives affected with the disease has been derived from data from the population-based, case-control Cancer and Steroid Hormone (CASH) Study, which can be used for individual risk assessment (Figs 7.1 and 7.2) (Claus et al., 1994, Claus et al., 1991, Colditz et al., 1996).

A clear example of a pedigree with an apparently autosomal dominant susceptibility to breast cancer was first clearly described in 1866 by Broca, whose wife's family contained 10 women in four generations who died of the disease (Broca, 1866; Lynch and Krush, 1971). There is epidemiological evidence for overlap between breast and ovarian cancer susceptibility. The overall age-adjusted RR for ovarian cancer in first-degree relatives of women with breast cancer has been estimated to be 1.7 (and 2.1 for breast cancer), and first-degree relatives of index cases of ovarian cancer have RR of 1.6 and 2.8 for breast cancer and ovarian cancer, respectively (Schildkraut et al., 1989). In one study, the RR for breast cancer in first-degree relatives of index cases ascertained because of colon cancer was estimated to be about 5 (Itoh et al., 1990), but in general, later studies of the risk of breast cancer after colorectal cancer, or colorectal cancer after breast cancer, have not supported this finding (Newschaffer et al., 2001). The only gene that might reasonably contribute to both breast and colorectal cancer in this context is *CHEK2* (Meijers-Heijboer et al., 2003), but this is probably only clinically relevant in the Netherlands and possibly Finland.

BRCA1 and BRCA2

The genes and the risks for cancer

Two genes in which germline mutations can cause a strong predisposition to breast cancer have so far been identified. The first of these was *BRCA1* on chromosome 17q12–23 (Miki et al., 1994, Futreal et al., 1994), which accounts for most families with inherited breast and ovarian cancer susceptibility and about 40 per cent of inherited breast cancer, particularly where the onset of breast cancer was at 45 years or younger. The cumulative risk of breast and ovarian cancer in BRCA1 carriers is shown in Figure 7.3.

A second breast cancer susceptibility gene, *BRCA2*, was subsequently identified (Wooster et al., 1995, Wooster et al., 1994), located on chromosome 13q12–13 (Collins et al., 1995; Miki et al., 1996). Germline mutations in this gene confer a strong susceptibility to breast cancer and a smaller risk of ovarian cancer than with *BRCA1* mutations. Gene penetrance for lifetime risk of breast cancer in *BRCA2*-mutation carriers are lower than in the case of *BRCA1* mutations, and results in later-onset disease: in cases unselected for family history, the average cumulative risks for breast cancer in *BRCA1*-mutation carriers by age 70 years was 65 per cent (95 per cent CI 44–78 per cent). In *BRCA2* carriers, the estimate was 45 per cent

Table 7.1. *RR estimates (95% floated CI) for mutation carriers, in BRCA1 and BRCA2 based on country and cohort-specific background rates (Antoniou et al., 2003)*

Age group	BRCA1		BRCA2	
	Breast cancer	Ovarian cancer	Breast cancer	Ovarian cancer
20–29 years	18 (4.4–75)	1.0	19 (4.4–82)	1.0
30–39 years	36 (25–52)	38 (17–88)	16 (9.3–29)	1.0
40–49 years	31 (25–52)	61 (38–99)	9.5 (5.9–15)	6.3 (1.4–28)
50–59 years	16 (9.6–27)	30 (14–65)	11 (6.6–17)	19 (9.1–41)
60–69 years	11 (5.0–25)	48 (22–109)	9.2 (5.1–17)	7.3 (1.8–30)

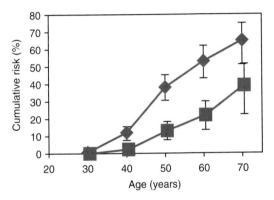

Fig. 7.3. Cumulative incidence of breast cancer (diamonds) and ovarian cancer (squares) in BRCA1-mutation carriers, to age 70. From Antoniou et al. 2003, with permission.

(31–56 per cent) (Antoniou et al., 2003). RR are shown in Table 7.1 above, and age-dependent penetrance is shown in Figure 7.3 (*BRCA1*) and Figure 7.4 (*BRCA2*). Mutations in *BRCA2* predispose to a wider spectrum of other cancers than do mutations in *BRCA1*. These cancer sites include: prostate, stomach, fallopian tube, pancreatic and male breast cancers (Breast Cancer Linkage Consortium 1999; Ford et al., 1995a; Couch et al., 1997). In this large international study, statistically significant increases in risks were observed for prostate cancer (estimated RR = 4.65; 95 per cent CI = 3.48–6.22), pancreatic cancer (RR = 3.51; 95 per cent CI = 1.87–6.58), gallbladder and bile duct cancer (RR = 4.97; 95 per cent CI = 1.50–16.52), stomach cancer (RR = 2.59; 95 per cent CI = 1.46–4.61) and malignant melanoma (RR = 2.58; 95 per cent CI = 1.28–5.17). The RR for prostate cancer for men below the age of 65 years was 7.33 (95 per cent CI = 4.66–11.52) (Table 7.2)

Table 7.2. *Risks associated with BRCA2 mutations: non-breast/ovary sites by age of onset*

Site	0–65 years of age		65–85 years of age	
	RR	95% CI	RR	95% CI
Buccal cavity + Pharynx	1.52	0.44–5.19	3.15	0.77–4.83
Stomach	2.57	1.13–5.84	1.93	0.77–4.83
Pancreas	5.54	2.72–11.32	1.61	0.45–5.72
Prostate	7.33	4.66–11.52	3.39	2.34–4.92
All except breast, ovary, prostate, pancreas	1.48	1.15–1.91	1.30	0.96–1.76

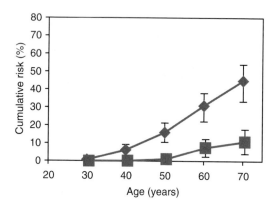

Fig. 7.4. Cumulative incidence of breast cancer (diamonds) and ovarian cancer (squares) in BRCA2-mutation carriers, to age 70. From Antoniou et al. 2003, with permission.

There was a significant reduction in risks for women in earlier birth cohorts. Particular mutations in *BRCA1* and *BRCA2* may confer higher RR of ovarian cancer than others (see p. 100). Of course, men may transmit breast cancer susceptibility, but the mutation is usually non-penetrant for breast cancer in males. Among families with male breast cancer, 80 per cent are linked to *BRCA2* and 20 per cent to *BRCA1* (Struewing et al., 1995b; Durocher et al., 1996; Couch et al., 1996; Narod et al., 1995a).

There is a high frequency of specific germline mutations in *BRCA1* and *BRCA2* in individuals of Ashkenazi Jewish origin (about 2 per cent; the 185delAG and 5382insC *BRCA1* and 6174delT *BRCA2* mutations), and up to 30 per cent of breast cancer cases in women from this ethnic group diagnosed with breast cancer under the age of 40 years, 40 per cent of breast cancer families, and 60 per cent of breast/ovarian families, carry one of these germline mutations (Tonin et al., 1996; Kirchoff et al., 2004). A high frequency of specific

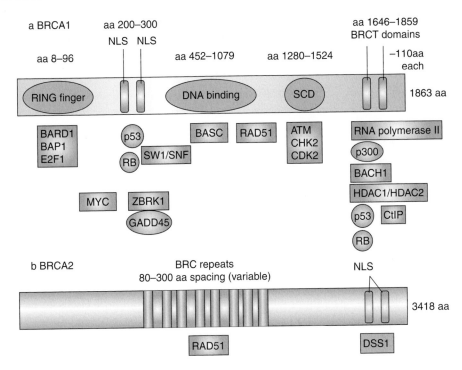

Fig 7.5. (a) BRCA1; (b) BRCA2

BRCA1/2 mutations have been found in other ethnic groups, probably due to a founder effect, for example the 999del15 *BRCA2* mutation in Iceland, detected in 0.6 per cent of the population, 7.7 per cent of female breast cancer patients and 40 per cent of males with breast cancer (Thoralacius et al., 1997). In one study from Poland, recurrent mutations were found in 33 (94 per cent) of the 35 families with detected mutations. Three *BRCA1* mutations – 5382insC, C61G and 4153delA – accounted for 51, 20 and 11 per cent of the identified mutations, respectively (Gorski et al., 2000). Mutations in *BRCA2* were rare. These observations simplify *BRCA1/2* genetic testing for individuals of Polish origin.

The proportion of breast cancer attributable to *BRCA1* mutations was estimated at 5.3 per cent in women diagnosed below the age of 40 years to 1 per cent in those diagnosed over the age of 70 years (Easton et al., 1995), and subsequent mutation analysis studies have proved these estimates to be approximately accurate (Whittemore et al., 2004b) (see Table 7.3).

BRCA gene function
BRCA1 and *BRCA2* are large genes with no known homology, containing 22 and 26 exons, respectively. Many, but not all of the functions of the BRCA1 and

Table 7.3. *Proportion of breast cancer due to germline BRCA1 or BRCA2 mutations by family history of breast cancer*

Breast cancer family history	BRCA1 (%)	BRCA2 (%)	Both (%)	Other genes (%)
2 cases <50 years	8	7	15	35
3 cases <50 years	15	13	28	39
4 cases <50 years	32	15	47	53
5 cases <50 years	47	13	60	40

Gareth Evans, derived from Collaborative group data (Easton) (Evans DGR, Kerr B, Lalloo F, Friedman J. (2004). *Risk Assessment and Management in Cancer Genetics*. Oxford University Press).

BRCA2 proteins have been established. BRCA2 is the larger of the two proteins and is 3418 amino acids in length.

BRCA2 facilitates homologous recombination, but little else is known about its function. In contrast, several known functions of BRCA1 could underlie its role in carcinogenesis. These roles include DNA repair, cell checkpoint control, protein ubiquination and chromatin remodelling. Both BRCA1 and BRCA2 are implicated in the repair of DNA through homologous recombination. BRCA1 is found in association with RAD51 in sub-nuclear clusters (Scully et al., 1997; Coene et al., 1997). RAD51 is a key component of DNA damage repair by homologous recombin-ation. When DNA is damaged, both BRCA1 and RAD51 become associated with DNA at the areas of damage. BRCA1 is phosphorylated during this process. The nature of the interaction between RAD51 and BRCA1 is unknown, whereas BRCA2 can interact directly with RAD51 via both the BRC repeats and a domain at the C-terminus (Mizuta et al., 1997; Sharan et al., 1997; Wong et al., 1997). BRCA2 exists in a complex with RAD51, holding it in an inactive state – when BRCA2 is absent, RAD51 foci do not form following DNA damage.

Cells defective in BRCA1 or BRCA2 are hypersensitive to agents that cross-link DNA strands, or that break double-stranded DNA, such as cisplatin and mitomycin C (Yuan et al., 1999; Moynahan et al., 2001; Tassone et al., 2003). In these cells, double-strand breaks are repaired in an error-prone fashion (e.g. via non-homologous end-joining) and errors can lead to chromosomal rearrange-ments (Patel et al., 1998; Zhong et al., 1999). It is believed that the chromo-somal instability is a cardinal feature of carcinogenesis. When cells are exposed to ionising radiation, both proteins (together with RAD51) initiate homologous recombination and the repair of double-strand breaks (Yuan et al., 1999). Not sur-prisingly, cells with mutated BRCA1 and BRCA2 are hypersensitive to ionising radiation and exhibit error-prone repair. The levels of expression of BRCA1,

BRCA2 and RAD51 increase in cells when they enter S phase, indicating that they function during or following DNA replication. So BRCA1 and BRCA2 function in a common pathway, which is responsible for the integrity of the genome and the maintenance of chromosomal stability (Venkitaraman, 2002). This may have clinical implications in terms of therapeutic response to chemotherapy and radiotherapy, and a trial of cisplatin treatment in BRCA1-mutation carriers with cancer is under way. Novel agents, such as PARP1 inhibitors, may also have an important role in the treatment of BRCA1/2-related cancers (Brody, 2005).

As well as having a clear role in the repair of double-strand break repair, BRCA1 has also been implicated in nucleotide excision repair. A recent study using human cells indicated that global genome repair, rather than transcription coupled repair, was deficient in cells that lacked BRCA1 (Hartman and Ford, 2002).

Another function of BRCA1 is that of checkpoint control. BRCA1 can exist as part of a BRCA1-associated genome–surveillance complex (BASC) (Wang et al., 2000). This complex includes proteins such as the Nijmegen breakage syndrome 1 protein, NBS1, RAD50-MRE11 (which has exonuclease activity at double-strand breaks), ataxia-telangiectasia mutated (ATM) (which acts upstream of BRCA1 in the double-strand break repair pathway) MLH1-PMS1, MSH2-MSH6, the Bloom syndrome protein BLM and DNA-replication factor C.

The BRCT motif at the carboxy terminus of BRCA1 is a common feature of proteins involved in DNA repair and/or in cell cycle checkpoint function (Callebaut and Mornon, 1997). Interestingly, unlike BRCA1, checkpoint function is remarkably well preserved in BRCA2-deficient primary cells (Patel et al., 1998).

Ubiquitylation is the process by which proteins are tagged for degradation by the proteasome. This is crucial in regulating the levels of proteins that might otherwise be unnecessarily retained. Many proteins that have ubiquitylation functions contain a RING finger motif. Both BRCA1 and its interacting protein, BARD1, possess a RING motif near the amino terminus, and it has been observed that the BRCA1–BARD1 complex (Wu et al., 1996) functions as a co-factor in the ubiquitylation process. However, disease-associated mutations of *BARD1* in *BRCA1/2*-negative breast cancer are uncommon (Hashizume et al., 2001; Ghimenti et al., 2002; Ishitobi et al., 2003).

BRCA1 can also act as a histone deacetylator (Yarden and Brody, 1999), and interacts with other proteins implicated in chromatin remodelling, such as BACH1 (Cantor et al., 2001), only serves to emphasise the importance of BRCA1 in processes that regulate DNA repair. Interestingly, a BRCA2-interacting protein, EMSY (Hughes-Davies et al., 2003) also has DNA repair functions and might provide a link between sporadic breast and ovarian cancer and alterations in *BRCA2*, which, heretofore, have been obscure. Thus mutations in EMSY have been shown to occur in somatic tissue where a single *BRCA2* mutation is present.

Other genes involved in breast cancer susceptibility

A number of studies have now tested for *BRCA1* and *BRCA2* mutations in population-based series of breast cancer cases, and thus the contribution of these two genes to familial aggregation can be assessed. Such a study (Peto et al., 1999) identified 30 mutations in 617 breast cancer patients diagnosed before age 46. Interestingly, only five of their mothers or sisters had had breast cancer, compared with 64 in the relatives of the 587 non-carriers. After allowing for the number of breast cancers that would be expected at population rates, and assuming a mutation sensitivity of 64 per cent, this would equate to approximately 16 per cent of the observed familial risk being due to *BRCA1* and *BRCA2*. In a previous linkage study, over 80 per cent of families with six or more cases of breast cancer were found to be linked to either *BRCA1* or *BRCA2*, but the proportion fell to 40 per cent in families with four or five cases, leaving room for other genes (Ford et al., 1998). *CHEK2* and *ATM* are candidates (where germline mutations confer a moderately increased risk) to fill the gap, but the identified mutations are either too low in frequency and/or of too low penetrance to account for more than a small part of the remaining familial cases, so other genes must also be involved (Narod and Foulkes, 2004).

Post-menopausal-onset familial breast cancer may not show 17q linkage. In one report it was shown to be linked to the oestrogen receptor (ER) gene in one family (Zuppan et al., 1991), and recent studies have suggested that variants in this gene could influence breast cancer risk in post-menopausal women (Gold et al., 2004).

Approximately 50 per cent of women with Li–Fraumeni syndrome (Hartley et al., 1986; see p. 215) develop breast cancer, particularly at young ages. The RR for breast cancer in women under 45 years of age in Li–Fraumeni syndrome families has been estimated at 17.9 (Garber et al., 1991). However, the proportion of cases of breast cancer overall is likely to be extremely small because fewer than 1 per cent of breast cancer cases can be demonstrated to have germline *TP53* mutations (Borresen et al., 1992), and even among early-onset breast cancer, *TP53* mutations have a minor role (Sidransky et al., 1992).

Genetic disorders which predispose to breast cancer are shown in Table 7.4.

Cowden Syndrome (p. 179) is associated with a substantially elevated risk of breast cancer (50 per cent or greater), especially at younger ages (Eng, 2003). The risk of breast cancer is also increased in Peutz–Jeghers syndrome (p. 241) (Lim et al., 2003). Both are rare causes of breast cancer overall.

Table 7.4. *Genetic disorders associated with breast cancer susceptibility*

1. Hereditary breast and ovarian cancer	(*BRCA1* and *BRCA2*)
2. Li–Fraumeni syndrome	(*TP53*)
3. Cowden syndrome	(*PTEN*)
4. Peutz–Jeghers syndrome	(*STK11/LKB1*)
5. Klinefelter syndrome	(*47XXY*)
6. Hereditary Cutaneous Malignant Melanoma	(*CDKN2A*)
7. Ataxia Telangiectasia	(*ATM*)

Epidemiological data have demonstrated an increased RR of early-onset breast cancer in the female relatives of cases of Ataxia Telangiectasia (see p. 169; Swift et al., 1991), and the proportion of breast cancer due to heterozygosity for *ATM* mutations has been estimated to be 7 per cent overall, a smaller proportion at later ages at diagnosis than at earlier ages (Easton et al., 1993a). However, since the *ATM* gene was characterised and it has been possible to look for germline mutations in affected women, the evidence suggests that only a very small proportion of breast cancer cases, even in radiosensitive subjects, are actually due to mutations in this gene (Wooster et al., 1993; Telatar et al., 1996; Khanna, 2000), so the original RR estimates may have been too high (Izatt et al., 1997). It is possible that truncating mutations are not pathogenic, but that certain missense mutations are (Gatti et al., 1999; Scott et al., 2002). One such mutation, *ATM*7271T* > G, probably originating in the Orkney islands north of Scotland, has been associated with a high risk of breast cancer in a few families (Stankovic et al., 1998; Chenevix-Trench et al., 2002), but it is not frequently implicated in hereditary breast cancer (Szabo et al., 2004). The most comprehensive study to date suggests that the RR for breast cancer in ATM carriers is 2.2 (95% CI 1.2–4.3), but is nearly 5 for those diagnosed under 40 years of age. There was no evidence for a difference in risk for carriers of missence or truncating mutations (Thompson et al., 2005).

It is thought that rare polymorphisms of certain genes can confer a small increase in relative cancer risk, and one rare allele of a microsatellite polymorphism of the *HRAS* proto-oncogene has been demonstrated in a meta-analysis to be associated with a 1.93 risk of breast cancer, and possibly to alter the ovarian cancer risk in *BRCA1* carriers (Krontiris et al., 1993; Narod et al., 1995b; Phelan et al., 1996). In addition, a common variant in the CASP8 gene, involved in apoptosis, may be associated with increased breast cancer risk (MacPherson et al., 2004). However, these associations have yet to be confirmed by further studies.

Histopathology of breast cancer and its relationship to genetics

Breast cancer histology is highly heterogeneous. Breast tumours are thought to be epithelial neoplasms originating in the terminal ductal structures. Ductal and lobular carcinoma in situ are by definition, non-infiltrating, and are often multicentric. Of infiltrating cancers, 70 per cent are ductal. Infiltrating duct carcinomas may be classified as papillary, medullary, tubular, mucinous, comedo and adenoid-cystic types – "not otherwise specified" is the largest sub-group however. There is substantial debate about whether there is a clear progression from more benign to more malignant phenotypes, but many consider atypical hyperplastic proliferative breast disease as a premalignant condition. Attempts to correlate histological type with family history in breast cancer initially demonstrated that all histological types may be found in both sporadic and familial cases of the disease (Rosen et al., 1982; Burki et al., 1987). Tubular and medullary histological types of breast cancer have been noted to occur more often in families showing the Li–Fraumeni spectrum of tumours (Birch et al., 1984). Breast cancers arising in *BRCA1*-mutation carriers can often be distinguished from cancers occurring in *BRCA2* or non-*BRCA1/2* carriers on morphological (Lakhani et al., 1998), immunopathological (Lakhani et al., 2002), cytogenetic (Tirkkonen et al., 1997; Wessels et al., 2002), gene expression (Hedenfalk et al., 2001; Van't Veer et al., 2002; Sorlie et al., 2003) and mutational (Greenblatt et al., 2001) grounds. *BRCA1*-related breast cancers are usually infiltrating ductal carcinomas of high grade. An atypical medullary phenotype is more common in *BRCA1*-related breast cancer than in matched controls (Lakhani et al., 1998; Chappuis et al., 2000). These findings suggest that *BRCA1* tumours develop along a distinct pathway. One characteristic of this pathway is the expression of basal keratins (Foulkes et al., 2003), such as cytokeratin (CK) 5 and 14, which are usually only expressed in normal basal cells of the breast and skin, but are also found in 5–15 per cent of all invasive breast cancers (Wetzels et al., 1989; Wetzels et al., 1991; Bocker et al., 1992). This basal character is associated with a specific pattern of genetic alterations in the breast cancers resulting in high-grade (Lakhani et al., 2002), tumours that do not express ER, HER2 or KIP1, but do express p53 and cyclin E (Foulkes et al., 2004). Ductal carcinoma in situ and lobular carcinoma are under-represented in *BRCA1*-mutation carriers (Sun et al., 1996; Breast Cancer Linkage Consortium 1997).

Benign breast disease may predispose to breast cancer, and may itself be a marker of familial disease. Seven per cent of patients with juvenile papillomatosis have been reported to have a family history of breast cancer, which is a higher percentage than would be expected (Rosen et al., 1985). Women with atypical hyperplastic proliferative breast disease have a significantly higher risk of developing breast cancer if they have a family history of breast cancer, and the RR of breast cancer in the presence of atypical lobular hyperplasia in a benign lesion is 3–4 (Dupont and Page, 1985; 1987). Twenty per cent of patients with atypi-cal hyperplasia report a positive family history of breast cancer, compared with 11.9 per cent of controls (Carter et al., 1988). Breast cancer can be multifocal, and malignant changes in the contralateral breast can be detected by biopsy at the time of surgery for invasive breast cancer in 7.5–18 per cent of cases (Forrest, 1990). The risk of a second primary cancer in the contralateral breast in a woman with breast cancer is four to five times the risk in unaffected women of comparable age in the general population.

Prognosis following familial and hereditary forms of breast cancer is contro-versial, but most studies point towards a similar or worse prognosis for cancer in *BRCA1*-mutation carriers (Chappuis et al., 1999; Evans and Howell, 2004) compared with age-matched non-carriers.

Genetic counselling

Genetic counselling for women with a family history of breast cancer requires an initial assessment of their lifetime risk of developing breast cancer on the basis of empirical data derived from taking a family history that includes infor-mation about cancer type and age at onset in all first-degree and second-degree relatives and as many more distant relatives as possible. It is important to try and confirm diagnoses whenever possible, since occasional cases of factitious family histories have been documented, and mistaken diagnoses can lead to erroneous advice being given. Such risk estimates can be obtained using epi-demiological data (Schwartz A.G. et al., 1985; Ottman et al., 1986; Gail et al., 1989; Claus et al., 1994), or with the help of computer programmes which cal-culate risks using these data, and can be expressed as a lifetime risk, or as a risk for developing cancer over a shorter time period, such as the ensuing 10 years (Antoniou et al., 2004). Programmes such as BRCAPRO can also calculate the probability of being a *BRCA1/2*-mutation carrier, although non-computer based methods may have some advantages (Apicella et al., 2003; Evans et al., 2004). Certainly the method cited by Evans et al. (2004) has the benefit of simplicity and user-friendliness, relying on a scoring system for the numbers of affected relatives, and avoids the need for a computer programme which may not be appropriate in the clinical setting. It is important to distinguish between systems which derive individual risks and those which assess the chance that there is a *BRCA1* or *BRCA2* mutation in the family. The relative accuracies of the latter are currently being assessed in the UK, comparing actual mutation detection rates with assessments using different programmes (Pharoah et al., 2001).

A woman whose mother has a germline breast cancer susceptibility mutation has a prior risk of 50 per cent of inheriting the susceptibility, so that her lifetime risk of developing breast cancer is about 40 per cent (assuming 80 per cent gene penetrance for breast cancer). However, if she remains healthy after the age of 50 years, her actual risk will have fallen because she has lived through a substantial amount of her risk period, most hereditary breast cancer occurring at a younger age. Thus, at the age of 50 years, a *BRCA1* gene carrier has a ~50 per cent chance of having developed breast cancer compared with a <2 per cent chance in the general population. Therefore, the risk that the daughter of a gene carrier who remains unaffected at 50 years of age has inherited the susceptibility has fallen to approximately one-third, and if she remains healthy, it is less likely that she has inherited the susceptibility the older she becomes. Predictive testing for the mutation would further define her risk.

The probability that the family is segregating for a *BRCA1* or *BRCA2* germline mutation may be derived from family history data, in order to give an indication as to the likelihood that the consultant could be offered a predictive test for such a mutation (Table 7.3). This chance is very dependent on age at diagnosis in the affected woman (there is a 17 per cent chance of a *BRCA1* mutation in breast cancer families with average age at diagnosis below 35 years, but a 1 per cent chance when the average age at diagnosis is over 59 years). A family history of ovarian cancer increases the chance of finding a *BRCA1* mutation, as does multiple primary breast or ovarian cancers in an affected woman of Ashkenazi Jewish origin (Couch et al., 1997).

In families in which the pedigree data suggest a high chance that a germline mutation will be detected, the consultant is asked whether she wishes to approach one or more of her close relatives affected with cancer of the breast or ovary and decide whether she would consider being tested for such a mutation. If so, blood is obtained from these relatives with full informed consent for such testing. This process is a lengthy and sensitive one, involving careful counselling and concerns for the maintenance of confidentiality. Affected relatives should have the benefit of full counselling about all the implications of the test before being tested, and psychological support should be offered if appropriate. If a pathogenic mutation is detected in an affected relative, predictive testing may be offered to the consultant, again with full counselling. The full implications of a positive or a negative result should be discussed, together with options for prophylactic and surveillance interventions before the test is undertaken, with additional discussions about insurance and employment issues (Collins, 1996; Friend, 1996). It is important that women seeking advice about genetic testing for breast cancer susceptibility should appreciate that a predictive test may not be available for them (Couch et al., 1997). The many potential psychological sequelae of predictive testing, particularly in relation to psychiatric morbidity and any effect on uptake of surveillance and prophylactic measures, need careful consideration (Lerman et al., 1996; Dudok-deWit et al., 1997a,b; Richards et al.,

1997; van et al., 2003), although it is fair to say that many of the initial fears surrounding testing have not been realised (Narod and Foulkes, 2004).

It is important to recognise that the detection of a germline *BRCA1* or *BRCA2* mutation in an affected woman can be of great psychological impact, possibly equivalent to the shock of the original cancer diagnosis, particularly as it indicates that she may have handed on the susceptibility to her children. There are also important management implications for her because there is a high risk of a second breast cancer, and possibly also of ovarian cancer developing.

While it may be expensive and time-consuming, *BRCA1/2* testing can be offered to women for whom the pathogenic mutation has not been defined in the family (in an affected relative). This is often simply a question of resource allocation. This process is much more straightforward for women from ethnic groups in which there is a high prevalence of certain founder mutations such as the Ashkenazim. Nevertheless, outside of these special situations, a positive finding of a germline mutation may be of uncertain significance (about 13 per cent of all Myriad Genetics Laboratories *BRCA1/2* tests in whites identify a variant of unknown significance – it is much higher (~40 per cent) in those with African origins), and a negative result may be meaningless as only a proportion of possible mutations will have been screened for. As stated, within specified populations, predictive testing for the common mutations does have some value, but the meaning of a "negative" result must be carefully explained as it would not rule out the possibility that the woman has a different germline mutation in a breast cancer susceptibility gene.

Screening and prophylaxis

Screening for breast cancer is based upon the detection of early cancer and not of a premalignant lesion (Smith et al., 2000). Despite a meta-analysis that concluded to a reduction up to 18 per cent of the breast cancer mortality among 40–49 years old women following regular mammographic screening, the effectiveness of this tool for the surveillance of pre-menopausal women remains debatable. Indeed, after decades of research, the "mammography debate" continues with much vitriolic comment (Rogers, 2003), and it seems unlikely that new data will help to resolve the issues easily (Goodman, 2002). The efficiency of screening should be higher if the women screened are at increased RR because of a family history of breast cancer, but as yearly mammography seems to be rather ineffective in *BRCA1/2* carriers (Brekelmans et al., 2001; Goffin et al., 2001; Tilanus-Linthorst et al., 2002), other screening modalities will be required.

The National Institute for Clinical Excellence (NICE) recently produced guidelines for screening and management of women with a family history of breast and ovarian cancer in the UK based on an analysis of published evidence, and a summary is presented in Table 7.5.

Table 7.5. *Example guidelines for the management of familial breast cancer*

Family history of breast cancer	Expected breast cancer cases between 40–50 years[a]	Lifetime risk[b]	GP clinical examination	Refer breast clinic[d]	Mammography[c]	Refer genetics clinic
1 relative						
1 relative >50 years	<1 in 75	<1 in 10	Yes	No	BSP at age 50	No
1 relative 40–50 years	1 in 50	1 in 7.5	Yes	No	BSP at age 50	No
1 relative <40 years	1 in 25	1 in 5–6	Yes	Yes	Yearly 40–50 years, then BSP	No
2 relatives						
2 relatives >60 years	<1 in 45	<1 in 7	Yes	Yes	Yearly from 40–50 years BSP at age 50	No
2 relatives 50–60 years	>1 in 25	1 in 4	Yes	Yes	Yearly 40–50 years, then NHS BSP	No
2 relatives average age <50 years	>1 in 17	1 in 3	Yes	Yes	Yearly 40–50 years, then NHS BSP	Yes
2 relatives average age <40 years	1 in 12	1 in 2.5	Yes	Yes	Genetics review	Yes
3 relatives						
Average age <60 years	1 in 10	1 in 2–3	Yes	Yes	Yearly from 40 years	Yes
1 or more relative ≤50 years + ≥1 relative with *ovarian* cancer	>1 in 17	1 in 3	Yes	Yes	Yearly from 40 years	Yes

(Continued)

Table 7.5. (*Continued*)

Family history of breast cancer	Expected breast cancer cases between 40–50 years[a]	Lifetime risk[b]	GP clinical examination	Refer breast clinic[d]	Mammography[c]	Refer genetics clinic
1 or more relative <40 years plus relative with childhood malignancy			Yes	Yes	Await genetics review	Yes

[a] Population risk for breast cancer age 40–50 years is 1 in 100 (1 per cent).

[b] Population lifetime risk (age 20–80) years is 1 in 12.

[c] Early screening mammography should start at age 40 years. However, women at very high risk may be screened annually from 30 years and 18-monthly after 50 years of age.

[d] Some districts may have a facility at the breast clinic to review those at increased risk, some may not. Some patients only will benefit from referral to the genetics clinic.

"Relative" includes first-degree relative and their first-degree relatives (first-degree relatives – mother, father, brother, sister and child). A relative with bilateral breast cancer counts as two. A male relative with breast cancer counts as a young female (<45).

BSP: 3-yearly mammography from age 50 years; GP: primary care physician.

Referral to genetics centre advised if family contains bilateral breast cancer, male breast cancer, ovarian cancer, sarcoma diagnosed <45 years, glioma, adrenocortical tumour, Ashkenazi Jewish ancestry, multiple early-onset cancers or strong paternal family history.

Source: NICE Guidelines on management of familial breast cancer www.nice.org.uk

Magnetic resonance imaging (MRI) is a non-ionising imaging technique that has already been demonstrated to be sensitive for invasive breast cancer. Its sensitivity is less impaired than mammography by dense parenchyma. Preliminary results of a German prospective non-randomised pilot project (including 192 asymptomatic women proved or suspected to be *BRCA1/2*-mutation carriers) demonstrated that the sensitivity and specificity of breast MRI was superior to conventional mammography and high-frequency breast ultrasound (Kuhl et al., 2000). The triple assessment was performed yearly, plus an additional physical and ultrasound examination every 6 months. Among the nine breast cancers diagnosed (6 prevalent, 3 incident), 4 were detected and correctly classified by mammography and ultrasound combined. Two other lesions were visible, but were misdiagnosed as fibroadenomas. MRI identified and correctly diagnosed the 9 lesions. Of note, the 9 cancers were pT1 stage (mean size: 1.05cm) without axillary node involvement (pN0). The genetic status was not known for all patients, but among the 9 women who developed breast cancer 7 had mutations in *BRCA1* ($n = 6$) and *BRCA2* ($n = 1$). Only 5 false positive findings were noted with MRI, compared with 7 and 19 with mammography and ultrasound, respectively. Among 105 asymptomatic women with validation of the screening results after the first year, the positive predictive value for mammography, ultrasound and MRI was 30, 12 and 64 per cent, respectively. Much larger studies in North America and Europe have confirmed that MRI is superior to mammography for the detection of breast cancers in *BRCA1/2* carriers (Kriege et al., 2004; Warner et al., 2004). It is not known if this will translate to a better outcome.

For some women at very high risk of breast cancer (e.g. *BRCA1*- or *BRCA2*-mutation carriers, those with Cowden syndrome, Li–Fraumeni syndrome, dominant breast/ovarian cancer pedigree), prophylactic bilateral sub-cutaneous mastectomies may be the preferred option, but the women require careful counselling and a discussion of the residual risk of breast cancer following different types of surgical procedure (a sub-cutaneous mastectomy, leaving the nipple may have a measurable residual risk, and a total mastectomy is probably the preferred option). Information is still accumulating about the efficacy of such prophylactic surgery, but so far, no invasive breast cancers have been reported after a total mastectomy in a *BRCA1/2*-mutation carrier (Meijers-Heijboer et al., 2001; Rebbeck et al., 2004) by contrast, there are two reports of invasive breast cancer following subcutaneous mastectomy in BRCA1 (Rebbeck et al., 2004) and BRCA2 (Kasprzak et al., 2005) carrier. Contralateral mastectomy should also be considered for women likely to be *BRCA1/2*-mutation carriers who have had breast cancer because their risk of contralateral breast cancer is substantially increased to approximately 40 per cent at 10 years follow-up. Notably, the risk is reduced by tamoxifen and oophorectomy (Metcalfe et al., 2004).

At the current time, screening protocols for *BRCA1/2* carriers usually include ovarian cancer surveillance, but the true value, if any, of regular asessment with (CA)-125 and transvaginal ultrasound is unknown (see p. 102). In all cases, the advantages and risks of the chosen screening procedure must be carefully explained. The establishment of a genetic register facilitates the ascertainment of women at risk of breast cancer by virtue of their family history, but the initial contact should always be made by members of their own family.

The role of chemoprophylaxis is still unclear in women with a family history of breast cancer, but drugs such as tamoxifen may be considered for such at-risk women – the data are conflicting, but point towards a benefit even for women who are destined to develop an ER negative breast cancer. Although not enough is known about the effects of the hormonal contraceptive pill in susceptibility gene carriers to give confident advice, one very large case-control study showed that early use, use before 1975 and prolonged use (>5 years) was associated with significantly increased risks of breast cancer among *BRCA1*, but not *BRCA2*-mutation carriers (Narod et al., 2002). By contrast, a population-based study found no evidence for increased risk, and even some suggestion of a decreased risk for *BRCA1* carriers (Milne et al., 2005; Colditz et al., 1995). Prospective studies, with lower doses of oestrogen, are awaited with interest, but in the meantime, avoiding oral contraceptive pill use in young *BRCA1* carriers seems prudent. The UK NICE guidelines for classification and care of women at risk are given in Table 7.6.

Uterine tumours

Uterine neoplasias can arise from the endometrium or myometrium. The most common myometrial neoplasias are leiomyomas while the most common endometrial tumours are endometrial carcinomas.

Table 7.6. *The UK NICE guidelines for classification and care of women at risk of familial breast cancer in primary, secondary and tertiary care*

Main recommendations are:
1. Mammograms below the age of 30 years not recommended, and no routine mammograms between 30 and 40 years age, although some leeway allowed. Any mammograms that are offered should be with full information, be at National Breast Cancer Screening Programme standard, and audited.
   Any mammograms offered outwith these recommendations should only be as part of research protocols.
2. Full screening of *BRCA1* and *BRCA2* should be available.
   - Specific recommendations:
     – Healthcare workers should not actively seek to identify women with a family history of breast cancer.
     – Family history should include first- and second-degree relatives, and allow risk assessment and development of care guidelines.
     – Standard written information should be available for women at all levels of care.
     – Access to psychological support should be available.
     – Genetic testing should be offered by a multidisciplinary team.
     – Women should be assessed in primary care, and can be managed in primary care if (1) only one relative diagnosed >40 years age. (2) Only one second-degree relative affected (10-year risk <3 per cent between 40 and 50 years age, lifetime risk <17 per cent). No specific screening offered at this level of risk
   - Exclusions: Any of the following: bilateral or male breast cancer, ovarian cancer, sarcoma diagnosis <45 years age, glioma, adrenocortical cancer, jewish ancestry, multiple early-onset cancers, or strong paternal family history.

Table 7.6. (*Continued*)

- Management can be in secondary care if:
  - One relative with breast cancer diagnosis <40 years age.
  - Two first or one first and one second-degree relatives affected with breast cancer average age at diagnosis >50 years age.
  - Three relatives average diagnosis >60 years age with same exclusions as for primary care.
  - Lifetime risk 17–30 per cent (3–8 per cent between 40 and 50 years age).

Screening offered by annual mammography from 40 years age and subsequently national breast cancer screening programme from 50 years age (3 yearly).

- Any additional screening should only be performed as part of an audited ethically approved study.
- Criteria for referral to tertiary care:
  - >8 per cent risk 40–50 years age, >30 per cent lifetime risk or >20 per cent of BRCA mutation.
  - Two first-/second-degree relatives diagnosis <50 years with breast cancer.
  - Three first-/second-degree relatives diagnosis <60 years with breast cancer.
  - Four relatives diagnosis any age.
  - One ovarian cancer, and one breast cancer diagnosis <50 years or 2 relatives diagnosed <60 years or another ovarian cancer.
  - Bilateral breast cancer diagnosis <50 years.
  - Male breast cancer and one breast cancer diagnosis <50 years or 2 diagnosed <60 years and exclusion criteria families (above).
  - Breast cancer diagnosis need not be verified.

Recommendations include:

- Those re counselling and risk-reducing measures.
- Oral contraceptives increase breast cancer risk but reduce ovarian cancer risk.

Oophorectomy reduces risk of breast cancer by 50–75 per cent if done <40 years.

HRT (Hormone replacement therapy) may increase risk.

Tamoxifen – best effect in young women, reduces risk by 38 per cent (48 per cent ER+, none ER−).

- Screening:
  - Women from 40 to 49 years age.
  - Annual mammography, audited.
  - Part of NHS R&D Health Technology Audit evaluation if possible.
  - Written information given.
  - 50 years age: 3 yearly (only more frequent if part of audited research study).
  - Individualised strategies for high-risk women.
  - MRI not recommended.

Uterine leiomyoma

Leiomyomas are benign, smooth muscle tumours with some connective tissue elements. They are very common, occurring in about 20 per cent of women over the age of 35 years, and the incidence increases with advancing age. They occur more frequently in women of Afro-Caribbean origin. Uterine leiomyomas are probably more common in first-degree relatives of index cases than in the general population. Uterine leiomyomas are component neoplasias of at least two heritable neoplasia syndromes: hereditary leiomyoma–renal cell carcinoma syndrome (HLRCC), which is also known as multiple cutaneous uterine leiomyomatosis (MCUL), and possibly Cowden syndrome. HLRCC/MCUL is caused by germline heterozygous mutations in the gene encoding fumarate hydratase, *FH* (Alam et al., 2001; Tomlinson et al., 2002). *FH* is a nuclear gene encoding a mitochondrial enzyme involved in electron transport and the Krebs cycle (Eng et al., 2003). While germline heterozygous *FH* mutations cause HLRCC, germline homozygous mutations cause severe neurodegeneration (Eng et al., 2003). Because uterine leiomyomas are common in the general population, it is difficult to prove that they are true components of Cowden syndrome (see section below). Nonetheless, it would appear that multiple uterine leiomyomas occurring relatively young is quite common in this syndrome, and is considered a minor criterion for the clinical diagnosis of Cowden syndrome (Eng, 2000c) (www.nccn.org).

While few somatic intragenic mutations in *FH* have been found in sporadic uterine leiomyomas, biallelic inactivation by both genetic and non-genetic mechanisms occur with some frequency in these sporadic tumours (Kiuru et al., 2002; Lehtonen et al., 2004). A chromosomal translocation t (12:14) (q14–15; q22–24) has been demonstrated in a proportion of sporadic benign uterine leiomyomas (Heim et al., 1988). The breakpoints in chromosome 12q14–q15 cluster in a region known as ULCR12 (uterine leiomyoma cluster region of the chromosome 12 cluster region breakpoints), and this has been shown to coincide with breakpoints found in translocations in lipomas and pleiomorphic adenomas (Wanschura et al., 1996).

Carcinoma of the uterus

This is the ninth most common malignancy in women with an incidence of 13 per 100 000 of population in the UK. In the US, approximately 4 per cent of women will develop uterine cancer in a lifetime. The most common histological type is adenocarcinoma, and adenomatous hyperplasia (endometrial precancer, endometrial intraepithelial neoplasia) may be the premalignant lesion. Of all endometrial adenocarcinomas, the endometroid histology is the most common. Squamous cell carcinomas, leiomyosarcomas and mixed mesodermal tumours may occur, but are rare.

Epidemiological studies have shown a slight increase in RR for endometrial cancer in women with a family history of this cancer (Parazzini et al., 1992), leading to the conclusion that about 1 per cent of endometrial cancers may be explained by genetic factors. Endometrial adenocarcinoma is a component cancer of Lynch syndrome/hereditary non-polyposis colorectal cancer syndrome (HNPCC, p. 200) and of Cowden syndrome (p. 179). As part of the clinical spectrum of HNPCC, endometrial carcinoma occurs in 42 per cent of women with this condition, which in fact is a higher frequency than that for colon cancer in these women (Dunlop et al., 1997; Aarnio et al., 1999). It is currently unknown if the risk of uterine cancer may vary with the underlying mismatch repair gene mutation. Up to 16 per cent of patients with endometrial carcinoma have been reported to have a first-degree relative with uterine cancer, and this is probably caused by a proportion of cases being secondary to HNPCC (Lynch et al., 1996a). Endometrioid endometrial carcinomas occur in women with Cowden syndrome, with an increased, but unknown, frequency (Marsh et al., 1998; DeVivo et al., 2000; Eng, 2000c). It is considered a major criterion for the clinical diagnosis of Cowden syndrome (see Section below, p. 179).

Microsatellite instability (MSI) occurs in virtually all HNPCC-related endometrial cancer and in 20–30 per cent of sporadic endometrial carcinomas. (Baldinu et al., 2002; Lohse et al., 2002) Nonetheless, a major somatic genetic aetiology for endometrial carcinoma had eluded investigators for over a decade despite uncovering chromosomal rearrangements of chromosome 1 (deletion 1p or duplication 1q) and trisomies of chromosomes 10, 2, 7 and 12 as well as allelic losses at 10q (Nagase et al., 1996) and 17p. Recently, *PTEN* has been shown to play a major role in the pathogenesis of both HNPCC-related and sporadic endometrial adenocarcinomas (Mutter et al., 2000; Mutter et al., 2001; Zhou et al., 2002). In HNPCC-related endometrial cancers, the mismatch repair deficiency likely predisposes to subsequent somatic mutations in *PTEN* as the great majority occur in one of several coding short mononucleotide repeat tracts (Zhou et al., 2002). In contrast, somatic *PTEN* intragenic mutations occur very early in sporadic endometrial carcinogenesis, being present at the precancer stage or even in normal appearing glands (Mutter et al., 2001; Zhou et al., 2002). Indeed, in the sporadic setting *PTEN* mutations can often precede MSI (Zhou et al., 2002).

Clinical surveillance for uterine malignancies in individuals at risk for endometrial cancers should be considered for all at-risk individuals. Indeed, the US-based National Comprehensive Cancer Network (NCCN) practice guidelines recommend annual uterine surveillance by blind repel biopsies of the endometrium from the age of 30 years for women with HNPCC and from the age of 35–40 years for women with Cowden syndrome (www.nccn.org (Eng, 2000c; Pilarski and Eng, 2004)). After menopause, surveillance would change to annual endometrial (transabdominal or transvaginal) ultrasound with biopsy of suspicious lesions.

Because the risk for endometrial cancer is higher than that for even colorectal cancer in women with HNPCC, such individuals should consider the option of concomitant prophylactic hysterectomy when they undergo bowel surgery for neoplasia.

Choriocarcinoma

This can follow pregnancy (of any type), and may be secondary to hydatidiform mole (which is thought to result from the fusion of two male gametes without the participation of an ovum). Invasive moles occur with a frequency of 1 in 15 000 pregnancies in the US; there is marked geographical variation, with a 10-fold higher incidence in South East Asia and the Far East. Hydatidiform mole can be familial and a locus has been mapped to 19q13 (Moglabey et al., 1999). The gene, *NALP7*, was recently identified (Murdoch et al., 2006). The protein is involved in the intracellular regulation of bacterial – induced inflammation, and is a negative regulation of IL-1β.

Fallopian tube carcinoma

This cancer is extremely rare, but has been reported in women with germline mutations in *BRCA1* or *BRCA2*, suggesting that a large proportion of these cancers arise in women with a genetic susceptibility to this type of cancer (see p. 70) (Rebbeck et al., 2002; Rutter et al., 2003). Hence prophylactic removal of the Fallopian tubes should be undertaken at the time of phophylactic oophorectomy.

Ovarian cancer

Ovarian tumours may develop from germ cells, epithelial or granulosa/theca cells. Germ cell tumours include dermoid cysts, teratomas and gonadoblastomas. Sex cord tumours may develop from the mesenchyme, may include granulosa cell tumours, and may be hormone secreting. Benign serous and mucinous fibromas and cystadenomas are also seen. Most ovarian tumours are serous and mucinous adenocarcinomas. Carcinoma of the ovary is almost always derived from the epithelial cells and may originate more widely from coelomic epithelium (i.e. peritoneal carcinoma). Teratomas, embryonal carcinomas, sex cord stromal tumours, choriocarcinoma and dysgerminomas are much less common.

Genetic disorders associated with ovarian neoplasms are listed in Table 7.7.

Ovarian carcinoma

The incidence of ovarian carcinoma is about 15 per 100 000 females in the UK; the lifetime risk to age 70 years is about 1.5 per cent in the UK and North America, slightly less in Southern Europe (Parkin et al., 1997), making it the fifth most common malignancy in females in Western Europe and North America. The disease has a very high mortality and is the most frequent cause of death from

Table 7.7. *Ovarian cancer as a feature of hereditary genetic syndromes*

Syndrome	Gene	% hereditary OC	Risk of OC by age 70 (%)	Other clinical features
Hereditary breast-ovarian cancer	BRCA1	60	20–50	Breast, fallopian tube cancer
HNPCC	BRCA2	25	10–30	Breast, prostate, pancreas, head and neck cancer
	MLH1 MSH2 MSH6 PMS2	10	≤10	Colorectal, endometrial, stomach, urinary tract, small bowel cancer
Peutz–Jeghers Syndrome	STK11	<1	<5	Mucocutaneous melanin spots; GI hamartomatous polyps; adenoma malignum of uterine cervix; breast, GI, pancreas cancer
Cowden disease	PTEN	<1	<3	Multiple hamartomas; mucocutaneous signs; breast, thyroid cancer
Nevoid basal cell carcinoma (Gorlin) syndrome	PTCH	<1	<2	Basal cell nevi/carcinoma; palmar/plantar pits; skeletal abnormalities; odontogenic keratocysts; medulloblastoma
Multiple enchondromatosis (Ollier disease)	?	<1	<2	Osteochondromatosis; hemangiomata
Epidermolytic palmoplantar keratoderma	KRT9	<1	<2	Epidermolytic hyperkeratosis

AD: autosomal dominant; GI: gastrointestinal; OC: ovarian cancer. There may be an increased risk for ovarian cancer in Carney Complex (Stratakis et al., 2000), but the numbers are too small for accurate risk assessment.

gynaecological malignancies in the Western world. Worldwide, one of the highest incidence for ovarian cancer is seen in Israeli Jewish women who were born in North America or Europe – these are highly likely to be Ashkenazi Jews (13.5 per 100 000, cumulative incidence, 1.55 per cent (to age 74). Interestingly, in Israeli non-Jews, these figures are 3.0 per 100 000 and 0.32, respectively (Parkin et al., 1997). These observations fit with the finding that up to 30 per cent of unselected Ashkenazi Jewish women with ovarian cancer carry mutations (Moslehi et al., 2000). This is a much higher figure than that observed in other groups. Early data suggested that for *BRCA1* in unselected non-Ashkenazi women with ovarian cancer, between 4 and 9 per cent can be expected to carry a *BRCA1* mutation, and between 0 and 4 per cent will carry *BRCA2* mutations, although this figure will be higher in certain founder populations, such as Iceland (Table 7.8(a)). The most recent data, using more comprehensive mutation analysis, has suggested that in a population unselected for ethnicity, about 15% of women with ovarian cancer carry a mutation in *BRCA1* (10%) or *BRCA2* (5%). Notably, half of all *BRCA2* carriers were diagnosed after 60 years of age, when 90% of *BRCA1* carriers were diagnosed under 60 years. Irrespective of family history between 20 and 25% of women diagnosed with ovarian cancer between the ages of 41 and 50 will carry a *BRCA1/2* mutation (Pal et al., 2005). These findings have important implications for referral guidelines to cancer genetics services. Among the Ashkenazim, these percentages are much higher, although some of the studies include selected cases (Table 7.8(b)). Overall, 25–30 per cent of all ovarian cancer in Ashkenazi Jewish women is attributable to one of the three founder mutations, with *BRCA1* mutation predominating at younger ages, and *BRCA2* at older ages. Ovarian cancer is diagnosed at a significantly younger age in *BRCA1* carriers than in the general population. *BRCA2*-related ovarian cancers tend to be diagnosed at an older age than both the aforementioned groups.

Women with ovarian cancer (carcinoma) are more likely than expected to have a family history of ovarian neoplasia, and first-degree female relatives of patients with ovarian cancer are at increased risk. A collection of studies from around the world are summarised in Table 7.9; as can be seen, the odds ratios for ovarian cancer in association with a positive family history of ovarian cancer vary substantially, but are usually greater if the index case was diagnosed at a young age. The risk of death from ovarian cancer is very much greater if two first-degree relatives are affected (Easton et al., 1996). In this study, relatives of ovarian cancer cases also had significantly increased mortality from cancers of the stomach and rectum, but interestingly, the observed increased mortality from colon cancer, breast cancer and pancreatic cancer failed to reach statistical significance.

Families in which there appears to be an autosomal dominant susceptibility to ovarian cancer, with a high penetrance of the cancer in predisposed females

Table 7.8. *Prevalence of BRCA1 and BRCA2 germline mutation in ovarian cancer*

Population studied	BRCA1/2 screening	Results (95% CI)	Reference
(a) Population- or hospital-based studies			
76 OC Japan	BRCA1: SSCA	4/76: 5% (1.5–13)	(Matsushima et al., 1995)
115 OC USA	BRCA1: SSCA	7/115: 6% (2.5–12)	(Takahashi et al., 1995)
50 OC Australia, UK, USA	BRCA2: HA, PTT	2/50: 4% (0.5–14)	(Foster et al., 1996)
38 OC Iceland	BRCA2: 999del5	3/38: 8% (1.7–21)	(Johannesdottir et al., 1996)
55 OC UK, USA	BRCA2: SSCA, PTT	0/55	(Lancaster et al., 1996)
130 OC USA	BRCA2: SSCA	4/130: 3% (0.8–7)	(Takahashi et al., 1996)
374 OC <70 years UK	BRCA1: HA	13/374: 3.5% (2–6)	(Stratton et al., 1997)
103 OC USA	BRCA1: sequencing	4/103: 4% (1–10)	(Berchuck et al., 1998)
116 OC USA	BRCA1: SSCA	10/116: 9% (4–15)	(Rubin et al., 1998)
	BRCA2: SSCA	1/116: 0.9% (0–5)	
615 OC Sweden	BRCA1 1675delA	13/615: 2% (1–4)	(Dorum et al., 1999)
	BRCA1 1135insA	5/615: 0.8% (0.3–2)	
107 OC USA	BRCA1: CA	2/107: 2% (0.2–7)	(Janezic et al., 1999)
101 OC <30 years UK	BRCA1: HA	0/101	(Stratton et al., 1999b)
	BRCA2: PTT	0/101	
113 OC French Canadians	7 FC founder mutations[a]	8/113: 7% (3–13)	(Tonin et al., 1999)
116 OC Japan	BRCA1: YSCA	7/116: 6% (2.5–12)	(Yamashita et al., 1999)
90 OC Hungary	BRCA1: 185delAG, 300T → G, 5382insC	10/90: 11% (6–19)	(Van der Looij et al., 2000)
	BRCA2: 6174delT, 9326insA	0/90	
233 OC Finland	All cases	Overall	(Sarantaus et al., 2001)
	12 BRCA1 and 8 BRCA2 Finnish founder mutations	BRCA1: 11/233: 4.7% BRCA2: 2/233: 0.86%	
	If family hx present BRCA1: PTT (exon 11)	No non-founder mutations identified, 12 of 13 mutations accounted for by one of 7 founders	
	BRCA2: PTT (exons 10 & 11)		

(Continued)

Table 7.8. (*Continued*)

Population studied	BRCA1/2 screening	Results (95% CI)	Reference
515 invasive OC Canada 134 LMP OC	Eleven most common mutations followed by	No mutations found in LMP OC	(Risch et al., 2001)
	BRCA1: PTT exon 11, DGGE	39/515: 7.5%	
	BRCA2: PTT exons 10 and 11	21/515: 4.1%	
478 invasive OC Norway 190 LMP OC	Norwegian founder mutations BRCA1: 1135insA, 1675delA, 816delGT, 3347delAG	No mutations found in LMP OC BRCA1: 19/478: 4.0%	(Bjorge et al., 2004)
413 OC USA, non-Hispanic Whites (non-AJ)	BRCA1: SSCP Two-stage testing strategy	High risk: 16/95: 17% (10–26%) Others: 13/216: 6% (3–10%)	(Whittemore et al., 2004b)
209 invasive OC Tampa area, USA	Full sequencing plus re-arrangement panel (Myriad Genetics Laboratory)	30/209 BRCA1: 9.5% (1–14) 12/209 BRCA2: 5.7% (0.3–10)	(Pal et al., 2005)

(b) Studies among Ashkenazi Jewish patients			
79 OC Israel	BRCA1 185delAG	15/79: 19% (11–29)	(Modan et al., 1996)
31 OC USA	BRCA1 185delAG	6/31: 19% (7–37)	(Muto et al., 1996)
21 OC Israel	AJ panel[b]	185delAG: 7/21 33% (15–57) 5382insC: 0/21 6174delT: 6/21 29% (11–52)	(Abeliovich et al., 1997)
29 OC Israel	AJ panel[b]	185delAG: 8/29 28% (13–47) 5382insC: 4/29 14% (4–32) 6174delT: 5/29 17% (6–36)	(Beller et al., 1997)
22 OC Israel	AJ panel[b]	185delAG: 5/22 23% (8–45)	(Levy-Lahad et al., 1997)

(*Continued*)

Table 7.8. (*Continued*)

Population studied	*BRCA1/2* screening	Results (95% CI)	Reference
		5382insC: 2/22	
		9% (1–29)	
		6174delT: 3/22	
		14% (3–35)	
59 OC Israel	*BRCA1* 185delAG	17/59: 29% (18–42)	(Gotlieb et al., 1998)
	BRCA2 6174delT	2/59: 3% (0.4–12)	
15 OC UK	AJ panel[b]	185delAG: 1/15	(Hodgson et al., 1999)
		7% (0.2–32)	
	+ *BRCA1* 188del11	5382insC: 1/15	
		7% (0.2–32)	
		6174delT: 1/15	
		7% (0.2–32)	
		BRCA1 188del11: 0/15	
32 OC USA	AJ panel[b]	185delAG:	(Lu et al., 1999)
		8/32 25% (11–43)	
		5382insC: 0/32	
		6174delT: 6/32	
		19% (7–36)	
208 OC l	AJ panel[b] + PTT	185delAG:	(Moslehi et al., 2000)
North America,		43/208 21%	
Israel		(15–27)	
		5382insC: 14/208	
		7% (4–11)	
		6174delT: 29/208	
		14% (9–19)	

[a] French Canadian founder mutations: BRCA1: C4446T, 2953del3 + C, 3768insA; BRCA2: 2816insA, G6085T, 6503delTT, 8765delAG.
[b] AJ panel: BRCA1: 185delAG, 5382insC; BRCA2: 6174delT.
AJ: Ashkenazi Jewish; CA: cleavage assay; HA: heteroduplex assay; SSCA: single-strand conformation assay; OC: ovarian cancer; PTT: protein truncation test; YSCA: yeast stop codon assay; OC: ovarian cancer; PTT: protein truncation test.
(We have used the original nomenclature in this table to avoid confusion.)

have been recognised for years, and the identification of *BRCA1* and *BRCA2* has permitted more precise estimates of age-dependent cumulative incidence (i.e. penetrance). A recent analysis of 22 studies suggested that the risk of ovarian cancer among *BRCA1/2* carriers who were not selected on the basis of family history of breast or ovarian cancer is very low before age 40 (below 2 per cent for both genes), but rises substantially with age in the case of *BRCA1*, and is above 1 per cent per year from age 45 onwards, reaching 2.5 per cent per year by age 65. For *BRCA2*, the risks are lower, start to rise at later ages and never reach 1 per cent per year (Antoniou et al., 2003) (Table 7.9).

The ovarian tumours in *BRCA1/2* carriers cases are carcinomas, with a predominance of serous papillary cystadenocarcinoma, but they do not differ histologically from sporadic tumours (Fraumeni et al., 1975), although mucinous and borderline ovarian carcinoma may be under-represented (Bewtra et al., 1992; Piver et al., 1993; Rubin et al., 1996).

The frequency of *BRCA* mutations in the general population is estimated to be about 1 in 800 for *BRCA1* and somewhat less for *BRCA2*, but it can vary significantly among some ethnic groups or geographic regions. Thus, the prevalence of the 3 *BRCA1/2* founder mutations among the Ashkenazim is approximately 1 in 50 (Struewing et al., 1995a; Oddoux et al., 1996; Roa et al., 1996). The Icelandic population carries the founder *BRCA2* 999del5 mutation at a frequency of 0.4 per cent (Johannesdottir et al., 1996). The frequency of *BRCA1* and *BRCA2* mutations in unselected series of women with ovarian carcinoma has been extensively studied, particularly in so-called "founder populations". A founder effect can occur when a relatively small group is genetically isolated from the rest of the population, because of geographic conditions or religious belief. If an individual in that isolated population carries a rare genetic alteration, the frequency of this allele in the next generations could increase in the absence of selection. Specific *BRCA1* and *BRCA2* mutations have been identified in diverse populations, such as in Ashkenazi Jewish, Icelandic, Swedish, Norwegian, Austrian, Dutch, British, Belgian, Russian, Hungarian, French Canadian and Polish families (Gayther et al., 1995; Shattuck-Eidens et al., 1995; Andersen et al., 1996; Johannesdottir et al., 1996; Johannsson et al., 1996; Wagner et al., 1996; Dorum et al., 1997; Gayther et al., 1997a; Peelen et al., 1997; Ramus et al., 1997; Shattuck-Eidens et al., 1997; Tonin et al., 1998; Gorski et al., 2000). The knowledge of well-characterised founder mutations in individuals of particular ethnic origins can simplify genetic counselling and testing, as the mutation screening can be limited to specific panels of mutations.

As shown in Table 7.10, three founder mutations (*BRCA1* 185delAG and 5382insC in *BRCA1*, *BRCA2* 6174delT) have been identified in the Ashkenazi Jewish families of Eastern European ancestry (Friedman et al., 1995; Berman et al., 1996; Neuhausen et al., 1996; Tonin et al., 1996). These mutations are carried by about 2.5 per cent of the Ashkenazi Jewish population (Struewing et al., 1995a; Oddoux et al., 1996; Roa et al., 1996). These founder mutations are particularly common in Ashkenazi Jewish women with ovarian cancer, even without

Table 7.9. *RR of ovarian cancer associated with a family history of the disease in epidemiological studies, 1969–2000*

Relatives studied	Country	Age group (years)	Cases	Controls	Odds ratio (95% CI)	Reference
Any	USA	All	150	300	"no positive association"	(Wynder et al., 1969)
First- + second-degree	USA	<50	150	150	15.7 (0.9–278)	(Casagrande et al., 1979)
First-degree	USA	45–74	62	1068	18.2 (4.8–69)	(Hildreth et al., 1981)
First-degree	USA	18–80	215	215	11.3 (0.6–211)	(Cramer et al., 1983)
First-degree	Greece	All	146	243	∞ (3.4–∞)	(Tzonou et al., 1984)
First-degree	Japan	N/A	110	220	∞ (0.1–∞)	(Mori et al., 1988)
First-degree	USA	20–54	493	2465	3.6 (1.8–7.1)	(Schildkraut and Thompson, 1988)
Second-degree					2.9 (1.6–5.3)	
First-degree	USA	20–79	296	343	3.3 (1.1–9.4)	(Hartge et al., 1989)
First-degree + aunts	Canada	All	197	210	2.5 (0.7–11.1)	(Koch et al., 1989)
First-degree	Italy	25–74	755	2023	1.9 (1.1–3.6)	(Parazzini et al., 1992)
First-degree	USA	N/A	883	Population database	2.1 (1.0–3.4)	(Goldgar et al., 1994)
First-degree	USA	<65	441	2065	8.2 (3.0–23)	(Rosenberg et al., 1994)
First-degree	USA	All	662	2647	4.3 (2.4–7.9)	(Kerber and Slattery, 1995)

Second-degree					2.1 (1.2–3.8)	
Third-degree					1.5 (1.0–2.2)	
First-degree	Australia	18–79	824	860	3.9 (1.6–9.7)	(Purdie et al., 1995)
First-degree	Finland	<76	559	Population incidence rate	2.8 (1.8–4.2)	(Auranen et al., 1996)
First-degree	UK	<60	1188	Population incidence rate	SMR = 223 (155–310)	(Easton et al., 1996)
Any	Canada	20–84	170	170	1.9 (0.8–4.4)	(Godard et al., 1998)
Daughters (≤53 years)	Sweden	n/s	n/s	Population incidence rate	2.7 (1.9–3.7)	(K. Hemminki et al., 1998)
First-degree	USA Israel	All	213	386	3.2 (1.5–6.8)	(Moslehi et al., 2000)
First-degree	UK		≥2 ovarian cancer in 316 families	Population incidence rate	7.2 (3.8–12.3)	(Sutcliffe et al., 2000)

Three studies (Auranen et al., 1996; Easton et al., 1996; Sutcliffe et al., 2000) have a population-based cohort design, the others are case–control studies.

Table 7.10. *BRCA1/2 mutation and ovarian cancer penetrance: selected studies, 1994–2003*

Population studied	BRCA1/2 screening	Penetrance to (age 70–75)	Reference
33 early-onset BC (<60 years) and OC families	BRCA1 linkage	BRCA1: 44% (28–56%)	(Ford et al., 2004)
33 early-onset BC (<60 years) and OC families	BRCA1 linkage	BRCA1: 63%	(Easton et al., 1995)
237 early-onset BOC families	Linkage or sequencing	BRCA1: 42% BRCA2: 27% (0–47%)	(Narod et al., 1995a) (Ford et al., 1998)
14 AJ BOC families	Risk estimate for mutation carriers relatives	BRCA1 185delAG: 41% 5382insC: No data BRCA2 6174delT: 30%	(Abeliovich et al., 1997)
2 BOC families	BRCA2 linkage	BRCA2: 10% (at age 60)	(Easton et al., 1997)
25 AJ BOC families	AJ founder mutations[a]	BRCA1 (185delAG + 5382insC): 57% BRCA2 6174delT: 49%	(Levy-Lahad et al., 1997)
922 incident OC (population-based study)	Segregation analysis	BRCA1: 22% (5–60%)	(Whittemore et al., 1997)
5318 Jews (population-based)	3 AJ founder mutations[a]	16% (6–28%)	(Struewing et al., 1997)
412 AJ BC patients	3 AJ founder mutations[a]	12%	(Warner et al., 1999)
112 families with ≥2 relatives with OC, +/–BC <60 years	PTT, SSCA, sequencing	BRCA1: 53%	(Antoniou et al., 2000)
374 OC <70 years		BRCA2: 31% BRCA1/2: 68% (36–94%)	
191 AJ patients, OC <75 years	3 AJ founder mutations[a]	BRCA1 185delAG: 37% BRCA1 5382insC: 21% BRCA2 6174delT: 14%	(Moslehi et al., 2000)

Combined analysis of
22 studies, including some
of the above studies

Numerous techniques

Penetrance per year (%)
by 5 year age group

(Antoniou et al., 2003)

Age	BRCA1	BRCA2
20–24	.001	.001
25–29	.002	.002
30–34	.18	.004
35–39	.28	.01
40–44	.87	.08
45–49	1.49	.14
50–54	.96	.60
55–59	1.19	.75
60–64	2.26	.38
65–69	2.49	.42

[a] AJ founder mutations: BRCA1: 185delAG, 5382insC; BRCA2: 6174delT.
AJ: Ashkenazi Jewish; BC: breast cancer; BOC: breast-ovarian cancer; OC: ovarian cancer; PTT: protein truncation test; SSCA: single-strand conformation analysis and RR: relative risk.

a family history of breast/ovarian cancer. These results show that among women with ovarian cancer, *BRCA1* and *BRCA2* mutations are at least 3 times more likely to be found in Ashkenazi Jewish women than in non-Ashkenazi women.

Interestingly, among otherwise unselected, very young onset cases (under 30 years of age at diagnosis) *BRCA1/2* mutations have not been observed (Stratton et al., 1999b), even though from epidemiological studies, mutations in genes are likely to be playing an important role in susceptibility.

There is evidence for genotype–phenotype relationships for ovarian cancer in *BRCA1/2*-mutation carriers. Mutations in the 3' portion of the *BRCA1* gene (exons 13–24) was initially associated with a higher frequency of breast cancer relative to ovarian cancer in a series of 32 European families (Gayther et al., 1995). This observation has not been confirmed by most larger studies (Phelan et al., 1996; Tonin et al., 1996; Levy-Lahad et al., 1997; Shattuck-Eidens et al., 1997; Stoppa-Lyonnet et al., 1997; Ford et al., 1998), although one study provided non-significant evidence in favour of the original finding (Moslehi et al., 2000). In a series of 25 English breast/ovarian cancer families, ovarian cancer was more prevalent than breast cancer when *BRCA2* truncating mutations were located in a region of approximately 3.3 kb in exon 11 (the ovarian cancer cluster region (OCCR), nucleotides 3035–6629). Additional data from 45 *BRCA2* families ascertained outside the UK provided support for this clustering (Gayther et al., 1997b). The analysis of 164 families with *BRCA2* mutations, 67 of whose had mutations in the OCCR has been reported (Thompson and Easton, 2001). The odds ratio for ovarian versus breast cancer in families with mutations in the OCCR, relative to non-OCCR mutations was 3.9 ($P < 0.0001$), confirming the importance of the OCCR in terms of ovarian cancer risk, but the effect was lost when Ashkenazi Jewish cases were omitted (6174delT is an exon 11 mutation). Case reports of multiple-case ovarian cancer families with mutations outside the OCCR temper enthusiasm for the clinical utility of these observations (Al Saffar and Foulkes, 2002).

The existence of a premalignant lesion for epithelial ovarian cancer is uncertain (Scully, 2000). Careful histopathological analysis of prophylactic oophorectomy specimens among high-risk women, either because they have been identified as *BRCA1/2*-mutation carriers or based on their family history, gave conflicting results regarding the presence of histological alterations that could evolve towards invasive carcinoma (Tobachman et al., 1982; Deligdisch et al., 1999; Stratton et al., 1999a; Werness et al., 1999). Interestingly, there has been a report of a tiny carcinoma in situ identified in an otherwise normal prophylactic oophorectomy specimen from a woman with a *BRCA1* mutation (Werness et al., 2000). Carcinoma in situ is very rarely seen in ovarian tissue, and this finding has not been replicated.

The incidence of primary serous carcinoma of the peritoneum among *BRCA1/2* carriers, before or after oophorectomy is not known, but is likely to be substantially higher than in the general population. According to one population-based study in Israel (Rutter et al., 2003), the protection against gynaecological cancer afforded by preventive oophorectomy was substantially less than that seen in selected series (Rebbeck et al., 2002), implying that, among women who have undergone prophylactic surgery, this cancer may become one of the major threats to health among *BRCA1/2* carriers in their later years. Peritoneal cancer is indistinguishable histologically or macroscopically from ovarian cancer occurring among *BRCA1/2*-mutation carriers and represents a major challenge in terms of prevention of cancer in mutation carriers (Tobachman et al., 1982; Piver et al., 1993; Struewing et al., 1995b; Bandera et al., 1998; Berchuck et al., 1999; Karlan et al., 1999). The potential increased risk of malignant transformation of the entire peritoneal surface is thought to reflect the common origin of the ovarian epithelium and peritoneum from embryonic mesoderm. However, the peritoneum on the surface of the ovary may be particularly vulnerable to malignant transformation as a result of repeated injury following ovulation and/or high levels of local oestrogen exposure (Fathalla, 1971; Eisen and Weber, 1998). Preliminary evidence suggests that some peritoneal carcinomas may arise multifocally, particularly in the context of *BRCA1* mutations (Schorge et al., 1998) and there may be a unique molecular pathogenesis of *BRCA1*-related papillary serous carcinoma of the peritoneum (Schorge et al., 2000).

The natural history of *BRCA1/2*-related ovarian cancer is thought to be different from sporadic ovarian cancer. Forty-three serous ovarian adenocarcinomas (81 per cent of the total), had an actuarial median survival of 77 months, compared with 29 months for the age, stage and histological type-matched control group who were believed not to have mutations in *BRCA1* on the basis of family history ($P < .001$) (Rubin et al., 1996). This good prognosis was attributed partly to the relative youth of the patients (mean age 48 years) but was also thought to be directly related to the presence of a *BRCA1* mutation. This study was criticised on methodological grounds, but a second study from the senior author using a historical cohort approach (which is not susceptible to ascertainment bias) gave similar results (Boyd et al., 2000). Interestingly, the better survival in hereditary cases was particularly noted for those women receiving platinum-containing chemotherapy. A Japanese study also found a better outcome for hereditary ovarian cancer (Aida et al., 1998), although this study is open to criticism on the grounds of ascertainment bias. Other more recent studies have supported the notion that the prognosis is better for *BRCA1/2*-related ovarian cancer (reviewed in Foulkes, 2006).

Mutations in other genes can cause ovarian cancer (Table 7.7). HNPCC is one of the most common autosomal conditions predisposing to cancer, accounts for 5–8 per cent of all colorectal cancers (discussed on p. 200). Mutations in *MLH1* and *MSH2* are rare in ovarian cancers not selected on the basis of family history of cancer (Rubin et al., 1998; Fujita et al., 1993).

Very few cases of ovarian carcinoma have been reported in association with other inherited genetic syndromes (Table 7.7). There have been few reports of clear germline *TP53* mutations in women with ovarian cancer in a strongly famil-ial setting for example (Borresen 1992; Jolly et al., 1994), and ovarian cancer is not considered as a feature of the Li–Fraumeni syndrome (Buller et al., 1995; Kleihues et al., 1997; Birch et al., 1998). Ovarian tumours, including carcinomas, have been reported in Carney complex, but it is not known if the incidence is truly increased (Stratakis et al., 2000). Familial aggregation of ovarian germ cell cancer has been reported (Stettner et al., 1999), but must be very rare.

Prevention of hereditary ovarian cancer is a major topic and is beyond the scope of this book; suffice to say that medically, the oral contraceptive pill is likely to offer significant (40 per cent of more) risk reduction (Narod et al., 1998; Whittemore et al., 2004a). Surgically, ovarian removal (Rutter et al., 2003) as well as tubal ligation (Narod et al., 2001) are options. Prophylactic salpingo-oophorectomy is often offered to women with germline *BRCA1* or *BRCA2* mutations, as the evidence is that it very much reduces the risk of ovarian cancer and also reduces the risk of breast cancer to 50 per cent in pre-menopausal women (Rebbeck et al., 1999; Rutter et al., 2003). While surgery clearly is effective in preventing serous papillary cancers arising from the ovary, the peritoneum remains at risk, as discussed above.

The early detection of carcinoma at a stage in which it might be surgically cur-able, or more amenable to chemotherapeutic agents, would have a significant impact on prognosis. The traditional screening methods for ovarian carcinoma are the measurement of the serum tumour marker, CA-125, transvaginal ultrasono-graphy and clinical examination. None of these methods alone achieve the required level of sensitivity; for example, CA-125 detects only about two-thirds of stage 1 ovarian tumours (Mackey and Creasman, 1995). In the general population, clini-cal examination, transabdominal (Campbell et al., 1989), transvaginal (Kurjak and Zalud, 1992; van Nagell et al., 2000) ultrasound and serum CA-125 screening tests (Cuckle and Wald, 1990) either alone or in combination (Jacobs et al., 1993) have all been assessed as potential screening tests in various settings. However, no test or combination of tests has yet proved to be effective for population screen-ing. In a longer term follow-up of their previous study (Jacobs et al., 1993), Jacobs and colleagues showed that although the median survival in the screened group was significantly better than for the control group, the number of deaths from an index cancer did not differ significantly between the two groups (18 deaths in 10 977 controls versus 9 in 10 958 screened women, RR 2.0 (95 per cent CI 0.78–5.13) (Jacobs et al., 1999).

For women at high risk of ovarian carcinoma, in the absence of good data, it has been recommended that they have an annual pelvic examination, vaginal ultrasonography and serum CA-125 measurement every 6 or 12-month intervals from their mid-20's or 5 years less than the earliest age of onset of ovarian cancer in the family (Burke et al., 1997). In the absence of better data, it may be appropriate to restrict these tests to a research setting. Trials are underway in the USA and in Europe both in high-risk individuals and in the general population. A worrying feature of hereditary ovarian cancer is the possibility that high-grade cancers can arise in very small foci that would not be detectable by ultrasound. A case report of a case of ultimately fatal advanced ovarian cancer diagnosed in a woman referred for a prophylactic oophorectomy was an early suggestion that delaying surgery could be dangerous (Rose and Hunter, 1994). Studies among proven *BRCA1/2* carriers have supported this finding. Three of 33 women with *BRCA1/2* mutations were found to have early ovarian cancer lesions on examination of prophylactic oophorectomy specimens. Notably, two of the three cases were bilateral at diagnosis, and both were only noted on histopathological review and not in the operating room (Lu et al., 2000). Similarly, high-risk lesions, or frank cancers can be found in the fallopian tubes of *BRCA1/2* carriers at preventive oophorectomy (Colgan et al., 2001; Leeper et al., 2002; Carcangiu et al., 2004; McEwen et al., 2004). In the latter study, 5 of 60 consecutive *BRCA1/2*-positive women undergoing preventive oophorectomy were found to have occult ovarian or fallopian cancer: one death had occurred at 4 years follow-up. In a similar study from the USA, 5 of 30 *BRCA1/2* carriers had cancer at surgery: one was a primary peritoneal cancer, three had tubal cancer and one had ovarian adenofibroma with adjacent areas of low malignant potential carcinoma (Leeper et al., 2002). Taken together, these studies suggest that screening for ovarian cancer by ultrasound and CA-125 will prove to be insufficiently sensitive for routine use in *BRCA1/2* carriers, but the results of controlled trials are awaited. The situation may be different for other inherited syndromes such as HNPCC (Hogg and Friedlander, 2004), but as ovarian cancer is less frequent in other syndromes than in *BRCA1/2*-mutation carriers, the specificity is likely to be a significant problem.

Other ovarian neoplasms (Table 7.7)

Non-epithelial ovarian tumours are found with increased frequency in Peutz–Jeghers syndrome (sex cord, granulosa cell tumours which are often hormone secreting) (Dozois et al., 1970) and Gorlin syndrome (ovarian fibroma) (Berlin et al., 1966), and Ollier disease and Maffucci syndrome have both been associated with ovarian granulosa cell tumours with precocious pseudopuberty (Vaz and Turner, 1986). A family has been described in which ovarian germ cell tumours were found in two daughters of a woman who herself had had an ovarian tumour in childhood, and her third child had a soft tissue sarcoma. Mutations of *TP53* could have been responsible for this, but were not looked for (Weinblatt and Kochen, 1991). There is a single case report of a mixed ovarian germ cell tumour occurring in a *BRCA2* carrier – interestingly, no LOH was seen and thus it is possible that this was an unrelated, chance finding (Hamel et al., 2006). Ovarian fibromas have been reported in a family in which the condition could have been inherited as an autosomal sex-limited dominant trait (Dumont-Herskowitz et al., 1978).

Occasionally, ovarian teratomas and dermoid cysts (usually bilateral and often in young individuals) have been reported to occur in more than one member of a family, suggesting that genetic factors may be important in the development of this type of tumour, but such reports are rare (Simon et al., 1985; Stettner et al., 1999). Teratomas are thought to be pathogenic, arising from a single female germ cell after the first meiotic division (Linder et al., 1975).

Gonadoblastoma is a dysgenetic gonadoma which itself does not metastasise but which may be associated with dysgerminoma and other malignant germ cell elements. The overwhelming majority (96 per cent) of gonadoblastomas develop in dysgenetic gonads of 46XY individuals. Most patients with this tumour are phenotypic females, the rest are phenotypic males with abnormalities of the genitalia and undescended testes. Further details of gonadal tumours in intersex conditions are described on p. 106. Familial ovarian arrhenoblastomas have (rarely) been described to occur with an apparent autosomal dominant predisposition, associated with nodular thyroid disease (O'Brien and Wilansky, 1981).

Cancer of the cervix

Carcinoma of the uterine cervix affects about 1 per cent of women (with an incidence of 8 and 12.5 per 100 000 population in Canada and the UK, respectively, but much higher incidence rates in some countries such as 67 per 100 000 in Zimbabwe, and 34 per 100 000 in Columbia) (Parkin et al., 1997). It is strongly linked to human papillomavirus (HPV), indeed infection with this virus is almost always a requirement for squamous cell carcinoma of the cervix (Lehtonen et al., 1996). The E6 and E7 viral proteins are consistently retained and expressed in these tumours, and can be demonstrated to bind to the p53 and Rb protein products, respectively. The viral proteins may thus interfere with the normal tumour suppressor function of the cellular proteins (Vousden, 1989). Host factors may also have a role in the pathogenesis of cervical carcinoma as women with HLA-DQw3 appear to be at increased risk of developing this tumour (Wank and Thomssen, 1991). Other HLA haplotypes have also been associated with increased risk (Apple et al., 1995).

There is a documented increased incidence of cervical cancer in women who were exposed to diethylstilboestrol in utero (Robboy et al., 1984). Although cervical cancer may occur as a complication of the genetic skin conditions ectodermal dysplasia and dyskeratosis congenita, a genetic predisposition to this cancer is rare.

Family history studies of women with cervical cancer have not shown a striking excess of cervical cancer in female relatives, although some familial aggregation has been observed (Ahlbom et al., 1997; Magnusson et al., 2000; Horn et al., 2002), as might be expected, especially if the HLA data are taken into consideration. A substantial fraction of the familial factors appear to be non-genetic, but this may depend on the relationship studied: in the Magnusson study, shared environments explained concordance between sisters, but not between concordant mothers and daughters. Similarly, cigarette smoking-associated cancers (lung, larynx, lip and cervix) were inter-associated in one systematic study (Goldgar et al., 1994). Nevertheless, the Breast Cancer Linkage Consortium did identify an excess of cervical cancer in *BRCA1*-mutation carriers (RR = 3.72, 95 per cent CI = 2.26–6.10, $P < .001$) (Thompson and Easton, 2002).

Screening for cervical cancer is offered as part of the population screening programme in the UK, and no particular addition to this has been suggested for women families with hereditary cancer syndromes, except Peutz–Jeghers syndrome, where adenoma malignum is seen (Spigelman et al., 1995). It is aetiologically distinct from squamous cell carcinoma. The excess of cervical cancer in *BRCA1* carriers is of interest, and deserves further attention in a prospective study. Primary melanoma of the cervix is very rare, and does not seem to be related to mutations in *CDKN2A* or *BRCA2*.

Other tumours of the female reproductive system

Cancer of the female genital organs other than of the uterus, cervix and ovary has an incidence of about 3.6 per 100 000 (Duggan and Dubeau, 1998)

Cancer of the external genitalia

Cancer of the external genitalia is rare. Squamous cell carcinoma of the cervix and external genitalia may complicate dyskeratosis congenital and ectodermal dysplasia. Vulval carcinoma may complicate vulval lichen sclerosis (which can occur rarely as a familial condition, see p. 157; Vanin et al., 2002). Vulval neoplasia is generally "non-genetic" and is associated with HPV infection and smoking (Edwards et al., 1996; Daling et al., 2002; Engelman et al., 2003). There is a possibility that genetic polymorphisms in genes altering susceptibility to cancer in smokers may also alter susceptibility to vulval and anal cancer (Chen et al., 1999). It can arise in Paget disease of the vulva and in Bowen disease of the vulva. Paget's disease of the vulva is a rare intraepithelial cancer of the apocrine glands and is occasionally associated with an underlying adenocarcinoma (Tinari et al., 2002). Chromosomal 11p abnormalities have been described in the latter (Swanson et al., 1997). Abnormalities of the *PRAD1* gene and *TP53* have been described in vulval carcinomas (Kurzrock et al., 1995). Vulvar carcinoma occurs with increased frequency in Fanconi anaemia (FA) (Alter, 1996) and Morris syndrome (Esposito et al., 1995). It appears that this increased prevalence in FA patients may be related to an increased susceptibility to HPV, and in FA patients an increased proportion of patients with FA and squamous cell carcinoma of the vulva are homozygous for Arg72, a TP53 polymorphism which is thought to be associated with increased susceptibility to HPV infection (Kutler et al., 2003).

Primary malignant melanoma of the vulva is the second most common vulvar malignancy, an aggressive cancer, usually occurring on non-hairy skin, thus non-ultraviolet (UV) light-associated (Ragnarsson-Olding, 2004). A family history of cutaneous melanoma is found in 15 per cent of cases, and a germline mutation in the melanocortin type 1 receptor has been described in one case (Wechter et al., 2004).

Vaginal carcinoma

An increased occurrence of this squamous cell cancer is associated with maternal ingestion of diethylstilboestrol during pregnancy (Robboy et al., 1984). In situ and invasive epithelial vaginal cancers have many of the same risk factors as cervical cancer, including a strong relationship to HPV infection (Daling et al., 2002)

Rare types of cancer of the vagina that have been reported are Brenner tumours (Ben-Izhak et al., 1998) and leiomyomas. The latter has been reported to occur as part of a dominantly inherited syndrome of multiple adult-onset schwannomas, multiple naevi and multiple vaginal leiomyomas (Gorlin and Koutlas, 1998). The naevi appear to be congenital in this condition. Giant hypertrophy of the labia minora and with neoplastic fibroblast and epithelial proliferation has been described in Ramon syndrome of arthritis, deafness and pigmentary changes in the retina (De Pina Neto et al., 1998)

Primary vulval and vaginal extraosseous Ewing sarcoma and peripheral neuroectodermal tumour has been described (Vang et al., 2000).

Prostate cancer

Prostate cancer is the most common cancer and the second most common cause of cancer death in North American men. Population prostate cancer risk is approximately 0.5 per cent by the age of 65 years and 2 per cent by the age of 75 years. The aetiology of prostate cancer is unknown, but androgen stimulation is implicated by observations of a low incidence in males castrated before the age of 40 years, and a high-fat diet has also been implicated. Evidence for a genetic contribution was provided by genetic epidemiological studies in Mormon families that suggested that the inheritability of prostate cancer was greater than that of breast or colorectal cancer (Cannon et al., 1982). A case-control study by Steinberg et al. (1990) found 15 per cent of prostate cancer patients had an

Table 7.11. *Cumulative risks of prostate cancer according to ethnicity, age and family history (adapted from Nieder et al., 2003).*

Group	Cumulative risk of prostate cancer by age		
	50 years	60 years	70 years
White men			
No family history in (%)	0.2	2	7.5
One FDR in (%)	0.4	5.2	19
Two or more FDR in (%)	0.8	10	38
Black men			
No family history in (%)	0.4	3.6	10.6
One FDR in (%)	1.1	9.2	27.1
Two or more FDR in (%)	2.1	18	34

FDR: first-degree relative.

affected father or brother, compared to 8 per cent of controls. Furthermore, the RR increased: (i) with the number of affected relatives such that men with one, two and three affected first-degree relatives were at twofold, fivefold and 11-fold increased risk for developing prostate cancer, respectively; and (ii) the younger the age at onset of prostate cancer in the proband. Meikle and Smith (1990) reported a 17-fold increase in RR of prostate cancer in brothers of men developing prostate cancer between 45 and 50 years of age. Segregation analysis of the family histories of 740 prostate cancer patients suggested that familial clustering of the disease could be caused by a rare, highly penetrant, dominantly inherited predisposition gene (Carter et al., 1992). Under the most likely genetic model, 43 per cent of early-onset prostate cancer (in men <55 years) would occur in gene carriers, but only 9 per cent of cases in men aged <85 years. This proposed model of a rare dominant predisposing gene (or genes) was similar to that suggested for breast cancer. Johns and Houlston (2003) undertook a meta-analysis of 13 studies of prostate cancer risk in first-degree relatives. They found that the pooled RR in first-degree relatives was 2.5, and 3.5 in men with two affected relatives. Risks were also increased if the affected relative had early-onset disease (<60 years). Nieder et al. (2003) provided cumulative risks by age according to family history details and ethnicity (see Table 7.11). The clinical course of familial and sporadic prostate cancer appears to be similar although the disease may be more aggressive in African-Americans.

Multiple prostate cancer susceptibility loci have been mapped by family linkage studies (e.g. *CAPB, HPC1, HPC2, HPX, MSR1, PCAP, HPC20, RNASEL*), but none of these equate with major high penetrance susceptibility genes present in many populations (as for *BRCA1* and *BRCA2* in familial breast cancer). Although mutations in three candidate prostate cancer susceptibility genes have been reported: *RNASEL* (*HPC1*, 1q24-q25), *MSR1* (8p22–p23) and *ELAC2* (*HPC2*, 17p11), in most cases these genes do not appear to represent rare highly penetrant loci and familial risks of prostate cancer may be explained better by a model of multiple interacting moderate-risk genetic variants. Germline *BRCA2* mutations may account for a small but significant group (2–5 per cent) of familial prostate cancer clusters or early-onset cases (Gayther et al., 2000; Edwards et al., 2002) and the relative risk of prostate cancer in camers is increased signigicantly, higher at younger ages, in mutation camers (RR 4.71 (95% confidence interval: 1.87–12.25) (Kirchoff et al., 2004).

Men at increased risk of prostate cancer can be offered screening by annual measurement of prostate specific antigen (PSA) and digital rectal examination from age 40 years. Male BRCAIeBRCAZ mutation camers are eligible for screening by annual PSA between 40 and 69 years of age with prostate biopsy if PSA > 3mg/ml, under a research trial, IMPACT (www.impact-study.co.uk).

Testicular neoplasms

Testicular cancer accounts for only 1 per cent of all malignancy in males (with an incidence of 4 per 100 000 males), but is the most frequent carcinoma in the 15–35-year age group. Most tumours are of germ cell origin (seminoma, teratoma) but some arise from stroma (Sertoli cell), and gonadoblastoma contain germ cell and stromal elements.

Familial aggregation of testicular germ cell tumours accounts for up to 2 per cent of all adult cases. In a literature review, 24 father–son pairs, 45 pairs of non-twin brothers and 12 pairs of identical twins with testicular cancer were cited (Patel et al., 1990). Tumours are of the same histological type in 70 per cent of identical twin pairs, but were mostly of different histology in other degrees of relationship. Testicular tumours are bilateral in about 4 per cent of patients, which is suggestive of a genetic basis (Patel et al., 1990). In a Dutch single centre study, RR of testicular cancer was increased 9- to 13-fold in brothers (Sonneveld et al., 1999). In an analysis of the Swedish Family-Cancer Database, familial risks were increased to 3.8-fold for fathers, 8.3-fold for brothers and 3.9-fold for sons, and although seminomas showed a later age at onset than teratomas (30 versus 40 years) the familial risks were similar for the two tumour types (Dong et al., 2001). Forman et al. (1992) found that brothers of men with testicular cancer had a 2 per cent risk of developing testicular cancer by the age of 50 years, which corresponds to a 10-fold increase in RR. The mean age at diagnosis in familial cases was slightly younger than in sporadic cases (29.5 years versus 32.5 years).

Large families with a high incidence of testicular cancer have been described but are rare: Lynch and Walzak (1980) studied a large inbred Dutch kindred in which four individuals had histologically proven testicular cancers, and Goss and Bulbul (1990) reported a large cancer-prone family (including early-onset breast cancer) in which five males had testicular cancer. Nicholson and Harland (1995) and Heimdal et al. (1997) have suggested that familial clustering of testicular cancer might be attributable to a recessive gene. However familial testicular cancer appears to be genetically heterogeneous and an X-linked locus has been mapped (see below).

The principal risk factor for testicular cancer is cryptorchidism, which is associated with at least a 10-fold increase in risk, and orchidopexy should be performed in early childhood for boys with cryptorchidism if this risk is to be diminished. Genetic factors have been implicated in cryptorchidism because up to 14 per cent of cryptorchid males have an affected relative, but it is unclear to what extent this might explain the familial occurrence of testicular tumours. Patients with X-linked ichthyosis (steroid-sulphatase deficiency) appear to be at increased risk of cryptorchidism and testicular tumours.

Klinefelter syndrome has rarely been reported to predispose to testicular tumours, but in some cases this may be related to cryptorchidism. In one case, however, bilateral testicular teratoma occurred in a sib pair with Klinefelter syndrome (Gustavson et al., 1975). The risk of testicular cancer (seminoma, Sertoli cell, teratocarcinoma and embryonal cell carcinoma) is unequivocally increased in patients with the testicular feminisation syndrome, and prophylactic gonadectomy is usually performed after pubertal growth. Gonadoblastoma occurs in XY gonadal dysgenesis (see below), and also in patients with the WAGR syndrome (Wilms tumour-aniridia-genital abnormality-mental retardation, see p. 113). A sub-class of Sertoli cell tumours (large-cell calcifying) can be familial and can be associated with cardiac myxoma, endocrine activity and pigmented skin lesions in Carney complex (NAME syndrome) (see part three).

Chromosomal analysis of germ cell testicular tumours has implicated isochromosome of 12p as a specific finding. Although various associations between HLA haplotypes and testicular cancer have been proposed, HLA class I analysis of affected sib pairs provided no evidence of a HLA-linked testicular cancer susceptibility gene (Forman et al., 1992). However, Rapley et al. (2000) mapped a locus for testicular germ cell tumours (TGCT1) to Xq27 using families compatible with X inheritance. Cases linked to Xq27 were more likely to have undescended testis and bilateral disease. There was clear evidence of locus heterogeneity and autosomal susceptibility loci are likely. More recent data suggests that no one single locus can account for a significant fraction of familial testicular tumours (Crockford et al., 2006). Interestingly, a Y-chromosome locus involved in infertility known as the "gr/gr" deletion is a rare, low-penetrance susceptibility allele for testicle tumours (particulary seminomas) with a population frequency of −0.013 and an odds ratio of 3.0 for seminoma ($P = 0.0004$) (Nathanson et al., 2005).

The occurrence of testicular tumours in high-risk individuals can be prevented by appropriate measures. Cryptorchidism should be corrected early to avoid an increased risk of testicular tumours. Non-functioning testes that present a significant risk for tumorigenesis (as in the testicular feminisation syndrome or intersex states) should be removed. Individuals thought to be at high risk of familial testicular tumours can be monitored by regular self-examination and ultrasonography.

Testicular tumours in intersex states

Gonadoblastoma is a dysgenetic gonadoma which itself does not metastasise but which may be associated with dysgerminoma and other malignant germ cell elements. An overwhelming majority (96 per cent) of gonadoblastomas develop in dysgenetic gonads of 46XY individuals. Most patients with this tumour are phenotypic females, the rest are phenotypic males with abnormalities of the genitalia and undescended testes. The tumour is frequently bilateral, usually develops in the second decade, and may secrete oestrogens or testosterone.

Germ cell tumours are rarely seen in individuals with gonadal dysgenesis who do not have any Y chromosomal material present (Verp and Simpson, 1987). Thus, girls with Turner syndrome with the chromosomal constitution 45,X;45,X/46,XX;46,X,del(Xp) or 46,X,del(Xq) are not at an increased risk of this tumour, but in cases of gonadal dysgenesis due to chromosomal mosaicism such as 45,X/46,XY, or where a Y fragment is present, gonadoblastomas are a significant risk in the dysgenetic gonads, perhaps occurring in up to 20 per cent of cases. However in a population-based study of girls with Turner syndrome, analysed by PCR to detect Y-chromosome material, Gravholt et al. (2000) reported that although the frequency of Y-chromosome material is high in Turner syndrome (12.2 per cent), the occurrence of gonadoblastoma among Y-positive patients was less than in previous estimates (7–10 per cent), Gonadal extirpation has been suggested for such patients unless they have an almost normal male phenotype with scrotal testes. Nevertheless, even then careful follow-up (perhaps including testicular biopsy) is needed (Verp and Simpson, 1987). The report of an infant girl with Turner syndrome, gonadoblastoma and 46XY(del Yp) karyotype indicated that the genes on the Y-chromosome that induce gonadoblastoma are distinct from the sex-determining locus (Magenis et al., 1984), and detailed mapping of the Y-chromosome gonadoblastoma susceptibility region close to the centromere has been undertaken and candidate genes proposed (Tsuchiya et al., 1995; Lau, 1999).

There is probably no increased risk of gonadoblastoma in Klinefelter syndrome (47, XXY) or in the XYY syndrome. However gonadoblastoma is associated with sex reversal caused by 9p deletion (Livadas et al., 2003) and WAGR syndrome caused by 11p13 deletion (see p. 113).

Single gene defects can also cause gonadal dysgenesis, and gonadal tumours are found in at least 30 per cent of XY cases. The tumours are gonadoblastomas or dysgerminomas, which arise in the second or third decade. Autosomal recessive forms of XX gonadal dysgenesis are probably not associated with an increased risk for gonadoblastomas, but XY gonadal dysgenesis (Swyer syndrome), is frequently complicated by this tumour. Affected individuals are of normal stature and do not have the features of Turner syndrome, but have streak gonads. H-Y antigen may or may not be positive. It has been suggested that the risk of gonadoblastoma and dysgerminoma is confined to the H-Y antigen-positive cases. XY gonadal dysgenesis may also occur as an autosomal recessive condition, and gonadal tumours frequently complicate the familial testicular dysgenesis syndrome, one of this group of conditions. Again, H-Y antigen-positive cases appear to be the ones susceptible to gonadoblastomas, with a 55 per cent incidence (Mann et al., 1983; Muller, 1990). Gonadoblastoma may be associated with renal impairment and gonadal dysgenesis in Frasier syndrome (see part three).

The incidence of gonadal neoplasia in true hermaphrodites (individuals with both testicular and ovarian tissue) appears to be low, although both ovarian and testicular tumours have been reported. Complete testicular feminisation (X-linked recessive inheritance) is associated with an increased risk of testicular malignancy (about 5 per cent), most commonly seminoma. If malignancy develops, it is usually after the age of 25 years, so that orchidectomy can be delayed until after pubertal feminisation. The risk of neoplasia in incomplete androgen-insensitivity states, including Reifenstein syndrome, is considered to be low (Verp and Simpson, 1987).

In the syndromes of persistent Mullerian duct and pseudovaginal perineoscrotal hypoplasia, the abnormally situated testes are susceptible to the development of seminomas, choriocarcinomas, embryonal carcinomas, gonadoblastomas or teratocarcinomas. The incidence of gonadal neoplasia may be slightly increased – to up to 4 per cent in 46XX cases, and 10 per cent in 46XY cases.

In the conditions predisposing to gonadal tumours, it is advisable to remove the gonads prophylactically in the second decade.

Epididymal tumours

Benign epididymal cystadenomas occur in von Hippel–Lindau disease, when they are frequently bilateral. Although scrotal ultrasound scan can be useful for demonstrating sub-clinical involvement, the presence of epididymal cysts alone does not represent a reliable criterion for identifying gene carriers in von Hippel–Lindau disease families (Seizinger et al., 1991).

8

Urinary system

Renal neoplasms

Cancers of the kidney account for approximately 1.5 per cent of all cancers and cancer deaths (with an incidence of 5–8 per 100 000 population in the UK, and commoner in males). Three main types of renal cancer are distinguished: (1) Wilms tumour, (2) renal cell carcinoma (RCC) (adenocarcinoma) and (3) medullary and transitional cell cancers of the renal pelvis.

Wilms tumour

Wilms tumour is one of the most common solid tumours in children, with an incidence of approximately 10 per 100 000 live births, and accounting for 8 per cent of all childhood cancers. Both sporadic and familial forms occur, although the latter is uncommon and only 1 per cent of Wilms tumour patients have a positive family history (Breslow et al., 1996). Median age at diagnosis of Wilms tumour is 3–4 years and 80 per cent of patients present by the age of 5 years. Approximately 5 per cent of cases have bilateral tumours, and this subgroup has an earlier age at diagnosis (mean 30 months), and an increased incidence of renal blastemal rests and congenital abnormalities (Breslow and Beckwith, 1982). In contrast to retinoblastoma, the age at onset and proportion of bilateral tumours are not significantly different in familial and sporadic cases. There are important associations between Wilms tumour and sporadic aniridia, Beckwith–Wiedemann syndrome, hemihypertrophy, genitourinary abnormalities, Drash syndrome and Perlman syndrome, Frasier syndrome and Simpson–Golabi syndrome (see part three). In addition, Wilms tumour has been associated occasionally with neurofibromatosis type 1, *BRCA1* mutations and Bloom syndrome (Rahman et al., 1996). Familial Wilms tumour segregates as an autosomal dominant trait with incomplete penetrance (in a large kindred reported by Schwartz et al. (1991), there were six affected relatives and eight non-penetrant obligate heterozygotes).

Wilms tumour is thought to be derived from a mesenchymal renal stem cell or metanephric blastema. Islands of cells resembling metanephric blastema (nephrogenic rests) may persist into infancy and are found in 1 per cent of normal infant kidneys, but in up to 40 per cent of kidneys with unilateral Wilms tumour and in almost 100 per cent of bilateral cases (Beckwith et al., 1990). Nephrogenic rests have been categorised into perilobar and intralobar rests. It appears that tumours associated with intralobar rests have an earlier age at onset and higher frequency of associated congenital abnormalities than those associated with perilobar rests.

There is a high risk of Wilms tumour in isolated cases of aniridia, particularly when the patient also has genitourinary abnormalities and mental retardation, the so-called Wilms tumour–aniridia–genital abnormality–mental retardation (WAGR) syndrome. This represents a contiguous gene syndrome. Approximately 1 in 40 Wilms tumour patients have aniridia, compared to 2 per 100 000 of the general population (Shannon et al., 1982). Wilms tumour is associated with sporadic aniridia and generally not with familial aniridia. For patients with sporadic aniridia, the risk of Wilms tumour had been estimated to be as high as 1 in 3, but this appears to be an overestimate and the risk may be closer to 15 per cent (Muto et al., 2002). The association of Wilms tumour with aniridia results from a contiguous deletion of the aniridia (PAX6) and Wilms tumour 1 (WT1) genes. Most patients with Wilms tumour and aniridia have a cytogenetically visible chromosome 11p13 deletion, but the risk of Wilms tumour can also occur in those with submicroscopic deletions. Molecular cytogenetic and genetic analysis can be helpful in determining the extent of a deletion and hence the risk of Wilms tumour (Gronskov et al., 2001). Patients with intragenic PAX6 mutations are not at risk of Wilms tumour, but only about 50 per cent of patients with WT1 deletions develop Wilms tumour (Muto et al., 2002). Additional features of the WAGR complex include mental retardation, ambiguous genitalia and gonadoblastoma, and in some cases of obesity (Gul et al., 2002). There is a high incidence of bilateral tumours (36 per cent) and a younger age at diagnosis in children with Wilms tumour and aniridia compared to non-WAGR children. The association of Wilms tumour with genitourinary developmental abnormalities has led to the recognition that WT1 had a role in the development of the normal kidney and genitourinary system (Pelletier et al., 1991a,b). In addition, children with WAGR syndrome have a significant risk of renal failure, albeit it less than in Denys–Drash syndrome (38 and 62 per cent, respectively at 20 years) (Breslow et al., 2000).

Approximately 2–3 per cent of Wilms tumour patients have constitutional chromosome 11p13 deletions (Scott et al., 2006). The catalase locus also maps to this region, and reduced catalase activity was useful in indicating those aniridia patients at high risk for Wilms tumour and gonadal tumours prior to the availability of molecular techniques. Detailed molecular analysis of 11p13 deletions in patients with one or more features of the WAGR complex established the following gene order: centromere–catalase gene–WT1 gene–aniridia

(PAX6)–pter. The *WT1* gene encodes a zinc-finger protein that is primarily expressed in renal blastemal cells during a critical period in the development of the glomerulus. The *WT1* gene product has a critical role in normal genitourinary development (see Denys–Drash syndrome, Part three). Somatic *WT1* mutations occur in less than 10 per cent of sporadic Wilms tumours, and *WT1* mutations are rare in familial Wilms tumour. Pelletier et al. (1991b) reported a father–son pair with Wilms tumour (and hypospadias and cryptorchidism in the son) associated with a germline *WT1* mutation. However, the associated genitourinary developmental abnormalities seen in *WT1* mutation carriers reduce the chances of familial transmission. Severe genital developmental abnormalities are seen in Denys–Drash syndrome, which is associated with dominant negative-acting *WT1* mutations (see part three).

A second Wilms tumour gene *(WT2)* was mapped by loss of heterozygosity studies to chromosome 11p15 in the region of the Beckwith–Wiedemann locus (see p. 170). Chromosome 11p15.5 allele loss preferentially affects the maternal allele that is compatible with a genomic imprinting effect and would be consistent with *WT2* being a maternally expressed imprinted tumour suppressor gene. The *p57KIP2 (CDKN1C)* gene is a candidate imprinted tumour suppressor gene that is mutated in patients with Beckwith–Wiedemann syndrome but is apparently not mutated in sporadic Wilms tumours. Loss of *IGF2* imprinting associated with *IGF2* overexpression occurs in many Beckwith–Wiedemann syndrome patients (Maher and Reik, 2000), and in the majority of sporadic Wilms tumours.

Loss of heterozygosity studies in sporadic Wilms tumours have mapped a Wilms tumour suppressor gene to chromosome 16. However, genetic linkage studies in familial Wilms tumour kindreds excluded linkage to the *WT1* and *WT2* regions on chromosome 11 and to chromosome 16 (Schwartz et al., 1991). Rahman et al. (1996) mapped a familial Wilms tumour gene *(FWT1)* to chromosome 17q12–21. Kindreds linked to *FWT1* demonstrate a later age at onset than unlinked familial cases and sporadic cases and do not have developmental anomalies (Rahman et al., 1998). In addition there is evidence of incomplete penetrance (15–26 per cent) in FWT1 kindreds suggesting that familial WT1 may be underascertained (Rahman et al., 2000). A further familial Wilms tumour locus (FWT2) was mapped to 19q13.3–q13.4, but there is evidence for further locus heterogeneity (Huff et al., 1997; Rapley et al., 2000). Wilms tumour may also occur in children with biallelic *BRCA2* mutations (Fanconi anaemia Type D1 see p. 193).

All children at increased risk of Wilms tumour (e.g. with sporadic aniridia, hemihypertrophy, Beckwith–Wiedemann syndrome, etc.) should be followed up carefully. A typical surveillance programme would include 3-monthly renal ultrasound from birth to the age of 8 years. Despite regular screening, Wilms tumour may develop between ultrasound scans, and parents should be alerted to possible presenting symptoms or signs, and in some cases are taught how to perform abdominal palpation as an alternative approach.

RCC (adenocarcinoma, hypernephroma)

RCC accounts for almost 90 per cent of malignant renal tumours. Familial cases of RCC are infrequent, and are estimated to account for about 2 per cent of all cases. McLaughlin et al. (1984), in a population-based case–control study, found a family history of RCC in 2.4 per cent of affected patients, compared to 1.4 per cent of controls. Sporadic RCC is histopathologically heterogeneous. The most common form is clear cell (concentional RCC) which accounts for 75–80 per cent of all cases. The most frequent non-clear cell histopathology is papillary (~15 per cent) RCC which can be divided into types 1 and 2. Chromophobe RCC and oncocytomas each account for 4 per cent of cases. Generally, there is a good correlation between genetic causes of familial RCC and histopathological appearance. Thus von Hippel–Lindau (VHL) disease (see Part three) is the most frequent cause of renal carcinoma susceptibility and RCC in VHL disease invariably has a clear cell appearance. Conversely germline mutations in the MET proto-oncogene cause type 1 papillary RCC while RCC in hereditary leiomyomatosis patients with germline fumarate hydratase mutations (see Part three) is usually classified as Type 2 papillary RCC. RCC is a feature of Birt–Hogg–Dube syndrome and is most often a mixed chromophobe–oncocytoma appearance, but other types of RCC can occur (Part three).

Familial RCC is characterised by: (1) an early age at onset compared to sporadic cases; (2) frequent bilaterality and (3) multicentricity. In addition, features of a susceptibility syndrome (e.g. VHL disease, hereditary leiomyomatosis or Birt–Hogg–Dube syndrome) may be present. Mean age at diagnosis in familial cases is about 45 years, more than 15 years earlier than for sporadic cases (Maher et al., 1990a). In addition to the major RCC susceptibility syndromes described above, familial clear cell RCC may be associated with constitutional chromosome 3 translocation (see below), renal tumours (consisting of a mixture of epithelial and stromal elements) may occur in hyperparathyroidism-jaw tumour syndrome (see Part three) and occasionally in tuberose sclerosis (although the most common renal tumour in this disease is angiomyolipoma). VHL disease should be sought in all cases of inherited, young onset or multiple renal clear cell carcinoma. RCC is the presenting feature in only 10 per cent of patients with VHL disease, but in many families the risk of developing a RCC rises to 70 per cent by the age of 60 years. Further details of VHL disease and a comprehensive screening programme for affected patients and relatives at risk for this disease are provided in Part three. Multiple renal cysts are frequent in VHL disease and may suggest the diagnosis.

Familial non-syndromic RCC should be considered according to the histopathology of the renal tumours. Thus familial non-VHL clear cell RCC is generally characterised by susceptibility to RCC only. Mean age at diagnosis is younger than in sporadic cases (50 per cent diagnosed <50 years of age) and tumours may be bilateral or multicentric (Maher and Yates, 1991; Teh et al., 1997; Woodward et al., 2000). Mostly, familial non-syndromic RCC is considered to be autosomal dominant, but evidence for a recessive inheritance in some cases has been reported (Hemminiki and Li, 2004). The molecular basis of familial non-VHL clear cell RCC kindreds without a chromosome 3 translocation has not been defined except that there is no linkage to *VHL*, *MET* or chromosome 3p (Teh et al., 1997; Woodward et al., 2000). Familial clear cell RCCs can rarely be associated with translocations involving chromosome 3. The first such kindred was reported by Cohen et al. (1979) and contained ten affected patients in three generations. In this family, RCC segregated with a t(3:8)(p14.2:q24.1), and it was estimated that each translocation carrier had an 87 per cent risk of developing this cancer by 60 years of age. Subsequently an increased risk of thyroid cancer was also reported in the family. Six other chromosome 3 translocation-RCC families have been described, but the breakpoints and partner chromosome are heterogeneous. In the original t(3:8)(p14.2:q24.1) kindred the 3p breakpoint occurred at the fragile site and disrupts the fragile histidine triad (*FHIT*) tumour suppressor gene. However the precise role of *FHIT* (and the chromosome 8 gene *TRC8*) in RCC is unclear and it has been suggested that instability of the translocated chromosome may be an important factor in this and other chromosome 3 translocation-RCC kindreds. All patients with possible RCC susceptibility should be examined for chromosome 3 translocations. In addition, adult translocation carriers in kindreds with chromosome 3 translocations and RCC should be offered regular renal surveillance (e.g. annual renal MRI or ultrasound scans). There are relatively little data available for the risk of RCC in patients ascertained after the finding of a chromosome 3 translocation. However, in one study there was a substantial increased risk of RCC in translocation carriers (van Kessel et al., 1999). Thus regular renal ultrasound surveillance may be indicated in chromosome 3 translocation carriers, particularly those with pericentromeric translocations.

Familial non-syndromic non-clear cell RCC was not well defined until the mid-1990s when Zbar et al. (1994, 1995) described ten families with a dominantly inherited predisposition to papillary RCC. They noted that while familial papillary RCC was often bilateral and multiple, examples of non-penetrance were also apparent and screening of asymptomatic at risk relatives is important.

Familial papillary RCC is rare (prevalence ~1 per 10 million) and is caused by germline mutations in the *MET* proto-oncogene (Schmidt et al., 1997). The histopathology of papillary RCC can be sub-classified into two groups: Type 1 tumours which are usually multiple and low grade and Type 2 which are single of higher grade and have a poorer prognosis (Delahunt and Eble, 1997), and can be caused by mutations in the FH gene (Tomlinson et al., 2002). Patients with germline *MET* and mutations have Type 1 tumours (Lubensky et al., 1999). Germline *MET* mutations in familial type papillary RCC are activating missense mutations within the tyrosine kinase domain (Schmidt et al., 1997). Individuals with, or at risk for, HPRC1 should be offered annual renal imaging (by MRI or CT scanning) from age 30 years.

In a kindred with familial papillary thyroid cancer susceptibility mapping to chromosome 1q21, two family members developed papillary renal tumours suggesting a possible link between these tumour types Malchoff et al. (2000).

Cancer of the ureter and renal pelvis

Carcinoma of the renal pelvis accounts for approximately 10 per cent of all malignant renal tumours. Environmental causes of carcinoma of the renal pelvis include occupational exposure (as for bladder cancer), and prolonged excessive phenacetin ingestion.

Examples of familial ureteric and renal pelvis transitional cell carcinoma are rare. Lynch et al. (1979) described two families with a predisposition to carcinoma of the bladder and renal pelvis, and familial ureteric cancer (mother and son) was observed by Burkland and Juzek (1966). Cancer of the ureter and renal pelvis is a feature of hereditary non-polyposis colorectal cancer (HNPCC) syndrome (Lynch syndrome, see Part three) and urothelial cancers may cluster in some HNPCC families. It has been suggested that the presence of an inverted growth pattern (endophytic) in urothelial carcinomas of the upper urinary tract may serve as a marker for identifying tumours with a higher frequency of microsatellite instability and so help identify patients who should be offered testing for HNPCC (Hartmann et al., 2002).

Renal medullary carcinomas are very rare, highly aggressive tumours that occur in young patients with sickle cell trait or disease (Noguera-Irizarry et al., 2003).

Bladder cancer

Carcinoma of the bladder accounts for 4.6 per cent of all cancers (with an incidence in men of 30 per 100 000, and in women of 10 per 100 000 in the UK), is the fifth most common cancer in men, and has a peak prevalence in the seventh decade. Environmental agents, including tobacco, amine compounds used in the manufacture of dyes, and schistosomiasis have been clearly implicated in bladder tumorigenesis, but genetic factors may also be relevant. Ninety per cent of bladder tumours are transitional cell carcinomas, which may contain elements of squamous carcinoma or adenocarcinoma. Less commonly, sarcoma, melanoma or small cell undifferentiated carcinoma may occur.

Familial clusters of bladder cancer were reported by Fraumeni and Thomas (1967) and McCullough et al. (1975). In these reports, bladder cancer affected a total of ten individuals from two-generation families. Lynch et al. (1979) also described two families showing a predisposition to transitional cell carcinoma of the bladder and renal pelvis. One individual developed bladder cancer at the age of 24 years. Familial clustering of bladder cancer could reflect shared exposure to environmental hazards or genetic susceptibility. A role for genetic factors is indicated by the association of bladder and other urothelial cancers with Lynch syndrome, and by the suggestion that there is an increased risk of bladder cancer in patients with germline *RB1* mutations. Kiemeney and Schoenberg (1996) reviewed the literature on familial transitional cell carcinoma and concluded that genetic susceptibility was likely to be a factor in familial clustering, however, in a study of thirty families with two or three affected relatives with urothelial cancer of the bladder, renal pelvis or ureter Aben et al. (2001) did not detect any constitutional chromosome abnormalities.

The most important contribution of genetic factors to bladder cancer risk is probably in determining individual susceptibility to environmental carcinogens, such as tobacco, or occupational exposure to aromatic amine compounds. Hence genetic susceptibility to bladder cancer is likely linked to low-penetrance susceptibility genes rather than rarer inherited high-penetrance mutations. As some chemical carcinogens become hazardous as a result of host metabolism, interindividual variations in the activity of metabolic enzymes might influence individual susceptibility to urothelial cancer. Many studies have investigated possible associations between bladder cancer risk and genetic polymorphisms in metabolic enzymes. Although early studies employed phenotyping assays, these have been superceded by genotyping analysis as phenotyping studies may be influenced by host factors, such as, concomitant drug therapy, co-existing disease, smoking status and renal function. N-acetyltransferase-2 (NAT2) activity has been implicated in the metabolism of arylamines which, in addition to their role in occupational bladder cancer, are also found in cigarette smoke. In a meta-analysis of 21 published case–control studies of *NAT2* and bladder cancer, Johns and Houlston (2000) detected a modest association (pooled odds ratio 1.31) with slow acetylator status. Similarly in a meta-analysis of polymorphisms in glutathione S-transferases (*GST*) and human diseases, Habdous et al. (2004) observed significant associations between bladder cancer and the *GSTM1*0* null allele and *GSTP1* polymorphism in smokers. Further studies will enable the possible effects of interactions between polymorphic variants in different genes and exposure to potential environmental carcinogens to be elucidated.

Bladder tumours are frequently synchronous or metachronous. However, while these features are classical indicators of genetic susceptibility, molecular studies have suggested that multicentricity does not reflect a high incidence of multiple primary tumours, but rather that a single primary transformation event may seed other tumours by spread across the urothelium.

Individuals who are at increased risk of bladder cancer should be screened by 6-monthly urinalysis and urinary cytology, with cystourethroscopy when these tests are abnormal. Analysis of urine sediment by microsatellite DNA markers may provide a novel method for monitoring bladder cancer recurrence (Steiner et al., 1997).

9

Blood and lymph

Leukaemia

Leukaemia is responsible for approximately 2 per cent of all cancers, with an incidence of about 8 per 100 000 in the UK. Acute myeloid and lymphoblastic leukaemias (AML and ALL) account for about 1 per cent of all cancers and 1.5 per cent of cancer deaths. The age incidence of leukaemia shows two peaks, in childhood and in the elderly. Genetic factors are not considered to have a prominent role in the pathogenesis of acute leukaemias or in chronic myeloid leukaemia, but have been implicated in chronic lymphocytic leukaemia (CLL). Gunz et al. (1975) studied the incidence of leukaemia in relatives of 909 patients with leukaemia. The overall incidence of leukaemia in first-degree relatives was three times higher than expected although only 2 per cent of patients had a first-degree relative with leukaemia. Among the main subtypes of leukaemia, an increased risk to relatives was most marked in chronic lymphocytic leukaemia, less so in acute leukaemias and absent in chronic myeloid leukaemia. When familial clusters of leukaemia have been reported, the type of leukaemia in individual relatives is not always concordant (Lee et al., 1987). Familial leukaemia does not necessarily indicate a genetic cause, and shared exposure to an environmental leukaemogen also needs to be considered, particularly in childhood acute leukaemias. Genetic disorders that have been associated with a predisposition to leukaemia are shown in Table 9.1 and discussed in detail in part three. Genetic disorders are thought to account for only 3 per cent of childhood leukaemia.

Acute lymphoblastic leukaemia

The most common malignancy in childhood, ALL accounts for 80 per cent of leukaemias in the paediatric age group. ALL is less common in adults, in whom it constitutes approximately 15 per cent of acute leukaemias. ALL is caused by the malignant proliferation of lymphoblasts which are the precursor cells of B- and T-lymphocytes. ALL is a heterogeneous disorder and various criteria have been used for subclassification, for example morphological (e.g. French–American–British classification), immunophenotyping (e.g. T-cell, B-cell and various precursor B-cell subtypes) or cytogenetic criteria (e.g. t(9;22), t(4;11), t(1;19) and t(12;21)). Immunological classification can be refined by the molecular

Table 9.1. *Genetic disorders associated with leukaemia*

Ataxia telangiectasia
Blackfan–Diamond syndrome
Bloom syndrome
Fanconi anaemia
Biallelic mismatch repair gene mutations
Immune deficiency diseases (e.g. severe combined
    immunodeficiency, common variable immunodeficiency)
Incontinentia pigmenti
Kostmann syndrome
Li–Fraumeni syndrome
Lynch syndrome
N syndrome
Neurofibromatosis Type 1
Seckel syndrome
Shwachman syndrome
Trisomy 21
Wiskott–Aldrich syndrome
WY syndrome

characterisation of immunoglobulin heavy and light chain gene arrangements to define further the cell of origin of ALL.

Childhood leukaemia is associated with genetic abnormalities in about 3 per cent and radiation exposure in less than 8 per cent of cases, so that the vast majority of cases are unexplained, although an infective (e.g. viral) origin has been postulated. Gunz et al. (1975) found that only 2 per cent of patients with acute leukaemia had a first-degree relative with leukaemia, and Till et al. (1975) observed that only 1.4 per cent of children with ALL had a close relative with leukaemia or lymphoma. However, there is a significant risk of childhood leukaemia in twins, particularly monozygotic. Thus Miller (1971) estimated that acute leukaemia in an identical twin under 6 years of age is associated with a 1 in 6 risk that the co-twin will develop leukaemia. The risk of leukaemia in the unaffected twin is highest in infancy, decreases with age, and appears to be linked to a shared placental circulation. Thus it is suggested that the leukaemia lineage arises in utero in one twin and migrates to the other (Ford et al., 1993).

Familial clustering of adult ALL has been reported infrequently and might reflect shared environmental and/or genetic factors. De Moor et al. (1988) found 5 of 74 adult patients with ALL had a relative with acute leukaemia or lymphoma, and that this subgroup of patients with familial leukaemia had a greater than expected incidence of HLA-Cw3 antigen. Horwitz et al. (1996) noted evidence of anticipation in familial leukaemia, but for ALL this was based on only four pedigrees, each containing two affected individuals. In contrast to childhood ALL, twin-risks are not high in adult acute leukaemias. Specific genetic disorders associated with ALL include Down syndrome, chromosome breakage syndromes (ataxia telangiectasia, Bloom syndrome), Li–Fraumeni syndrome and immune deficiency disorders (severe combined, Bruton agamma-globulinaemia, adenosine deaminase deficiency).

Acute myeloid (myelogenous) leukaemia

Whereas ALL is the most common form of acute leukaemia in children, AML predominates in adults. The overall incidence of AML is 2.5 cases/100 000 per year, with the highest incidence in those over the age of 60 years. Genetic disorders which have been associated with a predisposition to AML include Down syndrome, Fanconi anaemia, neurofibromatosis type 1 (NF1) and Kostmann syndrome (see Part three). An autosomal dominant syndrome of cerebellar ataxia, hypoplastic anaemia and predisposition to AML (associated with monosomy 7 in bone marrow cells) was described in a single two-generation family by Li et al. (1981) and in a further family by Daghistani et al. (1990). Bone marrow monosomy 7 is a frequent finding in chronic myeloproliferative disorders and AML, and only a small proportion of paediatric cases will have the ataxia pancytopenia syndrome. However familial clustering of AML with monosomy 7 may occur (Kwong et al., 2000).

Dowton et al. (1985) reported an autosomal dominant disorder of thrombocytopenia and platelet dysfunction associated with a predisposition to haematological (AML, lymphoma) and other malignancy in a single large kindred. Eleven years later, Ho et al. (1996) reported linkage to chromosome 21q22.1–22.2 in this family and subsequently germline mutations in the haematopoietic transcription factor *CBFA2* (*RUNX1*).

In a kindred with familial AML associated with an inactivating *CEBPA* (CCAAT enhancer binding protein α) mutation, there were latent periods of 10–30 years before the onset of overt leukaemia in the three affected patients (Smith et al., 2004).

Najean and Lecompte (1990) suggested that dominantly inherited thrombocytopenia is not rare but that the long-term prognosis is good as there were only four cases of leukaemia in three of the 54 families ascertained. A possible association between myeloid leukaemia and Prader–Willi syndrome was suggested by Hall (1985), and Davies et al. (2003) reported an increased risk of myeloid leukemia (40-fold), but not other cancers, in individuals with Prader–Willi syndrome.

Familial AML is uncommon, but large pedigrees demonstrating autosomal dominant inheritance have been reported (see Horwitz et al., 1996). Evidence of anticipation in familial AML has been noted such that of 79 individuals in nine families transmitting the disease, the mean age at onset in the grandparental generation was 57 years, compared to 32 years in the parental generation and 13 years in the youngest generation (Horwitz et al., 1996). Subsequently suggestive linkage to 16q21–23.2 was described (Horwitz et al., 1997).

A rare form of AML, erythroleukaemia, (FAB-M6) that accounts for 5 per cent of cases, may be familial (Diguglielmo syndrome) in a minority of cases. Thus affected families were reported by Peterson et al. (1984) and Lee et al. (1987). A possible link between a missense mutation in the erythropoietin receptor and erythroleukaemia was reported by Le Couedic et al. (1996).

Chronic myeloid leukaemia

Chronic myeloid leukaemia (CML) results from the malignant transformation of a pluripotent bone marrow stem cell. Typically, the disease has a triphasic course with an initial chronic phase (median duration 3.5 years) followed by an accelerated phase and then, after 3–12 months, an acute blastic phase associated with a poor response to therapy. The hallmark of CML is the Philadelphia chromosome (Ph), which was the first consistent chromosomal aberration to be associated with human malignancy (Nowell and Hungerford, 1960). It is now recognised that the Ph chromosome is present in more than 90 per cent of patients with CML, and that a proportion of apparently Ph-negative CMLs have a variant Ph translocation not visible by cytogenetic techniques (Kurzrock et al., 1988). The Ph chromosome is not specific for CML, and it is also found (and is associated with a poor prognosis) in a small proportion of patients with ALL (20 per cent of adults, 5 per cent children) and AML (2 per cent of adults). The classic Ph+ chromosome results from a translocation involving chromosomes 9 and 22, (t(9; 22)(q34; q11)). The breakpoint on chromosome 9 involves the Abelson oncogene (*ABL*) and on chromosome 22 the breakpoints occur within a small region that was originally designated the breakpoint cluster region (*BCR*). The *BCR* is a central segment within a 90-kb gene, now named the *BCR* gene (Kurzrock et al., 1988). The 9;22 translocation results in the juxtaposition of proximal 5′ *BCR* gene exons (1, 2 ± 3) and *ABL* sequences (exons 2–11, ±exons 1a and 1b).

Environmental agents associated with CML include irradiation and chemical (e.g. benzene) exposure (Jacobs, 1989), but there is relatively little evidence for a genetic predisposition. Familial CML was reported by Lillicrap and Sterndale (1984) in a family with three affected individuals in three generations; two siblings of the proband had abnormal haematological investigations (evidence of a myeloproliferative disorder in one and an excess of lymphocytes in the bone marrow of another). Cytogenetic studies of CML were performed in two affected patients, one was Ph+ and the other Ph−. Nevertheless, familial cases of CML appear to be rare.

Chronic lymphocytic leukaemia

This is the most common form of leukaemia accounting ~30 per cent of all cases and occurs particularly in the elderly, with a peak incidence between 60 and 80 years of age. Most cases are B-cell type.

In contrast to the acute leukaemias and CML, there is abundant evidence for a role of genetic factors in CLL. Conley et al. (1980) reviewed 51 reports of familial CLL, including three pairs of monozygotic twins and one family with six affected members. An association between disordered immune function and lymphoreticular malignancy is suggested by the finding that in some reports of familial CLL, autoimmune or immunological disorders have been noted among unaffected relatives. Conley et al. (1980) found that in two families with CLL and autoimmune disease (pernicious anaemia, thyroiditis, vitiligo), individuals with CLL or autoimmune disease shared a common HLA haplotype, but the haplotype differed in the two kindreds. Neuland et al. (1983) described a family in which CLL developed in a father and all four of his children. There was no association with HLA haplotype, and in one patient there was a spontaneous regression. Linet et al. (1989) found a fourfold excess of haematoproliferative malignancies among siblings of patients with CLL. Cartwright et al. (1987) reported a fourfold excess of lymphoid leukaemia in the families of patients with CLL, and a series of cohort and case-control studies have revealed relative risks in relatives ranging from 2.3 to 5.7 (reviewed by Houlston et al. (2003)). Li et al. (1989) suggested that the vast majority of cases of CLL are sporadic but that there may be a strong genetic effect in a few families. Among familial cases of CLL the mean age at onset was ~10 years earlier than in sporadic cases and an increased risk of second primary tumours was noted (Ishibe et al., 2001). Among 18 affected individuals from seven pedigrees with dominantly inherited CLL, Horwitz et al. (1996) described evidence for anticipation in most cases and this has been confirmed by others. The age at diagnosis in the offspring appears to be ~20 years earlier than in affected parents. Most familial CLL kindreds are small and both rare high penetrance and more common lower penetrance susceptibility alleles might be implicated in familial CLL. Interestingly, Rawstron et al. (2002) detected subclinical levels of CLL-like cells in 14 per cent of relatives compared to <1 per cent of normal controls suggesting that although the lifetime risk of CLL in familial cases is 20–30 per cent, there may be a significant incidence of subclinical disease.

Somatic inactivation of the ataxia telangiectasia gene (*ATM*, see Part Three) occurs in ~20 per cent of CLL cases and in some cases a germline mutation is also present. However whilst heterozygous *ATM* mutations may confer an increased risk of CLL, it seems likely that germline *ATM* mutations do not make a major contribution to familial cases of CLL (Houlston et al., 2003). Wiley et al. (2002) reported that a loss-of-function polymorphism in the cytolytic P2X7 receptor gene was overrepresented in patients with CLL compared to controls. However in another study the P2X7 SNP was associated with survival but not risk of CLL (Thunberg et al., 2002).

Familial clustering (sibling or parent–child pairs) of hairy cell leukaemia, an uncommon subtype of CLL with a prevalence of 1 per 150 000, has been reported in at least 30 cases (Colovic et al., 2001; Cetiner et al., 2003). Linkage to specific HLA haplotype has been suggested, but the influence of genetic and environmental factors in familial cases is unclear.

Polycythaemia

Increased red cell mass may be a primary abnormality, as in polycythaemia rubra vera (PRV), or secondary to a variety of causes including hypoxia, renal cysts or tumours and genetic disorders (benign primary familial polycythaemia or familial erythrocytosis), such as inherited haemoglobin variants (e.g. haemoglobin Chesapeake), familial disorders of erythropoietin regulation (Kralovics et al., 1998) and recessive von Hippel–Lindau (*VHL*) gene mutations as in Chuvash polycythaemia (Ang et al., 2002). However there is evidence for further loci for autosomal dominant primary familial polycythaemia (Jedlickova et al., 2003).

PRV is an uncommon myeloproliferative disorder (five new cases/million per year) in which increased red cell mass is usually associated with increased white cell and platelet counts. PRV usually pursues a chronic course, but there is a significant risk of an acute leukaemic transformation occurring. Clonal cytogenetic abnormalities such as, del(20q), trisomy 8 and 9, del(13q) and dupl(1q), have been reported in a minority of patients with PRV, but are present in most patients with leukaemic transformation (Heim and Mitelman, 1987). Familial PRV is rare and must be distinguished from the more common benign familial polycythaemia which is not associated with leukaemia (Ratnoff and Gress, 1980; Friedland et al., 1981). Inheritance appears to be autosomal dominant with incomplete inheritance (Kralovics et al., 2003).

Thrombocythaemia

Primary or essential thrombocythaemia is a myeloproliferative disorder characterised by megakaryocyte hyperplasia and elevated platelet count. The main complications are bleeding and thrombotic events, and occasionally acute leukaemic transformation can occur. Familial essential thrombocythaemia has been reported twice. Familial cases may be inherited as an autosomal dominant trait and may be caused by mutations in the thrombopoetin gene or it's receptor c-Mpl (Kondo et al., 1998). Large families with multiple generations involved (and male-to-male transmission in some cases) have been described Eyster et al. (1986), Schlemper et al. (1994), Kikuchi et al. (1995), van Dijken et al. (1996).

Lymphoma

The two major categories of malignant lymphoma are Hodgkin disease (which accounts for just under half of the total) and non-Hodgkin lymphoma. The latter is a heterogenous group of disorders, most are of monoclonal B-cell origin and a lesser number are of T-cell or non-T non-B type. Genetic disorders that predispose to malignant lymphoma are listed in Table 9.2 and discussed in Part three. Clearly, there is a strong association between genetic disorders that cause clinical immunodeficiency and the development of malignant lymphoma. Furthermore, the incidence of lymphoproliferative disorders is increased among patients with immunodeficiency secondary to therapeutic immunosuppression or human immunodeficiency virus (HIV) infection. Although many lymphomas in immune-deficient individuals are of B-cell origin, some are derived from other cells such as T-lymphocytes.

Tumours, especially lymphoproliferative disorders, are the second leading cause of death in immunodeficient disorders and it is estimated that 15–25 per cent of patients with the three major immunodeficiency syndromes (Wiskott–Aldrich syndrome, ataxia telangiectasia and common variable immunodeficiency) develop cancer. Review of almost 500 cases of cancer notified to the Immunodeficiency

Table 9.2. *Genetic disorders predisposing to lymphoma*

Ataxia telangiectasia
Chediak–Higashi syndrome
Common variable immunodeficiency
HyerIgM syndrome
Hypogammaglobulinaemia
Severe combined immunodeficiency
Wiskott–Aldrich syndrome
X-linked lymphoproliferative disease

Cancer Registry revealed that almost 60 per cent of cancers reported in patients with primary immunodeficiency disorders are lymphoma (Kersey et al., 1988). Non-Hodgkin lymphoma is about six times as frequent as Hodgkin disease in patients with primary immunodeficiency.

Hodgkin disease

This has an incidence of 2–3 per 100 000 population in the UK. Analysis of the age at onset of Hodgkin disease reveals a bimodal distribution, with one peak around the age of 25 years, then decreasing to a plateau in middle age, after which rates increase with advancing age for the second peak. The disease is more common in males than in females. The aetiology of Hodgkin disease is unknown, but an infective agent has been suggested, particularly in the younger age group and in the nodular sclerosis subtype. An association between familial clustering of multiple sclerosis and young-adult-onset Hodgkin lymphoma has been reported and suggests that the two conditions share environmental and/or constitutional factors (Hjalgrim et al., 2004; Shugart et al., 2000).

Among siblings of young patients (less than 45 years) with Hodgkin disease, there is a sevenfold excess risk of the disease (Grufferman et al., 1977). In a total of 59 sibling pairs with Hodgkin disease diagnosed aged less than 45 years, 42 pairs were sex concordant, so that Grufferman et al. (1977) estimated that siblings of the same sex as an affected person had twice the risk of Hodgkin disease of siblings of the opposite sex (although this was not confirmed by Chakravarti et al. (1986), see below). This excess sex concordance was interpreted as supporting the concept that the increased risk of Hodgkin disease in siblings of affected persons is caused by shared aetiological exposure or transmission. In this series, there was a greater than expected incidence of nodular sclerosis type of Hodgkin disease among sibling pairs. However, there was no excess risk of Hodgkin disease for siblings of patients diagnosed after the age of 45 years. Ferraris et al. (1997) reviewed the literature on familial Hodgkin disease. They confirmed an excess of males in familial cases, but the male to female ratio (1.5:1) was similar in familial and sporadic cases, and that the age distribution of familial cases shows a single major peak between 15 and 34 years of age. Both genetic and environmental (e.g. viral infections) factors have been implicated in familial clustering of Hodgkin disease. Analysis of 432 sets of twins affected by Hodgkin disease revealed that 0 of 187 dizygotic twins were concordant for Hodgkin disease, compared to 10 of 179 monozygotic twins – expected cases = 0.1 for each group (Mack et al., 1995). The higher concordance in monozygotic twins compared to dizygotic twins clearly implicates genetic factors in familial clustering of Hodgkin disease in young adults. In a study of Hodgkin disease in Sweden, Shugart et al. (2000) estimated the heritability to be 28 per cent and suggested that there was significant evidence for anticipation in parent–child pairs with Hodgkin disease (mean difference 14 years) (Shugart et al., 2001).

Epidemiological evidence suggests that Hodgkin disease may be a rare out-come of a specific infective agent, possibly Epstein–Barr virus (EBV). However EBV infection is common and often asymptomatic suggesting that additional factors such as, inherited immune response variants might be implicated in sus-ceptibility to Hodgkin disease. Hence a number of groups have investigated the associations between Hodgkin disease and HLA loci. Conte et al. (1983) reported that in four families, each containing two individuals with nodular sclerosis Hodgkin disease, all affected patients had HLA-B18 antigen. Other reported HLA associations include A1 (relative risk 1.4), B5 and B8. Linkage studies in multiple-case families have confirmed an association with a suscepti-bility gene at the HLA locus, and are consistent with a recessive gene, which would account for a twofold increase in relative risk for siblings of patients with Hodgkin disease (Chakravarti et al., 1986). This HLA-linked recessive sus-ceptibility gene was estimated to account for 60 per cent of cases in multiplex families, with the remaining 40 per cent caused by other familial and/or environ-mental factors. Linkage to the HLA class II region has also been demonstrated (Klitz et al., 1994; Taylor et al., 1996), in particular alleles at the HLA-DPB1 locus have been implicated specific histological subtypes and an association with EBV-positive cases has been suggested (Taylor et al., 1999; Alexander et al., 2001). There is an increased incidence of Hodgkin disease in immunode-ficient patients, and it accounts for about 10 per cent of tumours associated with primary immunodeficiency disorders. The mean age at diagnosis of Hodgkin disease in immunodeficient patients is 10.9 years, although there was a wide range, from less than 1 to 73 years (Kersey et al., 1988). Compared to paediatric patients with Hodgkin disease and no immunodeficiency disorder, there is an excess of mixed cellularity and lymphocyte depletion subtypes. However, most lymphomas that occur in immunodeficient individuals are categorised as non-Hodgkin lymphoma.

Non-Hodgkin lymphoma

This is a heterogenous group of disorders with a wide range of histological, immunological and cytogenetic subtypes. Non-Hodgkin lymphoma is the most frequent tumour to complicate the primary immunodeficiency syndromes (see Table 9.2) and may also occur in families of patients with CLL.

The most frequent causes of non-Hodgkin lymphoma complicating primary immunodeficiency are ataxia telangiectasia, Wiskott–Aldrich syndrome, com-mon variable immunodeficiency and severe combined immunodeficiency (see

Part three; Kersey et al., 1988), and it is the predominant malignancy in each of these disorders. Mean age at diagnosis is 7 years (from range less than 1 to 75 years) and the brain and gastrointestinal tract are frequent presenting sites. Compared to non-Hodgkin lymphoma in non-immunodeficient patients, lymph node involvement is less common. Most non-Hodgkin lymphoma in primary immunodeficient children is of B-cell origin, but the lymphomas in ataxia telangiectasia are very heterogeneous, with all the major histological subgroups represented. There appears to be no relationship between the severity of immunodeficiency and the risk of malignancy (Kersey et al., 1988).

A tendency for familial aggregations of haematolymphoproliferative cancers is recognised. Pottern et al. (1991) found 4.5 per cent of patients with non-Hodgkin lymphoma had at least one sibling and 3.3 per cent had a parent with a haematoproliferative cancer, while only 1.7 per cent of controls had an affected sibling and 2.2 per cent had a parent with a haematoproliferative cancer. Cartwright et al. (1988) reported a fourfold excess of leukaemias and lymphomas among first-degree relatives of patients with non-Hodgkin lymphoma. When familial aggregations of haematoproliferative cancers occur, there is often no particular pattern of tumour type, so that although concordant cancers may occur, so may seemingly diverse cell types. Familial clustering of lymphoma is uncommon, but Lynch et al. (1989a) reported a single exceptional family with seven cases of malignant lymphoma (six non-Hodgkin lymphoma and one Hodgkin lymphoma) in three generations – consistent with autosomal dominant inheritance. However most family clusters are small. In familial clusters of non-Hodgkin lymphoma with vertical transmission, evidence for anticipation has been reported (Wiernik et al., 2000; Shugart et al., 2001). Thus median ages at onset in the child and parent generations of all families analysed by Wiernik et al. (2000) was 48.5 and 71.3 years respectively. In an analysis of the Swedish Family-Cancer Database, Altieri et al. (2005) found evidence in support of the hypothesis of an autosomal dominant component for diffuse large B-cell non-Hodgkin lymphoma and a recessive component for follicular non-Hodgkin lymphoma. The molecular basis for familial non-Hodgkin lymphoma is unclear, although Baumler et al. (2003) suggested reduced sensitivity to an apoptotic stimulus in lymphocytes from a subset familial lymphoma patients.

Myeloma

Reports of sibling pairs with multiple myeloma suggest that occasionally, genetic factors may predispose to myeloma and Hemminki (2002) reported that offspring of multiple myeloma cases had a fourfold increased risk of disease. Horwitz et al. (1985) reviewed 30 families with two affected siblings and a further nine families with three affected siblings. In two reports of twins with multiple myeloma (Judson et al., 1985; Comotti et al., 1987), one emphasised the contribution of shared environment and the other genetic factors. A 2 per cent incidence of plasma cell disorders in siblings of myeloma patients has been reported, but this may not be excessive (Horwitz et al., 1985). Lynch et al. (2001) described a large kindred with familial multiple myeloma in three cases and a monoclonal gammopathy of unknown significance in two further relatives. Although there is no case for routine screening of relatives of myeloma patients, when familial myeloma is found, first-degree relatives should be screened (by blood and urine electrophoresis) and those with benign monoclonal gammopathy kept under surveillance.

Waldenstrom macroglobulinaemia

Familial occurrences of Waldenstrom macroglobulinaemia are uncommon, with 57 individuals from 22 families reported (Renier et al., 1989). In 11 of the 22 families, two generations were involved, and three exceptional families each contained four affected individuals (Youinou et al., 1978; Blattner et al., 1980; Renier et al., 1989). It has been suggested that 4 per cent of relatives of affected persons have a monoclonal IgM component (Kalff and Hijmans, 1969). In the family of Blattner et al. (1980), all four affected relatives had a common HLA haplotype (A2, B8, DRw3). However, in the other two reports, no consistent HLA associations were found. The monoclonal IgM light chain type may differ between relatives with familial Waldenstrom macroglobulinaemia, as occurred in monozygotic twins with Waldenstrom macroglobulinaemia (Fine et al., 1986). Autoimmune disorders and immunoglobulin abnormalities are frequent in relatives of patients with familial Waldenstrom macroglobulinaemia, suggesting that in these families Waldenstrom macroglobulinaemia may be one manifestation of a genetic predisposition to abnormal immunoglobulin synthesis control mechanisms (McMaster, 2003).

Histiocytoses

This is a heterogeneous group of disorders characterised by abnormal proliferation of histiocytes and non-malignant histiocytic disorders are subdivided into two major types: (i) Langerhans' cell histiocytosis (including Histiocytosis X, eosinophilic granuloma, Letterer–Siwe disease and Hand–Schuller–Christian disease and are characterised by the presence of the Birbeck granule) and (ii) haemophagocytic syndromes (which include familial erythrophagocytic lymphocytosis, also known as familial lymphohistiocytosis or familial reticuloendotheliosis).

Langerhans cell histiocytosis (LCH) is considered a non-hereditary disorder but rarely may be familial (Arico et al., 1999). Most such cases are in monozygotic twins and the concordance rate is 85 per cent (this does not necessarily indicate genetic factors as in utero spread via intraplacental anastomosis cannot be excluded).

Familial haemophagocytic lymphohistiocytosis is a rare autosomal recessive disorder (1.2 cases/million children each year), which usually presents in early childhood (80 per cent by the age of 2 years) with failure to thrive, fever, anaemia and hepatosplenomegaly and, histologically, multisystem (liver, spleen, lymph nodes, bone marrow, central nervous system) lymphohistiocytic infiltrates (Loy et al., 1991). Without treatment the prognosis is very poor. Familial haemophagocytic lymphohistiocytosis is a heterogeneous disorder. Mutations in the perforin gene account for ~30 per cent of cases and about 10 per cent are linked to the chromosome 9 FHL1 locus (Goransdotter Ericson et al., 2001). Recently mutations in hMunc13-4, a member of the Munc13 family of proteins involved in vesicle priming function, were identified in a further subset of familial haemophagocytic lymphohistiocytosis (FHL3). Inactivation of hMunc13-4 causes defective exocytosis of perforin containing lytic granules (Feldmann et al., 2003).

10

Musculoskeletal system

Bone tumours

In general, sarcomas of bone, muscle or connective tissue are rare, especially in children. Bone tumours comprise about 5 per cent of childhood cancers (3 per cent osteosarcomas and 2 per cent Ewing sarcoma) and their incidence overall is about 10 per million persons in the UK. The age-standardised rate of malignant bone tumours for white children (0–14 years of age) in the SEER Registry, 1983–1992 was 6.4 per million. Soft tissue sarcomas are slightly more common (10 per million). The rates are similar for black children in the same registry, except for Ewing sarcoma, which is nine times less common in black children (Parkin et al., 1993).

Osteosarcoma

Osteogenic sarcoma is commoner in males than in females, and shows two age peaks, one at adolescence and a second, which parallels that of chondrosarcoma, in the sixth and seventh decades. The tumour has a predilection for rapidly growing bone and is commoner in Paget disease. One family with three siblings with Paget disease has been reported. Two developed fatal osteosarcoma (Wu et al., 1991). Children with osteosarcoma are significantly taller at time of diagnosis than are unaffected controls (Gelberg et al., 1997). A similar, but not significant difference is seen for children with Ewing sarcoma. Interestingly, large dogs, such as Great Danes are at higher risk for osteosarcoma than are smaller breeds (Owen, 1967). Familial aggregations of Paget disease are sometimes seen (see above) but the mode of inheritance is unclear and autosomal dominant or multifactorial aetiology has been suggested (Moore and Hoffman, 1988). Familial osteosarcoma is rare, but multiple cases have been described in a number of sibships (Goorin et al., 1985). Hillmann and colleagues gathered all known reports of familial osteosarcoma. They identified 59 affected individuals from 24 families. Pointing towards an underlying genetic or environmental aetiology, seven patients had Paget disease, three had a history of multiple fractures, two had bilateral retinoblastoma and one had an osteosarcoma at another site. Interestingly, of six patients diagnosed at over 40 years of age, five had

Paget disease and the other had had an osteosarcoma 25 years previously (Hillmann et al., 2000). Lynch reported on 10 sarcoma-prone families, some of which contained individuals with osteosarcoma and germline mutations in *TP53* (Lynch et al., 2003). It had previously been shown that about 3 per cent of children with osteosarcoma carry germline mutations in *TP53*, and many may not have a substantial family history consistent with Li–Fraumeni syndrome (Toguchida et al., 1992; McIntyre et al., 1994).

Osteosarcoma may occur as a second tumour in individuals with germline mutations of the retinoblastoma gene (relative risk up to 500 times normal control) (see p. 20; Sanders et al., 1988), in the Li–Fraumeni syndrome, in the multiple exostosis and multiple endostosis syndromes (see below), in Bloom syndrome (Fuchs and Pritchard, 2002) and in Rothmund–Thomson disease, several cases of which have been described associated with osteosarcoma (Starr et al., 1985; Cumin et al., 1996; Leonard et al., 1996). Truncating mutations in the causative gene, *RECQL4* (Kitao et al., 1999) appear to be more strongly associated with osteosarcoma than are other types of mutations (Wang et al., 2003b). However, mutations in *RECQL4* are uncommon in sporadic osteosarcoma (Nishijo et al., 2004). There has also been a report of an African–American family with Familial gigantiform cementoma, where one individual developed an osteosarcoma (Rossbach et al., 2005). An association between osteosarcoma and osteogenesis imperfecta tarda has been reported (Lasson et al., 1978) but may be a chance finding.

There is a risk of malignant degeneration in both monostotic fibrous dysplasia (which is invariably sporadic) and in polyostotic fibrous dysplasia, in which activating mutations of Gs proteins have been detected (McCune–Albright syndrome) (see p. 218; Alman et al., 1996). Patients with polyostotic fibrous dysplasia are at higher risk than those with monostotic lesions, which is thought to reflect their greater number of lesions rather than an increased risk per lesion. Somatic mutations in GSα have been found in both groups (Lumbroso et al., 2004). In genetically predisposed individuals (e.g. with Li–Fraumeni syndrome), a second osteogenic sarcoma may develop in the field of radiation delivered to the initial primary cancer (Li et al., 1978). Osteogenic sarcoma occurs as part of the OSLAM syndrome, described in a single report of autosomal dominant inheritance of multiple childhood osteo-sarcomas associated with erythroid mastocytosis and a megaloblastic marrow and abnormalities (Mulvihill et al., 1977).

Hereditary multiple exostoses (diaphysial achlasis) is an autosomal dominant skeletal dysplasia with an estimated prevalence of 9 per 10 00 000 population. It is characterised by the development of numerous cartilage-capped exostoses in actively growing areas of bone. The most common sites are the juxta-epiphyseal

regions of the long bones, the pelvis, scapula and ribs, but the skull and vertebrae are usually spared. A Madelung deformity of the forearm is common. The
multiple exostoses produce bony deformities, abnormal bone growth and mild
short stature. Penetrance is almost complete when patients are studied radio-
logically, which reveals many subclinical lesions. Growth of the exostoses is
maximal during childhood and adolescence and the diagnosis is usually made
during the first decade of life. The major complication of this disorder is malignant degeneration of the exostoses. Estimates of this risk are variable, but the
incidence is probably less than 10 per cent. Patients should be alerted to the significance of a rapid change in the rate of growth and the development of pain
and inflammation (Voutsinas and Wynne-Davies, 1983). Regular surveillance
to detect these changes is recommended. If osteosarcomas occur, they develop
at an earlier age than their sporadic counterparts, at a mean age of approximately 30 years (range 10–50 years) (Hennekam, 1991). The presence of multiple exostoses in a patient with a balanced translocation t(8; 11)(q24.11; p15.5)
led to the identification of one of three loci now identified in which mutations
can cause this disorder (Ludecke et al., 1991; Wuyts et al., 1996). Thus, hereditary multiple exostoses are genetically heterogeneous, with the three loci so far
identified on chromosomes 8q24.1, 11p13 and 19p. Germline mutations have
been identified in the *EXT1* (Ahn et al., 1995) and in *EXT2* (Stickens et al.,
1996), the two genes that are known to be responsible for the disease, although
multiple genetic events are necessary for the development of these tumours
(Hecht et al., 1997). Both genes encode glycosyltransferases that are involved in
heparan sulphate biosynthesis. However, the severity of disease is influenced by
the gene: the risk for sarcoma is greater for those with *EXT1* mutations than for
EXT2 mutations, but there those with more severe disease were not at higher
risk. Screening for sarcoma in *EXT1* gene carriers is justified (Porter et al.,
2004).

Multiple exostoses also occur in metachondromatosis, Langer–Giedion syndrome and exostoses–anetodermia–brachydactyly type E (probably an autosomal
dominant disorder characterised by a combination of macular atrophy, multiple
exostoses and brachydactyly) (Mollica et al., 1984). Metachondromatosis is
probably an autosomal dominant condition characterised by short stature, with
exostoses and enchondromas occurring in the hands and long bones. The
osteochondromas point towards the joint and there is a tendency for them to
regress and even disappear. Enchondromas may produce deformity and functional
impairment, but malignant transformation is not a feature (Bassett and Cowell,
1985). Langer–Giedion syndrome (tricho-rhino-phalangeal syndrome type II)
is characterised by postnatal short stature, sparse hair, an unusual facies with
pear-shaped nose and long philtrum, micrognathia and protruding ears and

multiple exostoses (Buhler et al., 1987). About 70 per cent of affected individuals are mentally retarded. A deletion in chromosome 8q24.1 has been described in isolated cases of the Langer–Giedion syndrome (Buhler and Malik, 1984), and the disease is a true contiguous gene syndrome, as the causative *TRPS1* gene is adjacent to *EXT1* on chromosome 8q24. A contiguous gene syndrome on chromosome 11p11, known as DEFECT 11 involves *EXT2*. In general, the multiple cartilaginous exostoses develop in the first few years of life and increase in number until puberty is complete. They cause deformity and asymmetry of growth and there is a small risk of osteosarcoma developing. Inheritance appears to be sporadic, except for reports of twins and a father–daughter pair.

Patients with hereditary retinoblastoma are at risk of developing osteosarcoma later, especially in the irradiation field (see p. 20; Mertens and Bramwell, 1995). That osteosarcoma occurs in patients with inherited retinoblastoma and the Li–Fraumeni syndrome might suggest that the retinoblastoma and *TP53* tumour suppressor genes may be involved in the pathogenesis of this tumour. Somatic mutations in one or other of these two genes occur frequently in sporadic osteosarcoma (Toguchida et al., 1989; Miller et al., 1990). In sporadic tumours, the finding that there is preferential initial mutation of the paternally derived retinoblastoma gene suggests that genomic imprinting effects may be involved (Toguchida et al., 1989).

Osteosarcomas may develop in the context of the Li–Fraumeni syndrome, but recent studies have suggested that only about 3 per cent of paediatric osteosarcomas occur in individuals with germline mutations in *p53* (McIntyre et al., 1994).

Chondrosarcoma

The incidence of this tumour increases with increasing age. Chondrosarcoma is described as a complication of multiple enchondromatosis (Ollier disease; see below), inherited multiple exostoses (diaphysial achlasis; see above), Maffucci syndrome (p. 189; Hecht et al., 1995) and other conditions in which exostoses occur (see above). The incidence of malignancy in these syndromes is difficult to estimate, but has been assessed as 18 per cent (Sun et al., 1985). Chondrosarcoma of the limbs has been described in three brothers with normal karyotypes (Mulvihill et al., 1977).

Multiple enchondromatosis (Ollier disease) is usually sporadic, although several families with affected siblings have been described, and in one family an affected grandfather was reported suggesting an autosomal dominant inheritance with reduced penetrance (Lamy et al., 1954). Deformities, particularly of the long bones, develop because of enchondromas, resulting in asymmetrical, bilateral limb shortening, bowing or deformation. The enchondromas tend to grow until adolescent growth is over. Sarcomatous degeneration (chondrosarcoma) can occur in the lesions in adult life, and intracranial gliomas have been described (Chang and Prados, 1994). Ovarian juvenile granulosa cell tumours and precocious puberty have also been described in this condition (Tamimi and Bolen, 1984).

Maffucci syndrome, characterised by multiple enchondromas and subcutaneous hemangiomas, is associated with a high risk of malignant transformation, a risk of 30 per cent for chondrosarcomas and other malignancies being reported (Albrechts and Rapini, 1995). Intracranial chordoma has also been reported in this syndrome (Nakayama et al., 1994). There was a suggestion that a single germline mutation in parathyroid hormone-related protein (*PTHR1*), c.448C > T, resulting in R105C could be an important cause of endochrondromatosis (Hopyan et al., 2002), but a subsequent study did not find this mutation, or any others, in *PTHR1* in patients with enchondromatosis (Rozeman et al., 2004).

Ewing sarcoma

This tumour has a peak age at onset in adolescence, is rare in black races, and is not radiation-induced. Its incidence is 1.7 per 10 00 000 per year. Familial cases are rare, and the tumour only rarely occurs as part of specific familial cancer syndromes. It is probably a member of a family of neoplasms that includes a skin tumours and primitive neuroectodermal tumours of bone and soft tissue. Retinoblastoma has been recorded as a first primary cancer in 10 cases of Ewing sarcoma, and Ewing has also occurred after leukaemia and lymphoma. A startling excess of inguinal hernias in children with Ewing suggest development may be abnormal in these children (Cope et al., 2000).

A t(11; 22)(q24; q12) translocation occurs in 83 per cent of Ewing sarcomas and also in primitive neuroectodermal tumours and peripheral neuroepithelioma. Some Ewing sarcomas without a t(11; 22) show more complex rearrangements or rearrangements involving 22q12 and other chromosomes so that, overall, 92 per cent of tumours have a 22q12 breakpoint and 88 per cent have a 11q23.3 breakpoint (Griffin et al., 1986). A der(16) t(1; 16)(q11; q11) has been observed in the later stages of tumour development (Mugneret et al., 1987). The result of the t(11; 22) is that an aberrant protein is produced (Granwetter, 1995). None of these genetic rearrangements are inherited.

Rhabdomyosarcoma

Soft tissue sarcomas account for 4–6 per cent of all childhood cancers and 2 per cent of childhood cancer deaths, have an incidence of 8 per 10 00 000 per year, and are more common in Africa (Williams and Strong, 1985). About half occur in children aged under three years, with an equal sex incidence. Rhabdomyosarcoma accounts for two-thirds of paediatric soft tissue sarcomas and most commonly arise in the head and neck (40 per cent), genitourinary tract (20 per cent) and

extremities (20 per cent) (Crist and Kun, 1991). On histological criteria, rhabdomyosarcoma may be classified into two main subtypes: embryonal and botyroid
(two-thirds of all tumours) and alveolar (one-third).

Most rhabdomyosarcomas are sporadic, but they complicate neurofibromatosis type 1 (NF1; see p. 230; Yang et al., 1995), the Beckwith–Wiedemann syndrome (p. 170), and the Li–Fraumeni syndrome (p. 218). Segregation analysis for
soft tissue sarcomas in the absence of a known genetic syndrome suggests a heritability of 0.13, due to a postulated rare autosomal dominant gene (population
frequency 0.00002) with a penetrance of 50 per cent and 90 per cent at ages
30 and 60 years respectively. This gene could be the *Tp53* tumour suppressor
gene, mutations in which cause the Li–Fraumeni syndrome. The risk to first-
degree relatives is significantly increased if the index case has two or more primaries (Williams and Strong, 1985; Burke et al., 1991).

Germline mutations in *TP53* may be detected in children with rhabdomyosarcoma, in perhaps 10 per cent of cases (Diller et al., 1995), most of those with
these mutations have orbital alveolar rhabdomyosarcomas. Embryonal rhabdomyosarcoma (which is associated with Beckwith–Wiedemann syndrome)
specifically shows chromosome 11p allele loss in the same region in which the
Beckwith–Wiedemann gene has been mapped to (11p15) (Cavanee, 1991). A translocation between chromosomes 2 and 13 (2; 13)(q37; q14)) has been described
specifically in rhabdomyosarcoma (Meddeb et al., 1996). Although it is most frequent in alveolar rhabdomyosarcoma, it has also been reported in embryonal
and undifferentiated types (Douglass et al., 1987).

Other sarcomas

Synovial sarcomas occur in adolescents and young adults, especially males, have
no racial predilection, and are not noted for familial occurrence. The tumours
have been shown to have X:18 chromosomal translocations t(X:18)(p11.2;
q11.2), involving a breakpoint at Xp11.2 (Gilgenkrantz et al., 1989; deLeeuw
et al., 1994; Carbone et al., 2002).

A study of the family histories of children with soft tissue sarcomas showed
an increased family history of the Li–Fraumeni syndrome, sarcomas, gastric
cancer and neurofibromatosis, and it was considered that one-third of cases had
a genetic susceptibility (Hartley et al., 1993).

Extraskeletal myxoid chondrosarcomas have been found to show a 9:22 chromosomal translocation: t(9; 22)(q31; q12.2).

Kaposi sarcoma (multiple idiopathic pigmented haemangiosarcoma) has rarely
been described in several members of the same family, suggesting an autosomal
dominant pattern of inheritance. The condition is characterised by red–purple
nodules, plaques and macules which are commonest on the extremities but can

occur at any site, including internally. Oedema is associated, due to tumour infiltration of lymphatics, and the lesions spread, often with metastatic dissemination,
usually with fatal results, although spontaneous regression has been described.
The condition is commoner in people of Italian or Jewish origin (Finlay and
Marks, 1979; DiGiovanna and Safai, 1981). Multifactorial inheritance is more
likely in the majority of cases, with a high incidence in patients with AIDS. A viral
etiology is now suspected.

Uterine leiomyomas (fibroids) are discussed on p. 87, where the role of *FH* is
discussed. A single two-generation family with vulval and oesophageal leiomyomas was described by Wahlen and Astedt (1965).

Sacrococcygeal teratoma

After the first few years of life, most teratomas are gonadal. Familial benign cystic teratoma of the ovary has been described in three generations of a family
(Brenner and Wallach, 1983). Adult testicular gonadal germ cell tumours tend
to be aneuploid, although infantile gonadal germ cell tumours may more often
be tetraploid or diploid, which suggests that they may have a different aetiology
(Silver et al., 1994). In fact, most teratomas develop in the sacrococcygeal area
and tend to be benign. There may be associated malformations of the sacrum,
vertebrae, and gastrointestinal or urinogenital tracts. Familial teratoma with an
autosomal dominant mode of inheritance has been described (Ashcraft et al.,
1975). There may be variable penetrance of an autosomal dominant gene, with
some affected individuals having anterior sacral meningocoele, sacral defects or
skin dimples without teratoma (Yates et al., 1983).

11

Skin

Genetic predisposition to skin cancer may involve a variety of mechanisms. Firstly, there is a group of genetic disorders associated with a predisposition to specific skin cancers, and in which the premalignant lesions are primarily confined to the skin (see Table 11.1). These disorders are discussed below under the specific skin cancer involved. A second group comprises hereditary skin disorders which (possibly by virtue of chronic inflammation) predispose to skin cancers (see Table 11.1). These are described after the specific skin cancers (p. 139). The final group includes genetic disorders which (i) predispose to both skin and systemic neoplasms, or (ii) predispose to systemic neoplasia but are associated with cutaneous stigmata. These conditions are discussed in part three and include the chromosome breakage disorders (Bloom syndrome (p. 174), Fanconi anaemia (p. 193), ataxia telangiectasia (p. 167), xeroderma pigmentosum (p. 259), Cowden syndrome (p. 179), dermatitis herpetiformis/coeliac disease (p. 178), Di George syndrome, familial hyperglucagonaemia, Gardner syndrome (p. 184), Gorlin syndrome (p. 196), haemochromatosis, multiple endocrine neoplasia type 2 (*MEN2B*, p. 224), neurofibromatosis type 1 (NF1, p. 230), porphyria (p. 243), tuberose sclerosis (p. 246) and tylosis (p. 252).

Specific skin cancers

With Julia A Newton-Bishop

Melanoma is a relatively uncommon cancer, with an incidence in most of Northern Europe of around 10 per 100 000 per annum (Parkin et al., 1997). In many countries, and particularly in the UK, it is more common in women. The incidence has increased markedly this century in white people in most Western countries (Parkin et al., 1997) and in Australia and New Zealand, which have the highest rates in the world (Jones W. et al., 1999).

The commonest type of melanoma is the superficial spreading type, which has the appearance of a mole progressively changing in shape, size and colour. The melanomas commonly have irregularly distributed hues of brown, black or red. These tumours are most frequent on the lower leg in women, and on the trunk

Table 11.1. *Inherited and congenital disorders associated with skin neoplasia*

Inherited disorders predisposing to cutaneous or subcutaneous neoplasms	Inherited disorders predisposing to skin and extracutaneous neoplasms
Albinism	Blue rubber bleb naevus syndrome
Bazex Dupré Christol syndrome	Chediak–Higashi syndrome
Chelitis glandularis	Chronic mucocutaneous candidiasis (CMC)
Multiple cylindromatosis (turban tumours)	syndrome
Ectodermal dysplasias (Clouston,	Congenital generalised fibromatosis
Touraine and Rapp–Hodgkin types)	Cowden syndrome
Epidermolysis bullosa (autosomal	Dyskeratosis congenita
dominant and autosomal recessive types)	Familial melanoma syndrome
Epidermodysplasia verruciformis	Fanconi Anaemia
Extramammary Paget disease	Gorlin syndrome
Familial lichen planus*	Hereditary multiple cutaneous leiomyomas
Familial benign symmetric lipomas	Klippel–Trenaunay syndrome
Familial multiple lipomas	Maffucci syndrome
Ferguson-Smith self-healing epithelioma	Mast cell disease*
Flegel disease	McCune–Albright syndrome
Hermansky–Pudlak syndrome	Muir–Torre syndrome
Juvenile hyaline fibromatosis	Multiple glomus tumours
Keratitis–ichthyosis–deafness	Multiple benign trichoepithelioma
(KID) syndrome	(of Brooke)
Lichen sclerosis et atrophicus	NAME syndrome; Carney complex
Melanocytic naevi-giant	Neurocutaneous melanosis
pigmented hairy naevi*	NF1
Pachonychia congenita	Rothmund–Thompson syndrome
Porokeratosis of Mibelli	Ruvalcaba–Myhre–Smith syndrome
Rombo syndrome	Sclerotylosis
Steatocystoma multiplex	Tylosis
	Xeroderma pigmentosum

*rarely familial.

in males. The prognosis is determined by the Breslow thickness in millimetres, which is the thickness measured by the histopathologist from the granular layer of the skin to the deepest part of the tumour. Earlier diagnosis with thinner tumours is associated with a better prognosis (Balch et al., 2001).

Epidemiological studies have established that the most potent phenotypic risk factor identified to date is the presence of numerous (Bataille et al., 1996) or clinically atypical naevi, or moles (Fig. 11.1) (Augustsson et al., 1990; Bataille

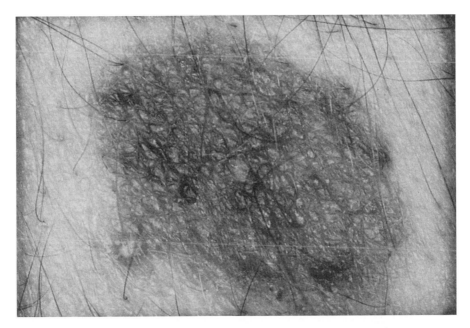

Fig. 11.1. Familial atypical mole-melanoma syndrome: a dysplastic or atypical naevus; note the irregular borders and pigmentation (courtesy of Julia Newton-Bishop).

et al., 1996). The presence of multiple naevi, some of which are clinically atypical, is called the atypical mole syndrome (AMS) phenotype (otherwise known as the dysplastic naevus syndrome (Greene et al., 1987) or the familial atypical mole and multiple melanoma syndrome (Bergman et al., 1992). It was thought originally that this phenotype was indicative of the inheritance of high penetrance melanoma susceptibility genes, but it is now recognised that the AMS is seen in 2 per cent of the general UK population (Newton et al., 1993). The odds ratio for melanoma in individuals with the AMS but no family history of melanoma is in the order of 10 relative to those who have very few naevi at all (Bataille et al., 1996). The absolute risk to such people is therefore moderate. Twin studies have shown that naevi are predominantly genetically determined (Zhu et al., 1999; Wachsmuth et al., 2001) and it is hypothesised that the AMS is indicative of low penetrance genetic susceptibility to melanoma but no such naevus genes have yet been identified.

Other risk factors relate to the presence of fair skin and hair, freckles and a reported susceptibility to sunburn, often referred to as people's "skin type" (Osterlind et al., 1988a; Elwood et al., 1990). A major genetic determinant of this phenotype (and a genetic risk factor for skin cancer) is the inheritance of common polymorphisms of the *MC1R* gene, which modulate the ratio of eumelanin (black pigment) to phaeomelanin (red pigment) in the skin and hair (Valverde et al., 1996; Bastiaens et al., 2001). Correspondingly, there is also an increased risk associated with environmental factors, such as a history of severe sunburn and sunbathing (Osterlind et al., 1988b). All of these risk factors are only moderate, in the order of relative risk 1.5–3.0 in most studies worldwide.

Genetic disorders associated with a considerably increased risk of melanoma include familial melanoma (in which there appears to be susceptibility to melanoma alone in most families; see below), hereditary non-polyposis colorectal cancer (HNPCC, p. 200), the Li–Fraumeni syndrome (p. 215), inherited retinoblastoma (p. 20) and xeroderma pigmentosum (p. 259). Inheritance of *BRCA2* mutations also appears to increase the risk of melanoma moderately (Liede et al., 2004).

Congenital anomalies such as neurocutaneous melanosis (p. 146) and giant congenital hairy naevi (p. 146) also predispose to melanoma.

Familial melanoma

Rare families exist in which there is an increased risk of melanoma and in which the tendency to melanoma appears to be inherited as an autosomal dominant with incomplete penetrance (Anderson and Badzioch, 1991), first recognised in the nineteenth century by Norris (1820). Within these families, the majority of melanomas are of the superficial spreading type, but there may be less common types such as nodular melanomas and lentigo malignant melanomas. Uveal melanomas may occur in some families, but this is very rare (McCarthy et al., 1993). In the UK families so far reported there is little evidence of increased susceptibility to other non-melanoma cancers (Newton Bishop et al., 1994). However, other groups have reported an association in particular with pancreatic carcinoma (Lynch and Fusaro, 1991; Borg et al., 2000; Lal et al., 2000; Goldstein et al., 2004), other gastrointestinal cancers (Bergman et al., 1986; Hayward, 2003) and breast cancer (Borg et al., 2000) (see below). In summary, insufficient numbers of families have so far been studied in order to quantitate the risk of non-melanoma cancers, but it is clear that some families have an increased susceptibility to gastrointestinal cancer as well as to melanoma, which is currently being explored by genoMEL the Melanoma Genetics Consortium (www.genomel.org).

Some melanoma families also have the AMS, but not all. In a proportion of families, this abnormal naevus phenotype in melanoma cases may be striking. It is characterised by the presence of clinically atypical moles (by definition more than 5 mm in diameter with an irregular or blurred edge and irregular pigmentation), numerous but otherwise banal moles, and moles in unusual places such as on the buttocks, in the iris and on the ears (Rodriguez-Sains, 1991; Newton et al., 1993).

The significance, even within melanoma-prone families, of this phenotype is unclear. Some families with melanoma do not have abnormal naevi at all. In the UK families so far described (Harland et al., 1997), the members of the largest family, with nine cases of melanoma, all had normal naevi. Overall, it is clear that although the AMS is associated in some way with familial melanoma, it is a poor indicator of gene carrier status and cannot be used even within these melanoma families to predict who is a gene carrier (Wachsmuth et al., 1998: Newton Bishop et al., 2000).

In deciding how AMS patients should be managed in terms of follow-up and risk estimation then, family history is the key. Patients with this syndrome without a family history should be taught how to self-examine their naevi and be given advice about sun protection, but long-term follow-up is not appropriate. Patients with a strong family history of melanoma with or without the AMS should retain long-term access to the pigmented lesion service. The screening of naevi in patients with the AMS and a family history of melanoma is a fairly specialised business and all such patients should be referred to the local Cancer Centre Pigmented Lesion Clinic, usually run by a dermatologist. In such clinics, the emphasis is on clinical examination of naevi, using photography for baseline documentation. Naevi are removed only if they appear to be changing and, therefore, if malignant change is suspected; they are not excised prophylactically.

Much progress has been made in understanding the genetic basis of high risk susceptibility. Initial reports of genetic linkage in melanoma families to chromosome 1p (Bale et al., 1989), have not been substantiated, so far, by other groups (van Haeringen et al., 1989; Cannon-Albright et al., 1990; Nancarrow et al., 1992). Strong evidence of linkage to chromosome 9p, reported by the Utah group (Cannon-Albright et al., 1992), was soon confirmed by others (Nancarrow et al., 1993; Goldstein et al., 1994), although genetic heterogeneity exists (Goldstein et al., 1994; MacGeoch et al., 1994). The tumour suppressor gene *CDKN2A*, which codes for the cyclin-dependent kinase (CDK) inhibitor p16, lies in the identified area of 9p (Kamb et al., 1994), and all groups working on familial melanoma have now identified germline mutations in this gene, so that to date the *CDKN2A* gene is the major identified cause of familial melanoma. Overall, germline mutations in this gene have been identified in around 40 per cent of families with three or more cases of melanoma (Holland et al., 1995; Dracopoli and Fountain, 1996; Della Torre et al., 2001), but much less frequently in families with only two cases (Harland et al., 1997; Holland et al., 1999; Della Torre et al., 2001). GenoMEL estimates an overall, *CDKN2A* mutation penetrance for melanoma of 0.30 (95 per cent confidence interval (CI) = 0.12–0.62) by age 50 years and 0.67 (95 per cent CI = 0.31–0.96) by age 80 years (Bishop et al., 2002). The CI for these estimations remain high. The Consortium will continue to improve its data. Geographical variation was demonstrated with, as expected, a higher penetrance in Australia (Bishop et al., 2002). It has also been demonstrated that penetrance is higher in mutation carriers who also have *MC1R* polymorphisms (and therefore a tendency to burn in the sun) (Box et al., 2001; van der Velden et al., 2001).

In some families with germline mutations in *CDKN2A*, there is also an increased susceptibility to pancreatic carcinoma, manifest in patients over the age of 45 years. This appears to be particularly seen in families with truncating mutations (Bartsch et al., 2002) such as the founder p16-Leiden mutation (Bergman et al., 1990), but is also seen in families with the founder mutation G101W, common in Italy and France (Ghiorzo et al., 2004). Most of these G101W families in which pancreatic cancer was seen also had melanoma, but rare families were reported with pancreatic cancer alone (Ghiorzo et al., 2004). In the p16-Leiden families the incidence of pancreatic cancer was reported to be 29 times greater than population levels (Bergman et al., 1990), and more recently a lifetime risk of 17 per cent was suggested (de Snoo et al., 2003). In the Italian G101W families a 9.4-fold risk (95 per cent CI 0.8–5.7) was reported (Ghiorzo et al., 2004). The elevated risk in the p16-Leiden families is sufficiently high that magnetic resonance imaging (MRI) screening is being investigated in clinical trials as a means of early detection.

There has been some suggestion of an increased risk of breast cancer in *CDKN2A* mutation positive women (Borg et al., 2000) but this is unsubstantiated as yet and the risks of this and other cancers will be addressed by the Melanoma Genetics Consortium. Although families are reported in which both uveal and cutaneous melanoma occur, there is little or no evidence of an increased risk of uveal melanoma in *CDKN2A* mutation carriers (Soufir et al., 2000). Very rare Danish families with uveal and cutaneous melanoma appear to be linked to a different locus on chromosome 9 (Jonsson et al., 2005).

Germline mutations have been identified in around 10–15 per cent of melanoma patients with multiple primaries (Monzon et al., 1998; Auroy et al., 2001). The prevalence of germline mutations in sporadic "population" melanoma cases is not yet known. In a population based study from Queensland only 9 per cent of highly selected samples deemed high risk on the basis of family history had identifiable mutations (Aitken et al., 1999).

Dracopoli Fountain (1996) identified two families with the same single base pair substitution in another gene: that coding for *CDK4* producing a protein anomaly at the site at which p16 binds (Zuo et al., 1996). Germline mutations in this gene are clearly extremely rare. To date, only three families worldwide have been described with these mutations (Zuo et al., 1996; Soufir et al., 1998).

However, the identification of the mutations strengthens the observation that the p16 protein is critical to melanoma carcinogenesis.

Reported evidence of linkage to 9p in melanoma families in whom *CDKN2A* mutations could not be identified suggested that *CDKN2A* mutations remained to be found. There was however no evidence for promoter mutations (Harland et al., 2000) except for a mutation of the CDKN2A5'UTR which creates an aberrant initiation codon (Liu et al., 1999) which has been identified in a number of families in North America, Australasia and Europe. Quite recently a deep intronic mutation creating an abnormal splice site was identified as a common mutation in UK families (Harland et al., 2001). It is possible that other intronic variants will be identified with time.

CDKN2A is an unusual locus with an alternative reading frame coding for another protein p14ARF, whose role in melanoma carcinogenesis remains of great interest. Families with a susceptibility to melanoma and neural tumours were described in whom there were germline deletions at 9p and the suggestion was that there was loss of CDKN2A and exon 1β, coding for p14ARF (Bahmer et al., 1990). More recently, a similar family was reported in which the deletion appeared to result in loss of exon 1β only, with no evidence of loss of CDKN2A (Randerson-Moor et al., 2001). Thus, the first evidence that p14ARF might be the third melanoma susceptibility gene was strengthened when a germline mutation in exon 1β, which creates an abnormal splice site was reported in a melanoma family (Hewitt et al., 2002) and a small deletion was reported in a Spanish melanoma family (Rizos et al., 2001).

Overall then, the consensus is that there are 3 high penetrance susceptibility genes: *CDKN2A* (p 16), *CDK4* and *p14ARF* and there is recent evidence for another at 1p22 (Gillanders et al., 2003). In the UK currently we have identified probable germline mutations in 53 and 68 per cent of 3 or more and 4 or more case families, respectively (Harland, Bishop and Newton Bishop unpublished). This figure is lower in some other centres particularly in areas of high incidence where lower penetrance genes may be more evident.

Gene testing within families with an identifiable mutation is just beginning. The majority of the *CDKN2A* mutations identified to date appear to co-segregate with the tumour and, from what is known about the structure of the p16 protein, it is to some extent possible to predict which mutations are real and which are silent. The p16 (INK4A) is a member of a family of CDK inhibitors, the other members of which are p15 (INK4B), p18 (INK4C) and p19 (INK4D). The members of the group have significant sequence homology and have a structure dictated by the presence of four or five so-called ankyrin repeats (Michaely and Bennett, 1993). Mutations which fall outside the ankyrin repeats are likely to be non-significant, like the common *CDKNA* polymorphism Ala148Thr. Some splice site variants outside these repeats are however increasingly being recognised (Harland et al., 2001; Loo et al., 2003). Mutations within the repeats are more likely to have an effect on protein function. In order to prove that identified mutations are significant, functional tests of the p16 protein have been developed. The test most widely used is a test of the ability of the mutant protein to bind to *CDK4* and *CDK6* (Harland et al., 1997). Using this test, defective binding to the *CDKs* can be demonstrated for most of the commonest described *CDKN2A* mutations, but not all. It is clear, therefore, that whilst this test may yield convincing evidence that a mutation is significant, it is not a comprehensive test of function. For mutations described in large families around the world such as Arg24Pro, Met53Ile and 23ins24, there is confidence that the mutations are real and that gene testing might be possible in the near future. For novel mutations, an abnormal functional test result would seem to be necessary before testing. GenoMEL holds a web-based database of mutations; a link to this is at www.genomel.org.

The value of gene testing however remains controversial (de Snoo et al., 2003) and the current view of genoMEL is that it is premature (Kefford et al., 2002).

Giant pigmented hairy naevus

One per cent of newborn infants have small congenital melanocytic naevi, but only 1 in 20000 infants have giant lesions. There does appear to be an increased risk of the condition in first-degree relatives of an index case, and autosomal dominant inheritance with very variable penetrance (e.g. only multiple small naevi in some affected patients) has been suggested in some families (Goodman et al., 1971). There may be a 10 per cent risk of melanoma developing in the large lesions (Makkar and Frieden, 2002; Swerdlow et al., 1995; Ruiz-Maldonado et al., 1992).

Intracranial melanomas and rhabdomyosarcoma have been described in this condition (Angelo et al., 2001; Hoanq et al., 2002).

Neurocutaneous melanosis

Congenital cutaneous melanosis is generally of sporadic occurrence, associated with meningeal infiltration by sheets of melanoblasts. About 10–13 per cent are reported to develop malignant melanoma; a higher proportion of cases with meningeal involvement show malignant degeneration (Fox et al., 1964; Arunkumar et al., 2001). All reported cases among twins have been discordant (including three pairs of monozygotic twins), and this disorder is probably caused by somatic mutations (Ferris et al., 1987; Hamm, 1999). Melanocytic infiltration of the meninges may cause hydrocephalus; and may be associated with Dandy–Walker syndrome and meningiohydroencephalocoele (Araim et al., 2004; De Andrade et al., 2004).

Basal cell carcinoma

This malignant epithelial tumour arises from the basal layers of the epidermis and its appendages. It is the most common skin tumour affecting light-skinned people, and appears predominantly in sun-exposed areas of the skin. It is more common in men than women, and rarely occurs before the age of 40 years. Arsenic is a known predisposing environmental agent.

There has been an increasing incidence of this cancer in recent years. The annual incidence of non-melanoma skin cancer is about 50 per 100 000 population in males and 40 per 100 000 in females in the UK. Genetic disorders associated with a predisposition to basal cell carcinoma include Gorlin syndrome (p. 196), xeroderma pigmentosum (p. 259), epidermolysis bullosa (p. 153), porokeratosis (p. 161), albinism (p. 148), Bazex syndrome (p. 150) and the rare Rombo syndrome (p. 162). Sporadic basal cell carcinomas show chromosome 9q allele loss, and mutations in the "Patched" gene, *PTCH*, which causes Gorlin syndrome (see p. 196) have been detected with high frequency in such tumours (Farndon et al., 1992; Quinn, 1996). This supports the view that the PTCH is a gatekeeper for common skin cancers (Sidransky, 1996). Individuals who have developed two basal cell carcinomas without syndromic features have an increased risk of germline mutations in *PTCH*. Multiple familial basal cell cancers including a case of segmental manifestations have been described (Guarneri et al., 2000). Familial (dominantly inherited) non-syndromic inherited cases have been described, with possible unilateral/segmental cases suggesting mendelian inheritance of susceptibility (Guarneri et al., 2000; Happle, 2000).

Squamous cell carcinoma

This tumour is derived from the epidermal keratinocytes. The incidence of squamous cell carcinoma shows marked geographical variation. It is most frequent in parts of the world where light-skinned people are exposed to large amounts of sunlight. Thus, it is much more frequent in southern than northern states of America, and the incidence is much higher in light-skinned than in dark-skinned races. Albino individuals are particularly at risk, especially if they live in the tropics. Arsenic, tar and oil derivatives and X-rays and gamma rays also predispose to squamous cell carcinoma. These cancers often arise in chronic scars, ulcers and sinuses. Squamous cell carcinomas appear to arise more readily in immunosuppressed individuals (Carrucci, 2004). In addition, any hereditary skin disorder that causes blistering and ulceration will predispose to squamous cell carcinoma (e.g. epidermolysis bullosa), and conditions associated with leucoplakia, such as dyskeratosis congenita and lichen sclerosis, and the keratitis–ichthyosis–deafness (KID) syndrome also have an increased risk of squamous cell carcinoma. Squamous cell carcinoma may also occur in the ectodermal dysplasias, the Rothmund–Thomson syndrome, sclerotylosis, Ferguson-Smith type self-healing squamous epithelioma, hereditary kerato-acanthoma and hyperkeratosis lenticularis perstans. Actinic keratosis is the most common epithelial precancerous lesion in light-skinned people. Genetic disorders predisposing to cutaneous squamous cell carcinoma may also predis-pose to squamous cell carcinoma in the mucous membranes, for example dyskeratosis congenita and ectodermal dysplasia can predispose to tongue, oesophageal and cervical carcinoma.

There is an increased risk of squamous cell carcinoma in first-degree relatives of cases (Tsai and Tsao, 2004).

Inherited conditions predisposing to dermatological malignancy

Albinism

Oculocutaneous albinism is a group of autosomal recessively inherited disorders of melanin synthesis, whose clinical manifestations are pale skin, white hair, nys-tagmus and photophobia. There is considerable genetic heterogeneity, at least 11 distinct types having been described (Kinnear et al., 1985; Griffiths 2002; Tsai & Tsao 2004; Orlow, 1997). Actinic skin damage, squamous cell carcinoma and basal cell carcinoma are well-recognised complications of oculocutaneous albinism; malignant melanoma is a much less common complication (Schulze et al., 1989).

Tyrosinase-negative albinism
This has a prevalence of about 1 per 39 000 in US whites and 1 per 28 000 in US blacks, about 1 per cent of whom will be heterozygotes. In this form of albinism, there is no detectable pigment in skin, hair or eyes. The skin is pink with no freckles or pigmented naevi, but vascular naevi do occur. The hair is white and the irides grey and translucent. There is severe photophobia and nystagmus, with poor visual acuity. Tyrosinase synthesis is absent; melanosomes do not develop beyond stage II and do not accumulate melanin.

Type 1 tyrosinase-negative oculocutaneous albinism may be due to mutations in the tyrosinase gene (Schnur et al., 1996). An overview of molecular aspects of ocu-locutaneous albinism is provided by recent reviews (Barsh, 1996; Summers et al., 1996; Rees, 2003; Tomita et al., 2003).

Variable tyrosinase test albinism

This includes the platinum and yellow mutant forms. In the platinum form, small amounts of pigment develop in childhood and strabismus is common. The yellow mutant form is common in the Amish; yellow-red hair and cream-coloured skin (which can tan) develop and pigmented naevi may be seen. Visual acuity improves with age.

A molecular defect in the tyrosinase gene has been detected (Spitz et al., 1990), both in the usual form of tyrosinase-negative albinism and in type 1B (yellow) oculocutaneous albinism, which are therefore allelic (Giebel et al., 1991). However tyrosinase-positive forms of albinism are not allelic.

Tyrosinase-positive oculocutaneous albinism

This involves the gradual accumulation of pigment with age. The hair may become yellow, the skin develops freckles and naevi, and can tan slightly. The irides are translucent but may become brown. Visual acuity is better than in tyrosinase-negative types. Mutations of the *P* gene encoding the tyrosine transporting membrane protein may underlie this form of albinism (Stevens et al., 1995).

Hermansky–Pudlak syndrome

This is a rare form of albinism with a haemorrhagic diathesis due to a platelet defect. The skin can be fair to dark. The bleeding tendency is usually mild, but can be life-threatening. Fibrosing alveolitis may occur. There is a deficiency of dense bodies (which normally store adenine nucleotides and serotonin) within platelets. In addition, there is an accumulation of a ceroid-like material in the reticuloendothelial system, oral, gastrointestinal and renal epithelium and cardiac muscle. The genes for this condition have been identified (Oh et al., 1996; Zhanq et al., 2002; Iannello et al., 2003).

Chediak–Higashi syndrome

This is a rare condition characterised by albinism and immunodeficiency, leading to a marked susceptibility to life-threatening infection with gram-positive organisms, and development of lymphoreticular malignancies in childhood. Most succumb to lymphomas or leukaemia by the age of 10 years. The skin is hypopigmented, but may develop papillary or hyperpigmented lesions after exposure to the sun; hair colour is light brown or grey, with slate-grey patches. Nystagmus and photophobia are present, there is uveal hypopigmentation, and the iris can be dark. Progressive peripheral neuropathy, mental retardation and seizures may develop. Less than 10 per cent survive beyond 20 years of life.

Giant lysosomal granules accumulate within leucocytes, Schwann cells, gastric mucosa, pancreas, conjunctiva, bone marrow and kidney. Neutrophils show reduced chemotaxis and bacteriocidal capacity, indicating an immune deficit. Natural killer cell activity is also impaired. There is a suggested defect of organelle membranes, which may also be responsible for the macromelanosomes observed. There may be a bleeding diathesis without thrombocytopenia. The gene for this condition has now been identified and phenotype–genotype correlations in respect of severity and age at onset are reported (Nagle et al., 1996; Karim et al., 2002; Shiflett et al., 2002; Ward et al., 2002).

Prenatal diagnosis of Chediak–Higashi syndrome is feasible by the detection of enlarged lysosomes in cultured chorionic cells by DNA analysis in certain families (Kahraman and Prieur, 1991; Barton et al., 2004).

Brown oculocutaneous albinism
This is a very mild form of albinism found in Nigerians.

Rufous oculocutaneous albinism
As its name implies, this is a condition, in dark-skinned people, in which the skin is red; and the hair may be light to dark. Visual acuity is quite good.

There are two further, very rare, forms of albinism described: the black locks-albinism deafness syndrome (BADS) of albinism with sensorineural deafness and scattered black locks of hair, and the Cross syndrome of hypopigmentation with microphthalmos, nystagmus, opaque cornea, athetosis, gingival fibromatosis and severe mental retardation. Single kindreds have been described in which oculocutaneous albinism segregates as an autosomal dominant trait.

Any patient with albinism is at an increased risk of cutaneous malignancies. This susceptibility to cancer appears to be related to the lack of skin pigmentation, and attests to the protective qualities of melanin. However, in patients with vitiligo or pibaldism, areas of skin where melanin (and melanocytes) is absent do not appear to be predisposed to malignancies in the same way (Fusaro and Lynch, 1982). Individuals with albinism should avoid sunlight exposure and use sunscreen creams when they are exposed to it.

Bazex syndrome (Bazex–Dupre–Christol syndrome)
This (probably autosomal dominant) trait (not to be confused with the non-genetic paraneoplastic acrokeratosis of the same name, in which psoriasiform changes develop on the hands, feet and face, with abnormalities of the nails associated with internal malignancy) is characterised by follicular atrophoderma, especially on the face, hands, feet and elbows, with the appearance of "ice-pick" marks (especially on the dorsum of the hands) but without palmar or plantar pits, and variable hypotrichosis. Facial hyperpigmentation and milia

occur. Multiple basal cell epitheliomas develop on the face from the second decade (Gould and Barker, 1978; Kidd et al., 1996). It is inherited as an X-linked dominant trait, with both males and females being affected, and is linked to DXS1192 at Xq14–q27 (Vabres et al., 1995).

Birt–Hogg–Dube syndrome

This autosomal dominant condition is characterised by skin fibrofolliculomas, lung cysts and a predisposition to spontaneous pneumothorax. These patients are at increased risk of developing renal neoplasms, most commonly chromophobe and oncocytic hybrid tumours. The gene responsible, *FLCL*, maps to chromosome 17p (see p. 173; Schmidt, 2004).

Chelitis glandularis

This rare condition, which can be inherited as an autosomal dominant trait, is characterised by diffuse nodular enlargement of the lower lip, with hypertrophy of the labial mucous glands, chronic inflammation and dilatation of the excretory ducts. There is a high risk of squamous cell carcinoma of the lower lip (Rada et al., 1985; Vernia, 2003).

Chronic mucocutaneous candidiasis syndrome

This is a rare condition characterised by chronic and recurrent *Candida* infections of the skin, nails and oropharynx from early childhood. There may be an underlying immune defect. In over 50 per cent of cases, there is associated endocrine disease. Several examples of familial chronic mucocutaneous candidiasis syndrome have been recorded, some showing an autosomal recessive and some an autosomal dominant mode of transmission; some cases are not associated with endocrinopathy (Buzzi et al., 2003). Late-onset cases may be sporadic. The condition can predispose to malignancy, especially of the oropharynx. The *Candida* endocrinopathy syndrome includes hypoparathyroidism, hypothyroidism, hypoadrenocortism and diabetes, usually autosomal recessive in inheritance (Wells et al., 1972; Ahonen, 1985; Coleman and Hay, 1997; Buzzi et al., 2003; Myhre et al., 2004). Vertical transmission of the syndrome with hypothyroidism has been described (Kirkpatrick, 1994), and a syndrome of immune deficit, mucocutaneous candidiasis and thyroid disease has been mapped to chromosome 2p in one family. A germline mutation in the *AIRE* gene has been described in a patient with this condition and muscular atrophy (Sato and Nakajima, 2002). An immune deficit causing dominant chronic mucocutaneous candidiasis and thyroid disease, maps to chromosome 2p in a single family.

Familial chronic nail candidiasis has been described with ICAM-1 deficiency with an autosomal recessive inheritance (Zuccurello et al., 2002).

Congenital generalised fibromatosis

This is a very rare, probably autosomal recessive, condition characterised by the development of multiple rubbery, firm, fibroblastic tumours of the skin, striated muscle, bones and viscera from infancy. Multiple subcutaneous nodules proliferate early in life, but tend to regress spontaneously if the patient survives. The visceral involvement may be fatal (Roggli et al., 1980). Some X-ray features resemble those of Ollier disease (Sty et al., 1996).

Dyskeratosis congenita

This is classically an X-linked condition (although other inheritance patterns have been described in some families, suggesting locus (genetic) heterogeneity; it comprises reticulated hyperpigmentation of the skin, with depigmented spots, nail dystrophy (in 98 per cent of patients and sometimes apparent at birth) and leucoplakia of the mucous membranes (87 per cent) with atrophy of the lingual papillae in affected males (Marrone & Mason, 2003). Signs of the condition develop in the first decade of life (Sirinavin and Trowbridge, 1975). There may be enamel dystrophy of the teeth. The skin changes are progressive, with development of poikiloderma, telangiectasia and atrophy. Hypertrophic squamous epithelium occurs in mucous epithelia. Bullous skin eruptions and hyperkeratosis, especially of the palms and soles, may occur, and atrophy of the skin of the palms may lead to loss of dermatoglyphics. Blepharitis, ectropion and nasolacrimal obstruction may occur and there are dental caries. Subnormal intelligence is sometimes a feature (in 42 per cent of cases). Leucoplakia develops, particularly of the oral mucosa, and also in the rectum and genitourinary tract (Davidson and Connor, 1988). There is thought to be an immune dysfunction, with reduced cellular immunity and T-cell function, leading to opportunistic infections. Complications include pancytopenia (due to bone marrow failure) (Fogarty et al., 2003) and squamous and basal cell carcinomas of the skin and mucous membranes, often developing in areas of leucoplakia, after the age of 20 years. Squamous cell carcinoma of the mouth, rectum, cervix, vagina, oesophagus and skin may occur, and there may be multiple primaries. An increased incidence of solid tumours (which can be multiple) has been claimed, with a total incidence of malignancy of 12 per cent (Kawaguchi et al., 1990). Clinical features of the condition are generally manifest by 10 years of age, but may not occur until puberty. Female carriers are generally normal. Linkage to markers at Xq28(D9S52) was demonstrated. Late-onset cases, or of aplastic anaemia may also be due to mutations in this gene (*TERC*) (Connor et al., 1986; Arngrimsson et al., 1993). Excessive spontaneous chromatid breaks have been reported in some cases of this condition, and an increased X-irradiation-induced chromatid breakage has been demonstrated in fibroblasts (DeBauche et al., 1988).

Mutations in the *KKC1* gene which encodes dyskeratin, a protein necessary for the function of telomerase, are now known to cause the majority of cases, accounting for the observed severe reduction in telomere length and reduced apoptosis in this condition, and disease anticipation has been shown to be associated with progressive telomere shortening (Montanaro et al., 2003; Shay and Wright, 2004; Vuilamy et al., 2004).

Ectodermal dysplasias

These conditions comprise a heterogeneous group of congenital diffuse disorders of the epidermis and appendages (Pinheiro and Freire-Maia, 1994). Three forms of autosomal dominant ectodermal dysplasia are described, and each of these may predispose to squamous cell carcinoma of the skin and nail beds (Mauro et al., 1972). The hidrotic type, Clouston syndrome, is characterised by thickened, deformed hypoplastic nails, thin sparse hair and thick dyskeratotic skin of the palms and soles. Areas of hyperpigmentation occur, especially in skin overlying joints (Escobar et al., 1983). A biochemical defect of keratin may be present, and ultrastructural abnormalities of the hair may be demonstrated. Hypohidrotic ectodermal dysplasia is rare, with hypodontia, hypotrichosis and variable hypohidrosis. The Rapp–Hodgkin syndrome comprises anhydrotic ectodermal dysplasia and cleft lip and palate. The hair in this condition is short and wiry, the teeth small and conical, the nails abnormal (Cirillo Silengo et al., 1982). Anhydrotic ectodermal dysplasia is an X-linked recessive condition; the cancer risk is not specifically increased in affected males.

The molecular basis of some of these are being identified – for instance, the X-linked form has been shown to be due to germline mutations in the gene encoding NEMO/1KK gamma, and an autosomal dominant form to germline I Kappa B alpha mutations (Courtois et al., 2003).

Epidermolysis bullosa

This is a heterogeneous group of inherited disorders characterised by extreme skin fragility and recurrent blisters. Classification is based upon the level at which blistering occurs (Pearson, 1988). Superficial blistering occurs in epidermolysis bullosa simplex, with breakdown occurring in the basal cells. This type is often inherited as an autosomal dominant trait, and is clinically mild, without scarring, and mucous membranes are spared. Nails may be mildly involved (Lin and Carter, 1989). The autosomal dominant Dowling–Meera form of epidermolysis bullosa simplex can be severe in infancy; the histology of this type is characteristic, and can be detected in foetal skin biopsies. In junctional epidermolysis bullosa, the split occurs in the lamina lucida, causing extensive blistering on the skin and mucosal surfaces. Severe scarring may occur. There are six clinical types of junctional epidermolysis bullosa, all inherited as autosomal recessive traits. Germline mutations in several keratin genes have been found to underlie the different forms of epidermolysis bullosa, the type of mutation correlating with phenotype (Corden and McLean, 1996; Jonkman et al., 2003; Porter and Lane, 2003; Uitto et al., 2002).

In dystrophic epidermolysis bullosa, blistering occurs in the dermis. Dominant and recessive forms are described, but the severe forms are usually recessively inherited. Bullae develop, particularly on the extremities, leading to severe mitten-like scarring and deformity (mutilans). Gastrointestinal involvement is common, leading to oesophageal strictures, erosions and webs, and life-threatening haemorrhage may occur. Chronic anaemia and hypoalbuminaemia occur. Dental enamel is defective, and there may be laryngeal involvement.

In epidermolysis bullosa, squamous cell carcinoma may develop in the scars, but this tendency is much more marked in the dystrophic type. These carcinomas may occur at multiple sites (70 per cent), mainly on the limbs (Mallipeddi, 2002; Tomita et al., 2003). They arise in young individuals (75 per cent develop in the 20–40-year age group), and are characteristically well or moderately well differentiated, but aggressive in behaviour and metastasise readily (Goldberg et al., 1988). The carcinomas may develop on mucosal surfaces, including oesophagus, stomach, bronchus, bladder and tongue (Tidman, 1990). Basal cell carcinomas may also develop in epidermolysis bullosa scars.

Simplex forms of epidermolysis bullosa are caused by mutations in the genes for the basal epidermal keratins *K5* and *K14* (Coulombe et al., 1991), and *K1* and *K10* mutations occur in epidermolytic ichthyosis (Smith, 2003). Dystrophic epidermolysis bullosa results from mutations in the anchoring fibril collagen gene *COL7A*, whereas the junctional form is due to mutations in laminin 5, alpha-3 and beta-3 subunits (Eady and Dunnill, 1994). Families with autosomal dominant epidermolysis bullosa simplex have shown linkage to the *K14* gene and others to the *K5* gene. Mutations in the *K14* gene have been demonstrated in affected individuals (Bonifas et al., 1991), and a mutation in type VII collagen has been demonstrated in a family with dystrophic epidermolysis bullosa (Ryynanen et al., 1991; Korge and Krieg, 1996; Bale and DiGiovanna, 1997). The genes in which mutations cause epidermolysis bullosa generally encode proteins in or around the hemidesmosome, the sited anchorage of the basal cell to the cell membrane, and the severity of disease determined by the functional position of the affected protein (Fuchs, 1996). Germline mutations in two adjacent genes (*EVER1* and *EVER2*) have been detected in individuals with this condition (Ramoz et al., 2002; Tate et al., 2004).

Prenatal diagnosis of epidermolysis bullosa may be offered, based on the histological findings at foetal skin biopsy at 18–20 weeks of gestation (Eady et al., 1985). The direct detection of mutations allows prenatal diagnosis of specific types of epidermolysis bullosa on chorionic villus samples when these mutations have been characterised in the family.

Epidermodysplasia verruciformis

This condition appears to be due to a genetic susceptibility (possibly recessively inherited, although the genetic basis for the disorder is not clear) to infection with human Papillomavirus, producing a verrucous, polymorphic, warty eruption, particularly affecting exposed areas of the face, neck, hands and the upper part of the back, where HPV4 is the infective agent, there is a high (20–25 per cent) risk of malignant transformation in the plaques (Jablonska et al., 1979; Orth et al., 1979; Lane et al., 2003; Majewski and Jablonska, 2004).

Ferguson-Smith type self-healing epithelioma (multiple self-healing squamous epithelioma)

This is a rare, dominantly inherited disorder, which is found in people of Scottish descent, and all cases of which are possibly descended from one individual. It is characterised by the post-pubertal appearance of multiple cutaneous keratoacanthomas, which enlarge, ulcerate and eventually heal, with calcification, to leave deep, pitted, irregular scars which can be very disfiguring. Most lesions occur on the head and neck, in exposed areas of skin, especially where pilosebaceous follicles are found. The lesions resemble squamous cell carcinomas, but metastasise only very rarely (to lymph nodes) and do not behave in a malignant fashion. In the past, treatment for the lesions (e.g. radiotherapy) has been as harmful as the lesions themselves. There is marked variation in the age at onset and number of lesions in different affected individuals (Ferguson-Smith et al., 1971). Linkage analysis has mapped the gene to chromosome 9q31–32 (Goudie et al., 1991; Richards et al., 1997; Bale, 1999). Although this disorder has phenotypic similarities to Gorlin syndrome (see part three) and maps to the same region of the genome, the two have not been shown to be allelic.

Flegel disease (hyperkeratosis lenticularis perstans)

This is an autosomal dominant condition characterised by punctate keratoses affecting the extensor surfaces of the legs and the dorsa of the feet, with palmar and plantar scaly papules and pits. Keratinosomes may be deficient. There is a risk of squamous and basal cell carcinomas (Beveridge and Langlands, 1973; Frenk and Tapernoux, 1974; Li T.H. et al., 1997; Miljkovic, 2004).

Juvenile hyaline fibromatosis

This is an autosomal recessive condition characterised by multiple subcutaneous fibromatous tumours, developing from the age of about 2 years, especially on the scalp. The tumours may be disfiguring, and there is associated gingival hyperplasia. Joint contractures and osteolytic bony lesions often occur. Excision of the tumours may be followed by recurrence (Fayad et al., 1987; Katagiri et al., 1996). The gene for this condition maps to 4q21, and mutations in *CMG2* (capillary morphogenesis gene-2) appear to cause both juvenile hyaline fibrosis and infantile systemic hyalinosis (Rahman et al., 2002; Paller et al., 2003).

KID syndrome

This rare condition is characterised by keratitis, ichthyosis and deafness. It usually occurs as a sporadic condition, but instances of vertical transmission have been described, indicating autosomal dominant inheritance (Langer et al., 1990). There are hyperkeratotic plaques on the skin and reticulated keratosis of the face, with keratoderma. Ichthyosis develops soon after birth, especially over extensor aspects of the skin. Sensorineural deafness is present from birth, and loss of visual acuity develops due to corneal vascularisation and opacification. Hair is sparse and the nails may be dystrophic. Recurrent *Candida* infection of the skin occurs in 50 per cent of cases, although no consistent immunological defect has been demonstrated. Cutaneous infections and abscesses may develop, and multiple squamous cell carcinomas ensue (Grob et al., 1987; Wilson et al., 1991). Germline mutations in the GJB2 gene encoding connxin 26 cause this syndrome (Yotsumoto et al., 2003; Janecke et al., 2005).

Klippel–Trenaunay syndrome

This is usually a sporadic condition, characterised by the triad of capillary or cavernous haemangiomas, hemihypertrophy and varicosities. Additional dermatological features include abnormal pigmentation, papillomas and varicose ulcers. Arteriovenous aneurysms and lymphatic abnormalities are common (Viljeon, 1988).

A de novo translocation t(8;14) (q22.3;q13) has been found in abnormal tissue in this condition (Wanq et al., 2001).

At least one gene (*RASA1*) in which germline mutations cause this syndrome has been identified (Eerola et al., 2003; Tian, 2003), although the latter finding has been recently thrown into doubt (Barker et al., 2006).

Lichen planus

This fairly common dermatological condition may predispose to cutaneous malignancy. Familial cases have been described, and in these cases the disease affects younger individuals and is a more widespread eruption (also spreading to involve nails and mucous membranes) than in isolated cases (Mahood, 1983; Sandhu et al., 2003). There may be genetic heterogeneity in aetiology in lichen planus, with idiopathic cases of cutaneous lichen planus showing some HLA associations (La Nasa et al., 1995; Sandhu et al., 2003).

Lichen sclerosis et atrophicus

This dermatological disorder is much more common in females than in males (10:1), has a predilection for the vulva, particularly in post-menopausal women, and is the most commonly encountered vulvar dystrophy. Extragenital lesions are most common on the trunk, arms, neck and face. The lesions are greyish, polygonal, flat papules, which may coalesce into plaques which atrophy. The vulvar lesions predispose to carcinoma of the vulva, with a reported incidence of up to 10 per cent of affected adult women. The lesions show elevated p53 levels, and 17p loss of heterozygosity (LOH). Several cases of familial lichen sclerosis with more than one affected generation have been described, including pre-menopausal women and children, but these are very rare (Friedrich and MacLaren, 1984; Shirer and Ray, 1987; Carlson et al., 1998).

Mast cell disease

This includes a wide spectrum of clinical entities, with urticaria pigmentosa with or without systemic lesions, and may rarely be associated with malignant mast cell leukaemia. Symmetrical hyperpigmented macules or papules may develop from infancy, most commonly on the trunk; they urticate on mild trauma. Vesiculation, erythema and telangiectasia may develop. Pruritus is common, and may be accompanied by flushing, tachycardia and malaise. Familial instances with autosomal dominant trait inheritance have been described (Shaw, 1968). A somatic point mutation in *KIT* may be detected in peripheral blood mononuclear cells in patients with mastocytosis with an associated haematological disorder (Nagata et al., 1995; Fritsch-Polanz et al., 2001; Ferger et al., 2002; Chang et al., 2001).

Multiple cutaneous leiomyomas

This is an autosomal dominant condition in which many small smooth muscle tumours develop in the skin. These tumours appear as single or multiple small, firm, painful dermal nodules, fixed to the skin, especially noted on the limbs, trunk and face, and develop more often in the third decade of life, although they can occur in childhood. Uterine myomas may be associated; 54 per cent of affected females in one family described in the literature had uterine myomas. These may rarely develop into leiomyosarcomas (Berendes et al., 1971), and there is also an increased risk of type II papillary renal cancer or renal cancer with collecting duct morphology. Affected individuals have reduced fumarate hydratase (FH) activity in lymphoblastoid cells. A case of 9p trisomy with 18p monosomy with this condition (with associated mental retardation) has been described (Fryns et al., 1985). Malignancy is rare. In about 75 per cent of cases the condition is due to germline heterozygous mutations in the *FH* gene, a component of the tricarboxylic acid cycle (Martinez-Mir et al., 2003; Tomlinson et al., 2002). Homozygotes (or compound heterozygotes for *FH* mutations) cause the fumarase metabolic deficiency syndrome characterised by developmental delay and death in the first decade (Tomlinson et al., 2002; Alam et al., 2003). However, not all mutation carrier parents of children with FH deficiency have a predisposition to leiomyomata.

Screening affected individuals should include regular abdominal ultrasound for renal abnormalities (Garman et al., 2003).

Multiple cylindromatosis (Brooke–Spiegler syndrome)

This is an autosomal dominant condition. It is characterised by multiple benign tumours of the skin appendages. These are smooth, dome-shaped, firm, pink tumours of the head (turban tumours), including syringomas and trichoepitheliomas, and sometimes spiroadenomas, which develop from early adulthood and may be very disfiguring. Basal cell epitheliomas may develop in the lesions, and radiation therapy may exacerbate this tendency (Welch et al., 1968; Szepietowski et al., 2001).

The tumours are of hairy skin, and are not associated with basal or squamous cell carcinomas. The condition has been linked to D16S411 and D16S416 on chromosome 16q12–13 (Biggs et al., 1995; Fenske et al., 2000), and mutations in the CYLD gene have been identified as causing the condition. Genotype–phenotype correlations have not been described until recently, when a family with mild disease (where the tumours tended to be small) the causative mutation was R758X in the *CYLD* gene (Oiso et al., 2004). Loss of the cylindromatosis tumour suppressor inhibits apoptosis by activating NF-kB. It has been suggested that, since aspirin also inhibits the action of NF-kB, it is a logical (topical) therapeutic agent for cylindromatosis, and phase 1 clinical trials of this are currently underway (Gutierrez et al., 2002; Bernends, 2003; Brummelkamp et al., 2003; Lakhani, 2004).

Multiple lipomatosis: familial

This rare autosomal dominant condition is characterised by the development of multiple, encapsulated, subcutaneous, non-tender, smooth lipomas on the forearms, trunk, thighs and arms. The lipomas are often symmetric, usually begin in early adulthood, and grow to a certain size and then stabilise; regression is rare, as is malignant degeneration. The distribution of the lipomas may follow that of the peripheral nerves (Leffell and Braverman, 1986). In one family the condition was linked to an *RBI* gene mutation with low penetrance retinoblastoma susceptibility (Genuardi et al., 2001).

Multiple lipomatosis: symmetric

This is a separate condition, predominantly occurring in adult males, and autosomal inheritance has been suggested (Enzi, 1984). The primary defect is thought to be in adrenergic-stimulated lipolysis. Clinically, lipomatous masses develop in a symmetric distribution at the back of the neck and shoulders, the breast areas, abdomen and pubic regions. There may be atrophy of uninvolved fat. Visceral lipomatosis can be life-threatening. Autonomic and peripheral neuropathy is associated, and alcoholism is thought to precipitate its development in many cases. The condition is probably heterogeneous, and may not be genetic, but may be confused with multiple lipomatosis (Gorlin, 1976). Autosomal dominant inheritance of multiple familial lipomatosis with polyneuropathy has been described (Wilson and Boland, 1994; Stoll et al., 1996; Nisoli et al., 2002), and mutations in the mitochondrial genome, possibly resulting in faulty noradrenergic modulation of proliferation and differentiation of brown fat cells (Gamez et al., 1998; Nisoli et al., 2002).

NAME syndrome: Carney complex

Carney complex is an autosomal dominant multiple endocrine neoplasia and lentiginosis syndrome characterised by spotty skin pigmentation, cardiac, skin and breast myxomas and a variety of endocrine tumours. The skin features include common and blue naevi and psammomatous melanotic schwannomas. Endocrine overactivity occurs. Pituitary tumours, adrenal cortical rest tumours, phaeochromocytoma, Leydig cell tumours, large cell calcifying Sertoli cell tumour of the testis, schwannomas and myxoid breast fibroadenomas and ductal adenomas have been described in this condition (Carney, 1995).

The condition is genetically heterogeneous. Mutations in the gene encoding the protein kinase A type 1-alpha regulatory subunit (PRKAR1A) on chromosome 17q have been identified in some affected individuals (Kirschner et al., 2000a and b; Veugelers et al., 2004); other families show linkage to chromosome 2p16 (Stratakis et al., 1996) and chromosome 2 abnormalities have been described in the tumours (Matyakhina et al., 2003).

This syndrome is distinct from the Carney triad, an association between stromal gastric sarcoma, pulmonary chondroma and extra-adrenal paraganglioma (Carney, 1999).

Pachyonychia congenita

This rare autosomal dominant condition is characterised by thickened nails (which are very difficult to cut), with yellow discolouration, follicular keratosis in 59 per cent, plantar keratosis in 72 per cent and leucokeratosis in 57 per cent of cases. The nail abnormalities may be seen soon after birth, and paronychial inflammation occurs. Subcutaneous hamartomatous cysts, bullae, ichthyosis and hyperkeratosis may develop. Blistering may occur over pressure areas, and there may be deafness, hair and dental abnormalities, hyperidrosis and corneal opacification. Oral leucoplakia is seen (Feinstein et al., 1988). Malignant changes may occur in the oral lesions, in cysts, or at sites of chronic plantar ulcerations, so that areas of chronic ulceration or bullous formation should be observed for the possible development of malignancy (Su et al., 1990). Steatocystoma multiplex is considered to be the same condition (Hodes and Norins, 1977; Stieglitz and Centerwall, 1983). Germline mutations in the *K17* gene may underlie certain types of this condition (Smith et al., 1997); others may be due to missense mutations in keratin 17 (Smith et al., 1997).

Pachyonychia congenita (PC) types 1 and 2 are described. These are similar but type 1 gets oral leucokeratoses whereas type 2 have premature dentition and multiple sebaceous cysts. Mutations in the keratin 17 (*K17*) gene can cause PC type 2 or steatocystoma multiplex PC types 1 and 2 → hypertrophic nil dystrophy, focal keratoderma and sebaceous cysts (Corello et al., 1998). PC type 1 is due to K6a and K16 mutations (Swenssen, 1999).

Palmar keratoses

It has been claimed that palmar and plantar keratoses are more common in individuals with bladder and lung cancer, occurring in 70–90 per cent of cases and in only 36 per cent of controls, but it is difficult to assess the significance of this finding since it is based on only a few studies (Cuzick et al., 1984). Keratin gene or connexin abnormalities may underlie this group of conditions (Bale and DiGiovanna, 1997; Kelsell et al., 2000; Kimyai-Asadi et al., 2002).

There are many subtypes, including palmoplantar keratoderma, the Clarke–Howel–Evans syndrome (see oesophageal cancer) (Malde, Meleda, Smith, 2003 subtypes).

Pilomatrixoma (benign calcifying epithelioma of Malherbe)

Pilomatrixomas appear in young adults, most commonly on the arms, face and neck, as asymptomatic, firm, lobular, bluish nodules, which may be painful and occasionally inflamed. They are usually sporadic, but have rarely been found to occur in families. They occur in both sexes, possibly with autosomal dominant inheritance (Duperrat and Albert, 1948). Multiple calcifying epitheliomas have been reported in association with myotonic dystrophy (Harper, 1972; Hubbard and Whittaker, 2004), and with Rubenstein–Taybi syndrome (Masuno et al., 1998). Activating mutations in CTNNBI are detected in a high proportion of tumours (Chan et al., 1999).

Porokeratosis of Mibelli

This is a rare, autosomal dominant defect of skin keratinisation. Centrifugally spreading patches are surrounded by horny ridges, and there is central atrophy. Onset is usually in childhood, and lesions may occur anywhere on the skin, enlarge slowly, and are usually asymptomatic. Squamous cell carcinoma, Bowen disease and basal cell carcinoma may develop in the keratoatrophodermic lesions, particularly on the extremities. X-ray treatment may increase the tendency to develop carcinoma (Goerttler and Jung, 1975; Gotz et al., 1999). There are other rare forms of porokeratosis: disseminated superficial actinic prokeratosis and porokeratosis plantaris, palmaris et disseminata, which are also inherited as autosomal dominant conditions predisposing to skin cancer, but which occur more in adults and are more likely to be symptomatic. Sporadic cases also occur, and malignancy may be more common in sporadic cases. Males are more often affected than females.

Proteus syndrome

This is a very rare condition (named after the Greek god Proteus) and is usually sporadic. Possible transmission of the condition from father to son has been described once (Goodship et al., 1991), but there is considerable debate about this in view of diagnostic pitfalls (Turner et al., 2001). Somatic mosaicism may explain some cases (Reardon et al., 1996). Congenital lipomas occur, sometimes with haemangiomatous or lymphangiomatous elements, and progress and are associated with partial or complete hemihypertrophy, asymmetry and disfiguration. Accelerated growth is seen in the first few years of life. Exostoses of the skull cause macrocephaly and skull asymmetry with frontal bossing. Localised deformities develop, especially of the hands and feet, and hemihypertrophy (segmental to total) is common. Dermatological features include pigmented naevi, diffuse areas of hyperpigmented and depigmented areas of skin, linear verrucose epidermoid naevi and massive cerebroid gyriform hyperplasia with rugosity of the soles of the feet is a characteristic feature. Bony and adipose overgrowth may lead to bizarre macrodactyly. Subcutaneous hamartomatous tumours, pigmented areas of skin, bony abnormalities and lung cysts have been described (Nishimura and Koslowski, 1990). Intelligence is usually normal (Gorlin, 1984). There is a theoretical risk of malignancy in this overgrowth syndrome, and a testicular mesothelioma at the age of 4 years has been described in a severe case (Barker et al., 2001).

Mutations in *PTEN* have been detected in a subset of cases, and are thought to be mosaic. In some cases the mutation was identical to a germline mutation found in an individual with Cowden syndrome, and in some, but not all cases, the second *PTEN* allele was shown to be inactivated in the abnormal tissue (Zhou et al., 2000, 2001a). These observations have been confirmed by Smith et al. (2002).

Rombo syndrome

This is a very rare syndrome, described in a four generation family, in which affected individuals developed follicular atrophy of the skin of the cheeks in childhood. In affected adults, telangiectasia and skin papules appeared, especially on the face, and the eyelashes and eyebrows were abnormal. Basal cell carcinomas occur frequently from the third decade (Michaelsson et al., 1981; Van Steensel et al., 2001).

Sclerotylosis (scleroatrophic and keratotic dermatosis of limbs; scleroatrophic syndrome of Huriez)

This rare autosomal dominant condition is characterised by scleroatrophy of the skin of the hands and feet, hypoplastic nails and palmoplantar keratoderma. Skin cancer (squamous cell carcinoma) and bowel cancer are said to be common in this condition (Fischer, 1978), and squamous cell carcinomas of the tongue and tonsil also occur. Linkage has been established with the MN blood group on chromosome 4q28–3. In the scleroatrophic syndrome of Huriez the histopathologic findings of an almost complete absence of epidermal Langerhans cells in affected skin may explain the susceptibility to squamous cell carcinoma in these lesions (Delaporte et al., 1995; Hamm et al., 1996; Downs and Kennedy, 1998).

Steatocystoma multiplex

In this condition, multiple, small, rubbery, elevated, cystic lesions develop, usually in adolescence. The lesions may become infected and this leads to scarring. Autosomal dominant inheritance is the rule (Kligman and Kirschbaum, 1964). Keratin 17 (*K17*) mutations can cause this condition and PC type 2 (Corden and McLean, 1996; Smith et al., 1997).

Syringomas

A rare condition with multiple facial syringomas, sometimes with neonatal teeth and oligodontia has been identified as an autosomal dominant condition (Morrison and Young, 1996; Metze et al., 2001).

Trichoepithelioma

This is an autosomal dominant inherited tendency to multiple, small, flesh-coloured, translucent tumours from childhood, mainly on the face. There is a risk of basal cell carcinoma developing in the lesions. The condition has been mapped to chromosome 9p21, close to D9S126 (Harada et al., 1996; Clarke et al., 2002).

Brooke–Spiegler (p. 158) syndrome is an autosomal dominant syndrome characterised by multiple cylindromas and trichoepitheliomas.

Tylosis

Tylosis, or focal epidermolytic palmoplantar keratoderma occurring after infancy, is associated with early-onset squamous cell carcinoma of the oesophagus in three families. The tylosis is characterised by abnormal thickening of the palmoplantar skin. Neonatal onset of palmoplantar keratosis is a different disorder and not associated with oesophageal cancer. The genetic locus for the tylosis oesophageal cancer (*TOC*) gene has been localised to 17q25 (Langan et al., 2004) (see section on oesophageal cancer).

Part three

Cancer-predisposing syndromes

12

Inherited cancer-predisposing syndromes

Ataxia telangiectasia

This autosomal recessive disorder, with a birth incidence of about 1 in 300 000, is characterised by the development of cerebellar ataxia in the first decade, along with choreoathetosis, dysarthria and abnormalities of ocular movements. Mental retardation is not usually a feature. The neurological features are progressive, leading to confinement to a wheelchair in the second decade of life. Oculocutaneous telangiectasia develops in childhood (often after ataxia is apparent) and then spread to involve other exposed cutaneous areas (see Fig. 12.1). Vitiligo, café-au-lait spots and macular hyperpigmentation may occur. The development of acanthosis nigricans is associated with the development of neoplasia. An immune deficiency occurs, with disordered B-cell and T-helper cell function, thymic hypoplasia and reduced levels of IgA (70 per cent) and IgE

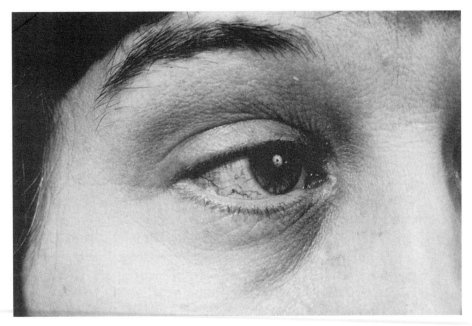

Fig. 12.1. The telangiectatic changes seen on the conjunctiva of an individual with ataxia telangiectasia.

(80 per cent), and reduced T-cells. Frequent bacterial (pulmonary or sinus) infections occur secondary to immunodeficiency. The serum alphafetoprotein is consistently elevated. There is an inconsistently increased incidence of spontaneous structural chromosomal aberrations (30–50-fold) (chromatid gaps, breaks and interchanges, and telomere fusions) in cultured white cells and fibroblasts, and this is markedly increased by exposure to X-radiation and radiomimetic agents. Peripheral blood lymphocytes may show abnormal clones of cells with a stable cytogenetic rearrangement, usually involving chromosome 14, particularly involving the T-cell receptor genes on 14q11, 7q14 and 7q35. Clones of cells with these translocations may develop into T-cell promyelocytic leukaemia. Other translocations involve the immunoglobulin genes in B-lymphocytes. In vivo sensitivity to X-rays is also observed (Tomanin et al., 1989), and this has been used as a basis for diagnosis and to define four complementation groups. Recombination is increased by a factor of 30–200 (Peterson et al., 1992; Viniou et al., 2001; Sun et al., 2002).

There is a 30–40 per cent risk of malignancy developing, most frequently Hodgkin and non-Hodgkin lymphoma (60 per cent), and lymphoblastic T-cell leukaemia (27 per cent) (Johnson, 1989). The lymphoreticular neoplasms develop before the age of 16 years, and epithelial carcinomas (including medulloblastomas; gastric, basal cell, hepatocellular, parotid, laryngeal, skin and breast carcinomas; uterine leiomyomas; and ovarian dysgerminoma) may develop in patients surviving longer (Spector et al., 1982). Severe reactions have been described to standard doses of radiotherapy in this condition.

A locus for ataxia telangiectasia (AT) was mapped to chromosome 11q22–23 by genetic linkage analysis (Gatti et al., 1988), and the *ATM* gene was cloned by a positional cloning approach in 1995 (Savitsky et al., 1995). The *ATM* gene encodes a serine–threonine kinase activated by exposure to X-irradiation, and is mutated in all complementation groups. McConville et al. (1996) and others have reported families with a milder clinical and cellular phenotype due to certain ataxia-telangiectasia mutations (Saviozzi et al., 2000; Meyn, 1999) causing reduced ATM function. Prior to the identification of the *ATM* gene, prenatal diagnosis of AT was achieved by detecting increased spontaneous and induced chromosome breakage in cultured amniocytes and chorionic villi (Schwartz et al., 1985). Prenatal diagnosis may be available by mutation analysis.

The AT carrier frequency is estimated to be about 1 per cent and it has been suggested that these heterozygotes have an increased risk of cancer, particularly breast cancer (Swift et al., 1987; Morrell et al., 1990). Some studies have suggested that the relative risk could be up to 15 for female heterozygotes and, if correct, AT heterozygotes would comprise a significant proportion (5–15 per cent) of sporadic breast cancer cases. The identification of the *ATM* gene provided opportunities unequivocally to identify AT heterozygotes. Although Athma et al. (1996) found an excess of breast cancer among proven heterozygotes ascertained via AT families, and this was confirmed in a larger study (RR~5 for breast cancer diagnosed under 50, see page 77) (Thomson et al., 2005). Fitzgerald et al. (1997) failed to demonstrate a significant excess of AT carriers among early-onset breast cancers. This might be due to sensitivity of the technique. In view of the reasonably established increased susceptibility to breast cancer, female heterozygotes should not undergo routine mammographic screening (Thorensten et al., 2003).

Ataxia-telangiectasia-like disorder (ATLD)

A small proportion of "AT" cases have mutations in the *MRE11* gene rather than *ATM*, causing a disorder known as ATLD. The lymphocytes of such patients show increased levels of translocations involving immune system genes, and chromosomal radiosensitivity is seen, but B-lymphocytes may not be affected and the cancer risk is less (Stewart et al., 1999; Duker, 2002; De la Torre et al., 2003).

Bannayan–Riley–Ruvalcaba syndrome (Bannayan–Zonana syndrome, Ruvalcaba–Riley–Smith syndrome)

Bannayan–Riley–Ruvalcaba syndrome (BRRS, MIM 153480), a rare autosomal dominant congenital disorder, is characterised by macrocephaly, lipomatosis, haemangiomatosis and speckled penis (Gorlin et al., 1992). Other features include Hashimoto thyroiditis, gastrointestinal (GI) hamartomatous polyposis most likely not associated with GI malignancy, hypotonia and variable mental retardation and psychomotor delay. While a lipid storage myopathy is still considered component to BRRS, its original aetiology, long chain acyl-coA dehydrogenase (LCHAD) deficiency has been questioned.

Germline *PTEN* mutations were originally found in two classic BRRS families (Marsh et al., 1997), and thus, a subset of BRRS is allelic to Cowden syndrome (see p. 179) (Marsh et al., 1999). Subsequently, 60 per cent of a series of BRRS probands were found to have germline *PTEN* mutations (Marsh et al., 1999). Of those that were mutation negative after PCR-based mutational analysis of exons 1–9 and flanking intronic regions, 10 per cent have been found to carry large deletions including or encompassing *PTEN* (Zhou et al., 2003a and b). Genotype–phenotype association analysis reveals that BRRS carrying germline *PTEN* mutations were at increased risk of neoplasia, especially malignant breast disease, and lipomatosis compared to those without *PTEN* mutations (Marsh et al., 1999).

Traditionally, medical management of BRRS has been symptomatic. However, given the genotype–phenotype association and that a subset of BRRS is allelic to Cowden syndrome, individuals with BRRS, especially those found to have germline *PTEN* mutations, should undergo similar surveillance and management to individuals with Cowden syndrome (p. 179). Because thyroid cancers can occur even in the teens in BRRS, it would be prudent to begin annual comprehensive physical examinations, paying particular attention to the neck, in the early teens.

Beckwith–Wiedemann syndrome (EMG syndrome and IGF2 overgrowth disorder)

This syndrome, with an estimated incidence of 1 in 14 000, is characterised by major (pre- and/or postnatal overgrowth, anterior abdominal wall defects (diastasis recti, umbilical hernia or exomphalos) and macroglossia) (see Fig. 12.2) and minor

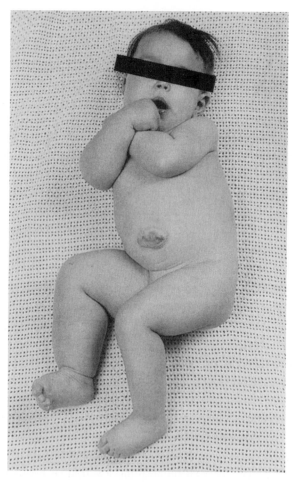

Fig. 12.2. Beckwith–Wiedemann syndrome.

features (earlobe grooves or helical rim pits, facial naevus flammeus, visceromegaly (liver, kidney, spleen), neonatal hypoglycaemia, hemihypertrophy, renal anomalies, cryptorchidism and, infrequently, cardiac defects) (Elliott et al., 1994). In addition embryonal tumours occur in about 8 per cent of patients. Strict diagnostic criteria were suggested by Elliott and Maher (1994) that required the presence of: (i) three major features or (ii) two major features plus three minor features (from ear creases or pits, hypoglycaemia, nephromegaly or hemihypertrophy). Less strict diagnostic criteria have also been proposed, for example at least two from: (a) positive family history, (b) macrosomia (height and weight >97 per centile), (c) anterior linear ear lobe creases/posterior helical ear pits, (d) macroglossia, (e) exomphalos/umbilical hernia, (f) visceromegaly involving one or more intra-abdominal organs including liver, spleen, kidneys, adrenal glands and pancreas, (g) embryonal tumour (e.g. Wilms tumour, hepatoblastoma, rhabdomyosarcoma) in childhood, (h) hemihypertrophy, (i) adrenocortical cytomegaly, (j) renal abnormalities including structural abnormalities, nephromegaly and nephrocalcinosis, (k) cleft palate (rare) and one from: (a) polyhydramnios, (b) neonatal hypoglycaemia, (c) facial naevus flammeus, (d) hemangioma, (e) characteristic facies, including midfacial hypoplasia and infraorbital creases, (f) cardiomegaly/structural cardiac anomalies/rarely cardiomyopathy, (g) diastasis recti and advanced bone age (Shuman and Weksberg http://www. geneclinics.org). However molecular genetic testing can diagnose most cases (Cooper et al., 2005). The characteristic craniofacial dysmorphological features of Beckwith–Wiedemann syndrome (BWS) are most apparent before the age of 3 years, and after the age of 5 years there are often only minor dysmorphisms. The differential diagnosis of BWS includes Perlman syndrome and Simpson–Golabi–Behmel syndrome and other overgrowth disorders, such as Weaver or Sotos syndrome.

The genetics of BWS are complex (Maher and Reik, 2000; Weksberg et al., 2003). Most published cases are reported to be sporadic, but approximately 15 per cent of cases are familial. Inheritance is as an autosomal dominant trait with parent-of-origin effects. Thus penetrance is more complete when the mother is the transmitting parent and examples of transmitting males with affected children are very rare (Koufos et al., 1989). As the features of BWS tend to vary there is wide variation in expression, and in some "sporadic" cases minor manifestations in relatives could have been overlooked. The penetrance of familial BWS is often incomplete. However, careful analysis of familial cases shows that siblings of affected individuals have a 50 per cent probability of being affected (full penetrance), whereas in sibships containing unaffected carriers penetrance is usually incomplete. Monozygotic twins discordant for BWS is well recognised. These clinical findings implicated genomic imprinting and molecular genetic studies have defined BWS as a model imprinting disorder. The finding of an increased incidence of BWS children conceived by assisted reproductive technologies suggested a link between these and genomic imprinting disorders (DeBaun et al., 2003; Gicquel et al., 2003; Maher et al., 2003).

BWS may result from chromosomal rearrangements, uniparental disomy or from mutations or epigenetic events involving imprinted genes at chromosome 11p15.5 (Maher and Reik, 2000; Cooper et al., 2005). Chromosome 11p15.5 was first implicated in BWS by the finding of paternally derived duplications of 11p15.5 in BWS patients. Subsequently maternally inherited balanced rearrangements of 11p15 were also demonstrated to be associated with BWS. It is estimated that up to 3 per cent of BWS patients have a chromosomal rearrangement. Chromosome 11 paternal uniparental disomy is found in ~20 per cent of sporadic cases and is invariably mosaic paternal isodisomy that includes the imprinted gene cluster at 11p15.5 that contains the maternally expressed genes *CDKN1C* and *H19* and the paternally expressed IGF2. Germline *CDKN1C* mutations occur in about half of familial cases and 5 per cent of sporadic cases (Hatada et al., 1996; Lam et al., 1999). Epigenetic errors at two putative imprinting control regions within 11p15.5 (IC1 and IC2) have also been implicated in BWS. Thus 5 per cent of BWS patients have an imprinting defect at the distal imprinting centre (IC1) such that as the maternal IGF2 and H19 alleles display a paternal epigenotype (hypermethylation and silencing of H19 and bi-allelic IGF2 expression). In 40 per cent of cases there is loss of paternal methylation at IC2 (KvDMR1) that is associated with silencing of CDKN1C expression and variable loss of imprinting (bi-allelic expression) of *IGF2*.

Genotype–phenotype correlations have been described for hemihypertrophy and exomphalos. Most cases with hemihypertrophy have mosaic uniparental disomy. There is a high incidence of exomphalos in patients with *CDKN1C* mutations and IC2 imprinting centre defects, but exomphalos is infrequent in patients with uniparental disomy or IC1 imprinting centre defects. In addition to patients with classical BWS, Morison et al. (1996) have reported that some patients with overgrowth and nephromegaly or Wilms tumour may have bi-allelic *IGF2* expression, and they coined the term "IGF2 overgrowth disorder" to describe these patients.

Patients with BWS have an increased risk of neoplasia. Wiedemann (1983) reviewed 388 children with BWS and found 29 children (7.5 per cent) with 32 tumours. Most tumours (26/29) were intra-abdominal (including 14 Wilms tumour, five adrenal carcinomas and two hepatoblastomas). Most tumours occur before the age of 5 years. A clinical association between hemihypertrophy and neoplasia in BWS was noted and among patients with BWS, the risk of Wilms tumour is highest in those with uniparental disomy and IC1 imprinting centre defect and the risk of Wilms tumour appears minimal in those with IC2 imprinting centre defects and CDKN1C mutations (Engel et al., 2000; Weksberg et al., 2001; DeBaun et al., 2002; Cooper et al., 2005). Thus in one study the risk of embryonal tumours was 9 per cent at age of 5 years in all cases (with a molecular genetic diagnosis) but 24 per cent in those with uniparental disomy (Cooper et al., 2005). Hepatoblastoma appears to be more common in children with IC2 defects so all cases of BWS should be offered screening for embryonal neoplasms. Thus it is recommended that abdominal ultrasound scans are performed in the neonatal period, then 3-monthly until 8 years of age. In those at increased risk of hepatoblastoma serum alphafetoprotein should be measured.

Birt–Hogg–Dubé syndrome

Following the description of familial renal oncocytoma (Weirich et al., 1998), it was reported that some familial renal oncocytoma kindreds contained affected individuals with rare hamartomatous tumours of the hair follicle known as fibrofolliculoma (Toro et al., 1999). Fibrofolliculomas are a characteristic feature of the dominantly inherited multisystem familial cancer syndrome Birt–Hogg–Dubé syndrome (Birt et al., 1977). Benign whitish-grey papular skin tumours develop on the face and upper body in the third decade and histological examination reveals fibrofolliculomas or trichodiscomas (Birt et al., 1977; Rongioletti et al., 1989). Additional features include lipomas and cystic lung lesions and pneumothorax. In some reports colonic polyposis is described, but Zbar et al. (2002) found a risk of renal cell carcinoma (RCC) but not colorectal cancer. A variety of histopathological subtypes of RCC have been described in Birt–Hogg–Dubé syndrome, but the most common (50 per cent) is a hybrid oncocytoma/chromophobe, 34 per cent are chromophobe RCC and 9 per cent clear cell (conventional) RCC (Pavlovich et al., 2002). The *BHD* gene maps to 17p11.2 and encodes a 64 kDa protein of unknown function (Nickerson et al., 2002). A mutation hotspot in a mononucleotide tract (C_8) in exon 11 has been identified. Interestingly two naturally occurring animal models of Birt–Hogg–Dubé syndrome, in the German Shepherd dog and rat, have been described (Jonasdottir et al., 2000; Okimoto et al., 2004). In view of the elevated risk of RCC in some BHD kindreds, it is suggested that affected individuals should be offered annual renal ultrasound scans from age of 25 years.

Blue rubber bleb naevus syndrome

This may occur as an autosomal dominant trait, but is usually sporadic and of unknown aetiology. Multiple vascular nipple-like lesions occur, especially on the trunk and upper arms and mucous membranes, and intestinal, hepatic and pulmonary angiomas may develop (Dobru et al., 2004). Bleeding from these lesions can lead to anaemia (Fukhro et al., 2002). Central nervous system (CNS) haemangioma and cerebellar medulloblastoma may also occur (Satya-Murti et al., 1986; Kim, 2000). It has been suggested that this syndrome is a variant of familial (autosomal dominant) venous malformations which has been mapped to chromosome 9p by linkage studies in two large kindreds (Gallione et al., 1995).

Blackfan–Diamond syndrome

This rare disorder (~1 in 250 000 births) is characterised by congenital hypoplastic anaemia with normal leucocyte and platelet counts. There is an increased risk of leukaemia (Alter, 1987). Gustavsson et al. (1997) estimated that 10–20 per cent of cases followed a recessive or dominant inheritance pattern, and they mapped a gene to chromosome 19q13 for both recessive and dominant forms. Subsequently Draptchinskaia et al. (1999) demonstrated germline mutations in the *RPS19* gene in Blackfan–Diamond anaemia (DBA). Overall about 25 per cent of DBA patients have *RPS19* mutations but a second locus has been mapped to 8p23 and there is evidence for further locus heterogeneity (Gazda et al., 2001).

Bloom syndrome

This rare autosomal recessive condition is much more common in Ashkenazi Jews than in other ethnic groups. It is characterised by low birth weight, growth deficiency and a sunlight-sensitive erythematous and telangiectatic rash, especially on the face from the first year of life. Sun exposure accentuates these changes, and may induce bullae, with bleeding and crusting on the face (especially the lips and eyelids). The nose is prominent in a long thin face, and there is clinodactyly. Spotty hypopigmentation and hyperpigmentation may be seen on the skin, and also "twin spots", which may be due to somatic recombination (Bloom, 1966). Adult height is usually less than 150 cm. Intelligence is normal. There is a severe immune defect with reduced gammaglobulin (IgA and IgM) levels, leading to a high incidence of chronic severe infections of the respiratory and GI tract. About 20 per cent of patients with Bloom syndrome develop neoplasms, half of these before the age of 20 years, and tumours may be multiple. Neoplasms are predominantly lymphatic and non-lymphatic leukaemia, lymphoma, and carcinomas of the mouth, stomach, oesophagus, colon, cervix and larynx. Early cervical screening should be offered to affected women. Screening for other cancers may be problematic, although regular oral examinations by a dental surgeon, and colonoscopy are also probably worthwhile. Myeloid leukaemia and myelodysplastic syndrome have been reported, often with monosomy for chromosome 7 (Aktas et al., 2000; Poppe et al., 2001). Wilms tumour has been described in four children with Bloom syndrome and one of these 4 children had a sib who developed a hepatocellular carcinoma at the age of 15 years (Cairney et al., 1987; Jain et al., 2001).

Few patients survive into adulthood, but in those that do, colorectal cancer has been reported. In one case, this occurred in the context of ulcerative colitis (Wang J et al., 1999), whereas in another case, an attenuated familial adenomatous polyposis (FAP) phenotype was observed (Lowy et al., 2001). Interestingly, a mucinous (i.e. hereditary non-polyposis colorectal cancer-like (HNPCC-like)) transverse colon cancer, with normal TP53 expression, has been reported in a 16-year old with Bloom syndrome. These observations led investigators to study the gene, *BLM*, identified by Ellis et al. (1995) (see Ellis and German, 1996) in individuals from the population with colorectal cancer. One mutation, *BLM: 2281del6ins7* is seen in approximately 1 in 110 Ashkenazi Jews, so this population was studied in detail. Overall, 1 in 54 Jews with colorectal cancer carried this allele, whereas the allele was seen in 1 in 118 controls (odds ratio: 2.76; 95 per cent CI: 1.4–5.5) (Gruber et al., 2002). This finding was supported by data showing that mice heterozygous for *Blm* developed twice the number of intestinal tumours when crossed with mice carrying a mutation of the *Apc* tumour suppressor gene (Goss et al., 2002). Somatic mutations in length repeats within *BLM* are also quite frequent in sporadic colorectal cancer (Calin et al., 1998), and interestingly, tend to be associated with mucinous colorectal cancers (Calin et al., 2000). Knocking-out *BLM* in karyotypically stable colorectal cancer cell lines results in increased sister chromatid exchange and homologous recombination (but without gross chromosomal rearrangements) (Traverso et al., 2003). Finally, in a murine model, chromosomal instability and tumour predisposition seems to correlate inversely with BLM protein levels (McDaniel et al., 2003). Taken together, these findings suggest that homozygous individuals are at considerably increased risk for colorectal cancer; and that heterozygosity for *BLM* can be added to the I1307 K *APC* allele as genetic risk factors for colorectal cancer in the Jewish population I1307K is at least 6 times as prevalent as *BLM^{Ash}*, and thus the clinical significance of the latter allele is very limited. Another possible founder mutation has been reported in Japan: *BLM: 631delCAA* (Kaneko et al., 2004), and studies of this allele in colorectal cancer in Japan would be of interest.

At the nuclear level, an elevated frequency of chromosomal breaks is observed, with an increase in sister chromatid exchanges, and an abnormal profile of DNA replication intermediates is reported in this condition (Lonn et al., 1990). The exact mechanism by which BLM maintains replication fidelity is debated. In a mouse model of Bloom syndrome, viable mice were prone to cancers at many sites, and cell lines showed elevated levels of mitotic recombination (and therefore loss of heterozygosity) (Luo et al., 2000). These data were supported by results in human cancer cells, as discussed above (Traverso et al., 2003).

There is a registry for cases of Bloom syndrome to help affected individuals and their families, and to assist in the assessment of the natural history of the disease. Although the registry is closed to accrual, follow-up continues. This registry is at the Laboratory of Human Genetics, New York, NY 10021, USA.

Carney complex (NAME syndrome, LAMB syndrome, Carney syndrome)

Carney complex (CNC) is a rare autosomal dominant heritable multiple neoplasia syndrome characterised by cardiac, endocrine, cutaneous and neural tumours, and a variety of mucocutaneous pigmented lesions. CNC is linked to at least two different loci. Germline mutations in *PRKAR1A*, on 17q22–q24, have been shown to cause a subset of CNC (Kirschner et al., 2000a and b). The gene on 2p15–p16 has yet to be identified. Some believe that a third minor locus might also be involved.

This rare condition is characterised by cardiac, breast and cutaneous myxomas, pigmented skin lesions and micronodular pigmented adrenal hyperplasia (Koopman and Happle, 1991). The tumours are commonly multicentric or bilateral, and the mean age at diagnosis of the first manifestation is 18 years. Most patients have two or more manifestations of the condition. Pituitary adenomas and testicular tumours (sertoli or Leydig cell in about 50 per cent of affected males) are associated, and the hormones secreted by these tumours cause characteristic phenotypic effects (Carney et al., 1986). Skin lesions include lentigines, blue naevi, dermal fibromas and myxoid neurofibromas. The pigmentation is spotty, particularly on the face (in 70 per cent of cases), hands and feet, and is similar to that seen in Peutz–Jeghers syndrome (PJS), although in the latter the lesions are seen more in the buccal region and palate, and the visceral lesions appear to be quite distinct in these two syndromes (Carney et al., 1985). Further, inner canthal pigmentation is virtually only seen in CNC. Eyelid myxomas are found in 16 per cent of affected patients. The tumours are usually benign, but liposarcomas and other malignant tumours may develop. The cardiac tumours are life threatening via embolism or directly.

CNC was found to be linked to 17q22–q24 and 2p15–p16. Germline loss-of-function mutations in *PRKR1A*, encoding the type 1A subunit of the protein kinase A receptor on 17q22–q24, have been found in a subset of CNC (Kirschner et al., 2000a and b). Nonsense-mediated decay of mutant transcript appears to be the mechanism leading to loss-of-function (Kirschner et al., 2000a).

As with other inherited tumour syndromes, mutation analysis should begin with a clinically affected individual. Once a family-specific mutation in *PRKR1A* is found, then predictive testing may be offered. Clinical and biochemical screening for CNC and medical surveillance for affected patients remain the gold standard for the care of patients with CNC. In brief, for post-pubertal paediatric and for adult patients of both sexes with established CNC, the following annual studies are recommended: echocardiogram, measurement of urinary free cortisol levels (which may be supplemented by diurnal cortisol or the overnight 1 mg dexamethasone testing) and serum IGF1 levels (Stratakis et al., 1999). Male patients should also have testicular ultrasonography at the initial evaluation; microscopic LCCSCT (large cell calcifying sertoli cell tumour) may be followed by annual ultrasound thereafter (Stratakis et al., 2001). Thyroid ultrasonography should be obtained at the initial evaluation, and may be repeated, as needed (Stratakis et al., 2001). Transabdominal ultrasonography in female patients is recommended during the first evaluation but need not be repeated, unless there is a detectable abnormality, because of the relatively low risk of ovarian malignancy (Stratakis et al., 2001). Because cardiac myxoma is responsible for a significant amount of morbidity and mortality, paediatric patients with CNC should have echocardiography during their first 6 months of life and annually thereafter; bi-annual echocardiographic evaluation may be necessary for patients with history of an excised myxoma.

Cockayne syndrome

This is a very rare autosomal recessive disorder characterised by growth failure leading to extremely short stature, lack of subcutaneous fat, cutaneous photosensitivity, deafness, progressive optic atrophy, neurological deterioration with a leukodystrophy and mental retardation. There is brain dysmyelination with calcium deposits. There is a typical "salt and pepper" retinitis and/or cataracts. These features develop from late infancy, but there is considerable variability of the phenotype, even within families (Mahmoud et al., 2002). Characteristic facial features include large ears, sunken eyes, and limbs that are relatively long. There is type II hyperlipoproteinaemia. There appears to be a deficiency of DNA repair after exposure to UV light, and deficiency in cellular repair of oxidative DNA damage. Death usually occurs before the age of 20 years and malignancy is not reported to be specifically increased in this condition. The disease is genetically heterogeneous, and genes for complementation groups CS-A and CS-B have been identified (Stefanini et al., 1996). The CS-B gene product is involved in transcription-coupled and/or global genome nucleotide excision repair of DNA damage induced by UV light, and other oxidative DNA damage (Mahmoud et al., 2002; Osterod et al., 2002; Tuo et al., 2003). Notably, in contrast to human Cockayne syndrome, homozygous knock-out mice for the murine orthologue of the human *CSA* gene ($Csa^{-/-}$) develop skin tumours after chronic exposure to UV light (van der Horst et al., 2002). The reason why humans with Cockayne syndrome do not develop skin cancer is not known. Interestingly, other cases of Cockayne syndrome with features overlapping with those of xeroderma pigmentosum (XP) are due to mutations in the *XPB*, *XPD* or *XPG* genes (Rapin et al., 2000). *XPG* and *CSB* mutations may also be responsible for the cerebro-oculo-facio-skeletal (COFS) syndrome (Graham et al., 2001). COFS is another autosomal recessive neurodegenerative disorder with growth failure, joint contractures, cataracts, microcornea and optic atrophy.

Coeliac disease

Patients with coeliac disease have an increased risk of oesophageal cancer (Harris et al., 1967), cancer of the mouth and pharynx, small bowel carcinoma and lymphoma (Holmes et al., 1989; Ferguson and Kingstone, 1996). Although non-Hodgkin lymphoma is the main cause of cancer death (Corrao et al., 2001), in a series of small bowel cancers, 13 per cent of adenocarcinoma cases and 39 per cent of lymphomas occurred in patients with coeliac disease providing evidence that coeliac disease confers susceptibility to adenocarcinoma of the small bowel, as well as lymphoma (Howdle et al., 2003). Small bowel adenocarcinomas associated with coeliac disease have a high frequency of microsatellite instability (MSI) and somatic inactivation of MLH1 or MSH2 (Potter et al., 2004). Although the absolute risk of malignancy in coeliac disease is small, those cases complicated by malignancy often appear to have been poorly controlled.

Coeliac disease itself shows familial aggregation, and a strong human leucocyte antigen (HLA) association (Houlston and Ford, 1996). Familial clustering appears to reflect multifactorial inheritance with major genetic risk factors (HLA-DQ2 and HLA-DQ8) and environmental triggers combining. Thus it appears that genes within the HLA class II DQ region are necessary but not sufficient for coeliac disease to develop. About 95 per cent of all patients have a DQ2 allele with DQ2 homozygotes being at highest risk. Of the remaining 5 per cent, most are DQ8 positive. It is estimated that HLA class II genes account for 50 per cent of genetic susceptibility to coeliac disease and non-HLA-associated genes are also implicated (Treem 2004 and references within).

Common variable immunodeficiency

This comprises a heterogeneous group of disorders characterised by hypogammaglobulinaemia, humoral immunodeficiency and susceptibility to infection. Some patients may also have defects in some aspects of cell-mediated immunity. Many cases are acquired, but genetic factors have been implicated in some cases and autosomal recessive inheritance proposed. There is an increased incidence of lymphoid malignancy in patients with common variable immuno-deficiency (Kersey et al., 1988).

Costello syndrome

This condition is also known as faciocutaneous syndrome, and is usually sporadic, possibly representing new mutations. The facial features are similar to Noonan syndrome, with increasingly coarse features with age, and nasal papillomata. There is excess skin on the hands. Developmental delay is usual. There is an increased risk of cancer, possibly up to 17 per cent, particularly rhabdomyosarcomas, neuroblastomas and transitional carcinomas of the bladder, and screening by 3–6 monthly abdominal ultrasound and 6–12 monthly urinary catecholamine estimations until 5 years of age and annual urinalysis thereafter until 10 years of age (DeBaun, 2002; Gripp et al., 2002). Most cases have heterozygous de novo activating mutations in the *HRAS* proto-oncogene (Aoki et al., 2005).

Cowden syndrome (multiple hamartoma syndrome)

Cowden syndrome (CS, MIM 158350) is an autosomal dominantly inherited multiple hamartoma syndrome characterised by an increased risk of breast, thyroid and endometrial cancer. Germline mutations in *PTEN*, encoding a lipid and protein phosphatase on 10q23.3, are associated with 85 per cent of CS (Eng, 2003; Zhou et al., 2003a and b; Enge and Peacocke 1998).

Clinical diagnosis is often a challenge, on account of the protean manifestations of CS, many of which can occur in isolation in the general population. For this reason, the true incidence is not known. After identification of *PTEN* as the *CS* gene (Liaw et al., 1997), a molecular-based study revealed the incidence to be at least 1 in 200 000 (Nelen et al., 1997; Nelen et al., 1999), although this is likely still to be an under-estimate. Because CS is under-diagnosed, the proportion of apparently sporadic cases and familial cases (two or more affected, related individuals) is not precisely known. As a broad estimate, perhaps 40–65 per cent of CS cases are familial (Marsh et al., 1998; 1999; Eng, unpublished observations, 2003).

The lack of uniform diagnostic criteria for CS prior to 1995, led to the formation of the International Cowden Consortium (C. Eng, Co-ordinator and Chair, engc@ccf.org), which represented a group of centres mainly in North America and Europe interested in systematically studying this syndrome to localise the susceptibility gene. The consortium arrived at a set of consensus operational diagnostic criteria based on published data and expert opinion (Nelen et al., 1996; Eng and

Parsons, 1998). These criteria have been revised annually in the context of new molecular-based data and are reflected in the practice guidelines of the US-based National Comprehensive Cancer Network Genetics/High-Risk Panel (NCCN, 1999; Eng, 2000a) (www.nccn.org for 2005 and 2006 revisions), as follows:

1. Pathognomonic criteria:
    - Mucocutaneous lesions:
        - Trichilemmomas, facial
        - Acral keratoses
        - Papillomatous papules
        - Mucosal lesions
    - Lhermitte–Duclos disease (LDD)
2. Major criteria:
    - Breast carcinoma
    - Thyroid carcinoma (non-medullary), especially follicular thyroid carcinoma
    - Macrocephaly (Megalencephaly) (≥97 centile)
    - Endometrial carcinoma
3. Minor criteria:
    - Other thyroid lesions (e.g. adenoma or multinodular goiter)
    - Mental retardation (IQ ≤ 75)
    - GI hamartomas
    - Fibrocystic disease of the breast
    - Lipomas
    - Fibromas
    - Genito-urinary tumours (e.g. RCC, uterine fibroids) or malformation

Operational diagnosis in an individual:

1. Mucocutaneous lesions alone if:
    (a) there are 6 or more facial papules, of which 3 or more must be trichilem-moma, or
    (b) cutaneous facial papules and oral mucosal papillomatosis, or
    (c) oral mucosal papillomatosis and acral keratoses, or
    (d) palmo plantar keratoses, 6 or more.
2. 2 Major criteria but one must include macrocephaly or LDD
3. 1 Major and 3 minor criteria
4. 4 minor criteria

Operational diagnosis in a family where one individual is diagnostic for Cowden:

1. The pathognomonic criterion/ia
2. Any one major criterion with or without minor criteria
3. Two minor criteria

More than 90 per cent of individuals affected with CS are believed to manifest a phenotype by the age of 20 years (Nelen et al., 1996; Eng, 2000c). By the
end of the third decade (i.e. 29 years), 99 per cent of affected individuals are
believed to have developed at least the mucocutaneous signs of the syndrome,
although any of a number of component features are manifest as well. The most
commonly reported manifestations are mucocutaneous lesions, thyroid abnormalities, fibrocystic disease and carcinoma of the breast, multiple, early-onset
uterine leiomyoma, and macrocephaly (specifically, megencephaly) (Starink et al.,
1986; Hanssen and Fryns, 1995; Mallory, 1995; Longy and Lacombe, 1996;
Eng, 2000c).

The two most well-documented component malignancies are carcinomas of
the breast and epithelial thyroid gland (Starink et al., 1986). In women with CS,
lifetime risks for breast cancer are estimated to range from 25 to 50 per cent
(Starink et al., 1986; Longy and Lacombe, 1996) in contrast to the 11 per cent in
the general population. The age at onset ranges between 14 and 65 years, with a
mean around 40–45 years (Starink et al., 1986; Longy and Lacombe, 1996).
The histopathology of CS breast cancer is adenocarcinoma of the breast, both
ductal and lobular (Schrager et al., 1997). Male breast cancer may be a minor
component of the syndrome (Marsh et al., 1998; Fackenthal et al., 2001). The
lifetime risk for differentiated thyroid cancer can be as high as 10 per cent in
males and females with CS. It is unclear if the age of onset is truly earlier than
that of the general population. Histologically, the thyroid cancer is predominantly follicular carcinoma although papillary histology has also been rarely
observed (Starink et al., 1986; Eng and Parsons, 1998; Eng, unpublished observations). Endometrial carcinoma may also be a component cancer of CS (Marsh
et al., 1998; DeVivo et al., 2000; Eng, 2000c). What its frequency is in mutation
carriers is as yet unknown.

The most common non-malignant component lesions include trichilemmo-
mas (hamartoma of the infundibulum of the hair follicle) and papillomatous
papules (90–100 per cent), thyroid adenomas and goitre (67 per cent), breast
fibroadenomas and fibrocystic disease (75 per cent), macrocephaly (>50 per cent),
and genito-urinary abnormalities (40 per cent) including uterine fibroids and
malformations. A rather striking non-malignant hamartoma is Lhermitte–
LDD or dysplastic gangliocytoma of the cerebellum (Eng et al., 1994a) which
usually manifests later in life at first as subtly as dysmetria on intent and progressing to frank ataxia.

CS was mapped to 10q22–q23 (Nelen et al., 1996). Germline mutations in
PTEN have been found in 85 per cent of CS probands, diagnosed by the strict
International Cowden Consortium criteria (Marsh et al., 1998; Zhou et al.,
2003b). These mutations result in loss-of-function and the majority occur in

exons 5, 7 and 8, which encode the phosphatase domain although mutations can occur throughout the gene including the promoter (Zhou et al., 2003b). Germline mutations in *PTEN* have also been found in approximately 60 per cent of individuals with Bannayan–Riley–Ruvalcaba syndrome, (BRRS) (p. 169) (Marsh et al., 1997; 1999). Thus CS and BRRS are allelic. Compared to *PTEN* mutations in CS, mutations in BRRS tend to occur in the 3′ half of the gene (Eng, 2003). There is a genotype–phenotype association in CS (Marsh et al., 1998): families found to have germline *PTEN* mutations have an increased risk of malignancy, in particular, breast cancer. The presence of CS and BRRS features in a single family, of glycogenic acanthosis of the oesophagus or of LDD increases (to >95 per cent) the prior probability of finding a *PTEN* mutation (Marsh et al., 1999; McGarrity et al., 2003; Zhou et al., 2003a).

Germline *PTEN* mutations have also been described in up to 20 per cent of Proteus syndrome and 50 per cent of a Proteus-like syndrome (Zhou et al., 2000; 2001a; Smith et al., 2002). Germline mutations in *PTEN* have been described in single patients with megencephaly and VATER association and with megencephaly and autism (Dasouki et al., 2001; Reardon et al., 2001). However, larger series of these two rare disorders need to be analysed further before firm conclusions can be drawn.

All individuals with or suspected of having CS or any PTEN-related disorder should be referred to cancer genetic professionals. *PTEN* mutation analysis is a useful molecular diagnostic test and in families with a known *PTEN* mutation, is a good predictive test.

Surveillance recommendations are based on expert opinion, governed by the component neoplasias, breast carcinoma, epithelial thyroid carcinoma and adenocarcinoma of the endometrium (Eng, 2000c; Pilarski and Eng, 2004) (www.nccn.org). Males and females should undergo annual physical examinations paying particular attention to the neck (thyroid) beginning at age of 18 or 5 years younger than the youngest diagnosis of thyroid cancer in the family. A single baseline thyroid ultrasound examination is recommended. Females should begin annual clinical breast examination and breast self examination around the age of 25 or 5 years younger than the youngest age at diagnosis of breast cancer in the family. Annual mammography should begin at 30–35 years or 5 years younger than the earliest age of breast cancer diagnosis in the family. The endometrium should be clinically screened beginning at the age of 35–40 or 5 years younger than the earliest age of endometrial cancer diagnosis in the family: annual blind repeal biopsies prior to menopause and transabdominal ultrasound after menopause. Clinicians who look after CS patients should be mindful to note any other seemingly non-component neoplasias, which might be over-represented in any particular family as well.

Patients carrying the clinical diagnosis of CS and any individual with a germline *PTEN* mutation, regardless of clinical diagnosis, should undergo surveillance.

Denys–Drash syndrome

This is a rare disorder characterised by male pseudohermaphroditism, Wilms tumour and characteristic glomerulonephropathy causing progressive renal failure. Not all patients have the complete triad, and nephropathy plus Wilms tumour or urogenital abnormalities are sufficient to make the diagnosis. Wilms tumour in Denys–Drash syndrome (DDS) presents early (at a mean age of 18 months) and is usually bilateral (Jadresic et al., 1991). Gonadoblastoma may also occur. The nephropathy is characterised by the presence of focal or diffuse glomerulosclerosis and usually presents with proteinuria, progressing to nephrotic syndrome and hypertension, and then end-stage renal failure by 3 years of age (Coppes et al., 1993). Males (XY karyotype) with DDS usually have ambiguous genitalia or phenotypically normal female external genitalia (male pseudohermaphroditism). In addition, the internal genitalia are frequently dysplastic or inappropriate (Mueller, 1994). Screening for Wilms tumour is discussed on p. 114, but the risk of Wilms tumour in DDS is high enough for bilateral prophylactic nephrectomy to be performed in children with incomplete DDS (e.g. pseudohermaphroditism, hypogonadism and renal failure) (Hu, M et al., 2004). Molecular genetic analysis of patients with this syndrome has demonstrated de-novo germline *WT1* mutations in most cases (reviewed by Coppes et al., 1993; Mueller, 1994). The majority of mutations affect the zinc-finger domains and are thought to have a dominant negative effect on genital development (Little et al., 1993). DDS is allelic with Frasier syndrome which is characterised by focal glomerular sclerosis, renal failure and complete gonadal dysgenesis. *WT1* mutations causing Frasier syndrome alter the balance of WT1 isoforms (Klamt et al., 1998). Although the risk of Wilms tumour is much less in Frasier syndrome than in DDS, gonadoblastoma is frequent.

Down syndrome

The risk of acute leukaemia in Down syndrome (DS) (trisomy 21) is 20–30 times that of the general population. This increased risk relates both to acute lymphoblastic and acute myeloid leukaemia (AML), and transient leukaemia occurs almost exclusively in infants with DS (Hasle et al., 2000). About 1 per cent of infants with DS will be affected, most commonly with acute non-lymphocytic leukaemia subtype M7-megakaryocytic leukaemia, a type very rare in individuals with normal karyotypes (Zipursky et al., 1992; Shen et al., 1995). Acute megakaryolastic leukaemia (AMKL) is particularly prevalent, with an estimated 500-fold increased risk compared to the general population, and a transient form of AMKL (TL) is seen in about 10 per cent of cases with DS, which usually resolves, but about 20 per cent will develop AMKL within the first 4 years of life. Leukaemia comprises about 60 per cent of all malignancies and 90 per cent of all childhood malignancies in DS. The standard incidence rate (SIR) for leukaemia in DS is 56 at <4 years and 10 at 5–29 years of age. This risk is particularly pronounced for AML, usually early onset, 49 per cent developing below 1 year of age (Ragab et al., 1991; Hasle, 2001). AML-M after myelodysplastic syndrome is characteristic, as is trisomy 8 with reduced granulocyte lineage. The cumulative risk of leukaemia in DS is 2.1 per cent by age of 5 years and 2.7 per cent by age of 30 years. Leukaemic clones in DS are nearly always megaloblastic with GATA1 (Zinc finger transcription factor required for erythroid and megakaryocytic development) mutations conferring a clonal advantage (Groet et al., 2003). Leukaemic blasts in DS-AMKL harbour mutations in GATA1, which encodes a haematopoietic transcription factor. Most mutations cluster in exon 2 resulting in a truncated mutant protein, GATA1s, lacking the amino-terminal transcriptional activating domain. These mutations are also demonstrable at birth, thus representing an early intrauterine event, and a persistent subclone of TL cells may develop into AMKL as a result of additional mutations (Hitzler and Zipursky 2004). However, the overall occurrence of solid tumours (especially breast cancer) in DS is reduced, except for retinoblasoma and germ cell tumours (Look, 2003).

Familial adenomatous polyposis

This is the most common of the hereditary polyposis syndromes, with a prevalence of about 1 in 8000 (Alm and Licznerski, 1973). It is inherited as an autosomal dominant trait with high penetrance but variable age at onset, and the mutation rate is high (up to 30 per cent of cases are considered to be new mutations (Bussey et al., 1978) although this may be an overestimate, and some single generation cases may be due to bi-allelic germline mutations in MYH) (Sieber et al., 2003). FAP is characterised by the appearance of over a hundred, to thousands of adenomatous polyps in the colon (Bussey, 1975). Polyps usually develop in the teens and penetrance is almost complete by age of 40 years in classical cases (see Fig. 12.3). Progression to malignancy is inevitable, and colorectal carcinoma often develops in untreated cases by about the fourth decade or even in childhood, 20–30 years earlier than in non-familial colon cancer. Histologically, single crypt adenomas are a characteristic feature. Polyps also occur elsewhere in the GI tract. Gastric polyps in FAP are of two types: benign hyperplastic fundic gland

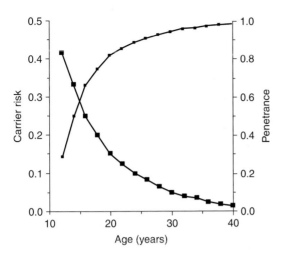

Fig. 12.3. Age-related carrier risk (larger squares) for relatives at 50% prior risk of FAP, that is an affected parent, and a negative bowel examination at that age. The age-related risk was derived from the age-related penetrance data (smaller squares). Adapted from Burn et al., 1991.

polyps occur in most patients, and adenomas may also occur, usually in the pyloric region of the stomach, but at a much lower frequency (Kurtz et al., 1987; Domizio et al., 1990). Gastric cancer may develop, even in young patients. Adenomatous duodenal polyps occur in most patients with FAP (over 80 per cent), are most numerous around the ampulla of Vater, and are associated with a significant risk of malignant transformation. Duodenal cancer is now the leading cause of death in this condition if colorectal cancer is prevented, and occurs in about 5 per cent of cases (Spigelman et al., 1995; Groves et al., 2002). There is some evidence that the administration of oral sulindac (a non-steroidal anti-inflammatory drug) or cyclo-oxygenase-2 (COX-2) inhibitors in general may cause regression of duodenal adenomas (Farmer et al., 1991; Oshima et al., 1996; Phillips et al., 2002). Carcinoma of the rectal stump may occur (in about 10 per cent of cases) after surgical removal of the colon and ileo-rectal anastomosis (Bulow, 1984), and COX-2 inhibitors may also be effective in reducing polyp recurrence in the colorectum (Steinbach et al., 2000). Carcinoma of the gallbladder and bile ducts also occurs (Walsh et al., 1987).

Extra-intestinal lesions develop in most patients with FAP, and may be apparent before the bowel lesions. Epidermoid cysts may occur in two-thirds of patients, and although they can develop anywhere on the body, they are most noticeable on the scalp. These are very rare in normal children before puberty. Osteomas of the mandible may be detected in more than 90 per cent of patients using orthopan-tomograms, and are uncommon in the general population (4 per cent). A third of patients may have impacted teeth, and dentigenous cysts, supernumerary and unerupted teeth may occur (Bulow et al., 1984). Exostoses may develop in the skull, digits and long bones, and cortical thickening is described. The association of FAP with sebaceous cysts, osteomas and supernumerary cysts is known as Gardner syndrome. Although older reports speculated that the two might be distinct diseases, careful review of large families demonstrated that both can occur within single kindreds. That FAP and Gardner syndrome are allelic disorders has been proven by the detection of *APC* gene mutations in patients with Gardner syndrome (see below).

The most common extra-intestinal manifestation of FAP is multiple areas of retinal pigmentation, said to indicate areas of congenital hypertrophy of the retinal pigment epithelium (CHRPE). These are found in about three-quarters of affected individuals. These are discrete, darkly pigmented, rounded lesions, 50–200 μm in diameter, and may have depigmentation around them (Fig. 12.4). Smaller, solitary, unilateral lesions may be seen in normal people, but it is rare for normal individuals to have more than three lesions (Burn et al., 1991). Most (although the exact proportion differs between series) patients with FAP have four or more CHRPEs and there are qualitative differences between areas of CHRPEs in FAP patients and normals: larger, oval, pigmented lesions with surrounding halo (type A lesions) are specific for FAP whereas CHRPEs in controls are usually small dots (type B) (Polkinghorne et al., 1990). Therefore, the presence of multiple bilateral, ocular lesions (four or more) in an asymptomatic individual at risk for FAP suggests that he or she has the condition. A CHRPE coefficient has been proposed, whereby type A lesions are given a score of 3 and type B lesions a score of 1; CHRPE-positive status is then defined as an individual who has a score of 3 or over (Olschwang et al., 1993). Histological information is scanty, but the larger lesions are probably congenital, and appear to be choristomas of myelinated axons; the small lesions may show enlarged retinal pigment epithelial cells with increased pigment (Parker et al., 1990). CHRPEs have been detected in infancy and are thought to be congenital; they can therefore be used as a biomarker for the *APC* mutation from birth (although there may be little indication to determine a child's status until he or she reaches an age at which screening is to commence). There are difficulties in using the presence of CHRPE as a marker for FAP in at-risk individuals. There are interfamilial differences in predisposition to CHRPE so that in some families multiple CHRPEs are usually present in affected individuals, whereas in other families gene carriers tend to have fewer than four CHRPEs (Romania et al., 1989; Maher et al., 1992). This heterogeneity of CHRPE expression is thought to be related to the position of the mutation in the *APC* gene, mutations distal to exon 9 being more prone to be associated with such lesions (Olschwang et al., 1993; Bunyan et al., 1995). However there are exceptions to this (Pack et al., 1996), and there is intrafamilial

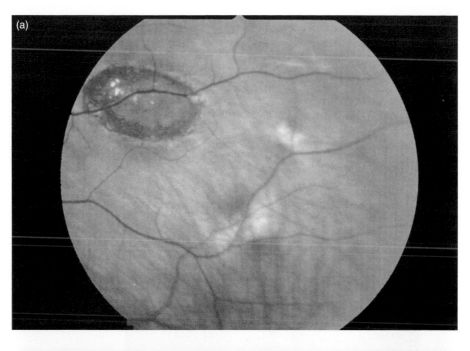

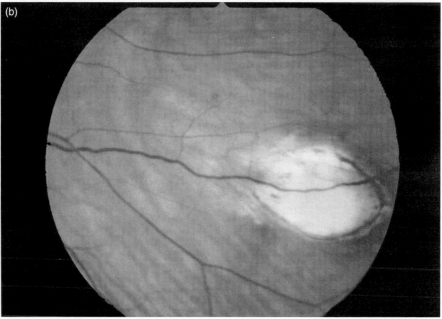

Fig. 12.4. FAP: (a) pigmented CHRPE, (b) depigmented CHRPE and (c) florid colonic polyposis.

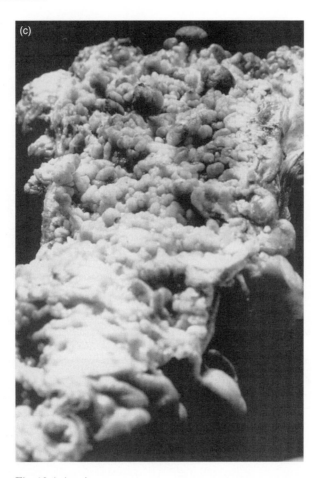

Fig. 12.4. (*cont.*)

variability in numbers of CHRPEs (Hodgson et al., 1994). Nevertheless, it has been estimated that in families in which CHRPEs appear to be a feature of the disease, the finding of fewer than three lesions in an individual at 50 per cent risk reduces the carrier risk whereas the presence of more than three lesions conveys a very high probability that the individual is affected (Burn et al., 1991).

Desmoid disease is common in FAP, occurring in about 5–10 per cent of cases. It is nearly twice as common in females as in males and occurs at an earlier age in females (Klemmer et al., 1987). Desmoids are more common in some families than in others. Histologically, they are composed of very vascular, fibrous tissue, and may be diffuse or encapsulated. They occur predominantly in the small bowel mesentery, peritoneum or abdominal wall, and often develop after a surgical procedure or pregnancy; 10 per cent resolve; 50 per cent may remain stable for prolonged periods; 30 per cent fluctuate; and 10 per cent grow rapidly. Desmoid tumours do not metastasise but do infiltrate locally and can cause major morbidity and death, being one of the three most common causes of death in FAP (with colorectal and upper GI cancer). They tend to recur after surgery so treatment with sulindac or cytotoxic chemotherapy with computerised tomography monitoring is preferable.

Extra-intestinal cancers associated with FAP include papillary carcinoma of the thyroid, brain tumours (medulloblastoma, astrocytoma) and hepatoblastoma). Papillary carcinoma of the thyroid, characteristically the cribriform variant, appears to occur at increased frequency in young women (under 35 years of age) with FAP and tends to occur in individuals with specific mutations in the *APC* gene, particularly at codon 1061 (Plail et al., 1987; Fenton et al., 2001). Brain tumours (especially astrocytomas) are rare overall, but the relative risk is high in individuals with FAP: 23 to age of 29 years for all brain tumours (7 for all ages), and 99 to age of 29 years for cerebellar medulloblastomas. Turcot syndrome is often due to *APC* mutations and is thus a variant of FAP in most cases (see p. 215; Kropilak et al., 1989; Hamilton et al., 1995). A number of cases of hepatoblastoma have been described in children at risk of inheriting FAP and although the absolute risk is small the relative risk is is high (>500) and screening might be considered in high-risk families (Garber et al., 1988; Hirschman et al., 2005).

Classically, the diagnosis of FAP is made clinically by a finding of more than 100 adenomatous polyps in the colon and rectum, with histological evidence of single crypt adenomas. The differential diagnosis is from other causes of intestinal polyposis, most importantly MYH-associated polyposis (p. 72 and p. 230) and other causes of inherited bowel cancer, such as HNPCC. Variable numbers of adenomatous polyps occur in families in which affected individuals have "flat adenomas", or "attenuated FAP" with multiple adenomas, usually fewer than 100, and such a phenotype may be caused by mutations in the first 4 exons of the *APC* gene (Leppert et al., 1990; Olschwang et al., 1993).

The FAP gene (*APC*) was localised to chromosome 5q21 following the serendipitous report of a mentally retarded man who had Gardner syndrome and a constitutional deletion of chromosome 5q (Herera et al., 1986). Characterisation of the mutation in the *APC* gene in an affected individual in the family (Groden et al., 1991; Kinzler et al., 1991) allows predictive testing to be made available to at-risk relatives. The gene is large, and has 15 exons, of which exon 15 is much the largest. Currently, it is possible to detect mutations in the *APC* gene in up to 82 per cent of families (Armstrong et al., 1997; Giardiello et al., 1997). Most mutations in FAP patients are frameshift (2/3) or nonsense (1/3) mutations which result in the production of a truncated protein (Nagase and Nakamura, 1993). Many different mutations have been described, but there are two common ones, at codons 1061 and 1309 in exon 15. The *APC* gene product appears to function as a tumour suppressor with subcellular location and interaction with catenins (Munemitsu et al., 1995). It contains a number of coiled-coil heptad repeats at the 5′ end that promote oligomerisation; the central part of the gene contains β-catenin-binding domains, involved in cell–cell interaction, and Armadillo repeats, and the 3′ end contains tubulin-binding domains, with properties of binding to microtubules (reviewed by Ilyas and Tomlinson, 1997; Fodde, 2001).

Phenotype–genotype correlations are apparent, with the common mutations (1309 and 1061) being associated with a severe phenotype (Nugent et al., 1994), mutations before exon 9 usually being associated with a lack of CHRPE, and mutations in the first 6 exons being associated with a more variable and often milder phenotype, including "attenuated FAP" (Foulkes, 1995). However, these correlations are not clear cut, and there is considerable intrafamilial variation (Bunyan et al., 1995) and the absence (in a cytogenetic deletion) of one whole APC allele causes a classical FAP, or possibly somewhat milder phenotype (Hodgson et al., 1993). *APC* mutations found in "attenuated FAP" most commonly occur in exon 4; however, the phenotype in different individuals with the same mutation may vary widely (Spirio et al., 1993), and many individuals with this "attenuated" form do not appear to have *APC* mutations; some may have MYH associated polyposis. The observation that very short variant proteins may result in a less severe phenotype tends to support the "dominant negative" theory, but large deletions of the gene may be found in individuals with a severe phenotype, so that other factors including the loss of the mild APC mutant allele (Spirio et al., 1998) or the effects of other polymorphic alleles such at the *NAT1* and *NAT2* genes (Crabtree et al., 2004) must also be involved in the pathogenesis of the disease process. Approximately one third of sporadic cases of FAP do not have detectable mutations in the *APC* gene, but as stated above biallelic MYH mutation accounts for a fraction of these.

Usually there is reasonable consistency with regard to severity of adenomatous disease in different individuals with FAP within a single family, but some worrying exceptions to this have been reported, with very variable age at onset of polyps in different cases, some presenting decades later than their affected relatives (Evans et al., 1993). This implies that great caution should be exercised when discharging "at-risk" patients with no detectable adenomas from follow-up.

The phenotypic effects of a germline *APC* mutation are not always consistent, thus the identical mutation may or may not be associated with extra-colonic features or medulloblastoma (Kinzler and Vogelstein, 1987), and the severity of polyposis is less concordant in the same family the more distantly related the affected individuals. FAP modifier genes have therefore been proposed, and one such gene has been delineated in the mouse model Mom[1] (modifier of the multiple intestinal neoplasia, MIN) phenotype, which encodes a secreted phospholipase A2. Other potential modifiers include genes encoding DNA methyltransferase and COX-2 (Fearon, 1997; Crabtree et al., 2002; 2003).

Acquired *APC* point mutations are found in adenomas and sporadic colon cancers (Bourne, 1991), demonstrating that loss-of-function of both *APC* alleles is an early event in colonic neoplastic change.

An apparently "benign" mutation in the *APC* was detected in an individual with a family history of colorectal cancer but not polyposis. Subsequent analysis suggested that this T–A mutation, germline mutation, predicted to result in a change from isoleucine to lysine position 1307 of the protein predisposed to the development of somatic mutations of the *APC* gene, and that gene carriers were therefore predisposed to colorectal cancer without florid polyposis. There is thought to be a twofold increase in risk of bowel cancer in mutation carriers (Rozen et al., 2002). This mutation is almost entirely restricted to the Ashkenazim (Laken et al., 1997), and there has been much debate about whether population screening for this mutation in Ashkenazim should be advocated, with colonoscopic surveillance for gene carriers. Currently the increase in risk is not thought to be sufficient for such a measure to be appropriate, but colonoscopy is in fact often offered to individuals when the risk is less than twofold elevated. Other germline variants such as *E1317Q* may be associated with an attenuated phenotype (Lamlum et al., 2000), but the evidence for this is much less clear (e.g Hahnloser et al., 2003).

Management

Patients with FAP should be offered total colectomy with ileo-rectal anastomosis or proctocolectomy with restorative ileo-anal anastomosis once colonic polyps have developed. The risk of colorectal cancer is significant once polyps have begun to develop, irrespective of polyp density (Phillips and Spigleman, 1996). After surgery conserving the rectal stump, subsequent management should include lifelong surveillance of the rectal stump by yearly sigmoidoscopy as there is a 3.5 per cent risk of colorectal cancer in it after 5 years, rising to 10 per cent at 10 years. Proctocolectomy removes this risk and may be done after 50 years of age. In addition, since upper GI cancer is reported to occur in 5 per cent of patients, with an estimated prevalence of duodenal dysplasia of up to 90 per cent, initial surveillance by means of upper GI endoscopy at about 25 years of age to give a baseline for subsequent follow-up is suggested (Arvanitis et al., 1990; Debinsky et al., 1995). Subsequent endoscopies every 2–3 years could be continued, depending upon the severity of duodenal disease. If adenomas are detected, they should be biopsied; larger adenomas may be removed and further surveillance continued with annual duodenoscopy, depending on the Spigelman severity score (Dunlop, 2002).

Palpation of the thyroid gland and possibly ultrasound in young women with FAP has been suggested, but the rarity of death from thyroid cancer in this disease makes this of questionable benefit unless there is a family history of thyroid cancer.

Relatives of affected individuals should be ascertained with the help of a genetic register, and those at risk of inheriting the disease should be offered screening and genetic testing if possible. Screening of at-risk relatives is usually commenced between the ages of 11 and 13 years by annual sigmoidoscopy because the rectum is involved by adenomas at an early stage and polyps rarely develop before 11 years of age (Alm and Licznerski, 1973). However, if symptoms arise, it may be necessary to arrange endoscopy earlier because there are case reports of colonic polyps developing in young children (Distante et al., 1996). In addition, once a child has been found to carry the APC mutation in the family, it is appropriate to consider colonoscopy in their early teens to establish the extent of polyposis. In an at-risk child where a predictive genetic test is not available, if polyps are found, these are biopsied (to confirm they are adenomatous and to exclude malignancy) and colonoscopy is arranged. Although small numbers of polyps can be managed by endoscopic resection, because of the inevitability of florid polyposis develop-ing and the risk of malignant change, definitive surgery (see above) is usually arranged at this stage. In the absence of positive findings, sigmoidoscopy is con-tinued annually, with colonoscopies with dye spray after 20 years of age, to exclude more proximal polyposis. This is continued to at least the age of 40 years, by which time the risk to an individual with an affected parent has fallen below 1 per cent (see Fig. 12.3). However, since very variable age at onset has been described in some families, it is advisable to continue screening well beyond this age (Evans et al., 1993). Endoscopic surveillance should also be offered to individ-uals with attenuated polyposis and their close relatives (Heiskanen et al., 2000).

Predictive testing based on mutation analysis (where the pathogenic nature of the mutation in the family can be confidently deduced either by demonstrating that it segregates with the disease in the family, or because it is a known patho-genic mutation in other families) may be available, and individuals who have not inherited the mutation can be discharged from follow-up. A more cautious approach to management is indicated where the predictive test was based upon linkage analysis, surveillance being indicated until the estimated chance that the individual is affected is calculated as below 0.1 per cent on Bayesian risk analysis combining clinical and molecular data. Prenatal diagnosis is available by mutation or linkage analysis in informative families, although the uptake rate appears to be low. The acceptability of such testing in a disorder such as FAP is a very per-sonal matter, and the decision about whether to opt for such testing should be one made by the family after non-directive genetic counselling. Many parents wish their children to be tested at a very young age, but there are arguments for delaying such testing until clinical screening would normally be instituted, since, until this time, clinical management would not be affected (Hyer and Fell, 2001).

The effectiveness of intervention strategies, such as the administration of non-steroidal anti-inflammatory drugs (e.g. COX-2 inhibitors, Steinbach et al., 2000) or of adding non-absorbable starch to the diet, which may lead to adenoma regression, are being evaluated (Mathers et al., 2003), but are not sufficient to obviate the need for colectomy in affected individuals once polyps have developed.

Fanconi anaemia

Fanconi anaemia (FA) is an autosomal recessive chromosomal instability disorder which is characterised by congenital abnormalities, defective haemopoiesis and a high risk of developing AML and certain solid tumours. The birth incidence of FA is around 3 per million. Affected individuals can have mild growth retardation (63 per cent) and median height of FA individuals lies around the 5th centile. Other clinical features include areas of skin hyper- and hypo-pigmentation (64 per cent), skeletal defects (75 per cent) including radial limb defects (absent thumb with or without radial aplasia), abnormalities of ribs and hips and scoliosis, and cardiac (13 per cent) and renal (34 per cent) malformations. Other associated anomalies include micropthalmia (38 per cent) and developmental delay (16 per cent). The phenotypic abnormalities are variable and there is marked variability between affected individuals in the same sibship. Importantly, up to one-third of FA cases do not have any obvious congenital abnormalities, and are only diagnosed when another sibling is affected or when they develop a haematological problem. However most FA cases do have some subtle clinical features, such as dermatological manifestations.

The pancytopenia usually develops between the ages of 5 and 9 years (median age 7 years), and symptoms due to this develop progressively. The cumulative incidence of any haematological abnormality in FA is up to 90 per cent and the cumulative incidence of leukaemia is around 10 per cent by age of 25 years. The crude risks (irrespective of age) for MDS are around 5 per cent and for leukaemia is 5–10 per cent (Alter et al., 2003). FA patients that survive into early adulthood, are around 50 times more likely to develop solid tumours compared to the general population and in one study 29 per cent developed a solid tumour by the age of 48 years (Rosenberg et al., 2003). In particular, there is a high risk of hepatic tumours (which may be related to androgen use) but also squamous cell carcinomas of the oesophagus, oropharynx and vulva (Alter, 2003, Rosenberg et al., 2003).

The hallmark feature of FA cells is chromosomal hypersensitivity to DNA cross-linking agents such as mitomycin C (MMC) or diepoxybutane (DEB) and the resulting increase in chromosome breakage provides the basis for a diagnostic test (Auerbach, 1993). The characteristic chromosomal findings are excess tri- and quadri-radial and complex interchanges. The basic defect appears to be a deficiency of the repair of DNA strand cross-links. The relationship between the DNA repair defects and chromosomal aberrations found in this condition and the susceptibility to cancer is not fully understood; an increased mutation rate or incidence of tumour-promoting translocations may be a factor.

There is some evidence that heterozygotes for FA have an increased risk of certain cancers, especially leukaemias, gastric and colonic cancers, with a relative risk of 3 reported, but this does not reach statistical significance (Swift et al., 1980; reviewed in Tischkowitz and Hodgson, 2003). A separate study of 125 relatives of FA patients failed to reproduce these observations (Potter et al., 1983). Chromosome breakage testing in FA heterozygotes is complicated by overlap with the normal range (Pearson et al., 2001).

Prenatal diagnosis has been achieved by demonstrating increased spontaneous and induced chromosome breakage in fetal cells (cultured amniocytes or chorionic villus cells) (Auerbach et al., 1985).

At least 11 complementation groups have been identified and the genes defective in *eleven* of these have been identified (Levitus et al., 2003) (see Table 12.1). *FANCA* mutations account for almost two-thirds of cases, *FANCC* and G for 25 per cent, and *FANCE* and *FANCF* for a further 8 per cent. Diagnosis by direct mutation detection is available. Molecular studies have established that a common pathway exists, both between the FA proteins and other proteins involved in DNA damage repair, such as NBS1, ATM, BRCA1 and BRCA2 (reviewed in Venkitaraman, 2004). *FANCB* has been localised to Xp22.31, and the protein it encodes is an essential part of the nuclear core complex responsible for monoubiquitination of FANCD2 (Meetei et al., 2004).

FANCD1 has been shown to be *BRCA2* (Howlett et al., 2002). FA cases due to bi-allelic *BRCA2* mutations are rare but seem to be associated with an increased risk of medulloblastoma or Wilms tumour that may precede development of aplastic anaemia (Offit et al., 2003) or an earlier onset of leukaemia (Wagner et al., 2004). A family history of breast or ovarian cancer might provide clues in these cases. At present it is not known whether such cases should have intensive screening for solid tumours or whether they would benefit from more aggressive treatment with earlier stem cell transplants. The finding that FA can be caused by bi-allelic *BRCA2* mutations should be taken into account when counselling *BRCA2* mutation carriers, particularly if their partner is from an ethnic group with a high incidence of *BRCA2* founder mutations, such as the *BRCA2*6174delT* in Ashkenazi Jews. Although interestingly no homozygosity for this mutation has been identified.

At diagnosis patients should have a full haematological assessment that should include examination of the bone marrow; HLA typing in anticipation of possible bone marrow transplantation should be performed. Other investigations

Table 12.1. *Complementation groups in Fanconi anaemia, with details of identified genes*
Note that *FANCD1* is caused by biallelic *BRCA2* mutations and *FANCJ* is also known as *BACM1* or *BRIP1*

Complementation group	Identified gene	Frequency in FA (%)	Chromosomal location	Exons	Amino acids
FA-A	*FANCA*	66	16q24.3	43	1455
FA-B	*FANCB*	<1	Xp22.31	10	853
FA-C	*FANCC*	12	9q22.3	14	558
FA-D1	*BRCA2*	<1	13q12–13	26	3418
FA-D2	*FANCD2*	<1	3p25.3	44	1451
FA-E	*FANCE*	4	6p21.3	10	536
FA-F	*FANCF*	4	11p15	1	374
FA-G	*FANCG*	12	9p13	14	622
FA-I	unknown	<1	?	?	?
FA-J	*FANCJ* *BACH1* *BRIP1*	<1	17q22–24		1249
FA-L	*FANCL*	<1	2p16	14	375
FA-M	*FANCM/HeF*	<1	14q21.3	23	2048

at presentation should include audiometry, ultrasound of the renal tract, an endocrine assessment, especially if there is evidence of growth failure, and an ophthalmology assessment. Referral to hand surgeons and plastic surgeons may be indicated to consider correction of radial ray defects with a view to improving function and appearance. It is important that siblings are also tested as they may not have any congenital abnormalities.

If there is no haemopoietic defect at time of diagnosis, haematological monitoring may only be required once per year but as the patient becomes older and develops haematological complications, haematologists play an increasingly central role. Many patients who develop bone marrow failure initially respond to treatment with androgens and haemopoietic growth factors. Eventually most patients become refractory to these therapies and the definitive treatment currently available for bone marrow failure is haemopoietic stem cell transplantation.

Gorlin syndrome (naevoid basal cell carcinoma syndrome)

This is an autosomal dominant condition with a minimal prevalence of 1 in 70 000 of the population. The main features of this syndrome are multiple basal cell carcinomas (BCC) of the skin (most common in sun-exposed areas) and palmar and plantar pits (occurring in 65 per cent of cases) (see Fig. 12.5(a)). The basal cell skin lesions arise as pink or brown papules from the age of puberty onwards. Only 15 per cent manifest before puberty, and 10 per cent or more of patients have no skin lesions at the age of 30 years. It is very rare to develop a first basal cell carcinoma after the age of 55. They mainly affect the thorax, neck and face. UV light increases the incidence of the BCC; they are more common in white-skinned patients, and therapeutic radiation is often associated with progression of BCC that are present within the radiation field. Only a small proportion of carcinomas become locally invasive, but they can cause severe destruction, particularly around the eyes and orifices. Metastasis is very rare. There are many associated non-dermatological features, including hypertelorism with a broad nasal bridge and frontal and parietal bossing and a prominent chin. Odontogenic keratocysts of the jaw are common (see Fig. 12.5(b)). These are multiple, usually bilateral, recurrent and slow growing and occur in 85 per cent of mutation carriers by the age of 40 years. Squamous cell carcinomas have been reported within keratocysts in patients with Gorlin syndrome who have been treated by radiotherapy for facial BCC (Moos and Rennie, 1987). Variable skeletal abnormalities are associated, including "bridging" of the sella with calcification of the falx cerebri (see Fig. 12.5(c)), bifid (usually third, fourth or fifth), absent or rudimentary ribs, fusion defects of the cervical spine, polydactyly or syndactyly, short fourth metacarpals, flame-shaped lucencies of the metacarpals and/or phalanges, and Sprengel deformity. Ocular abnormalities have been reported, including exotropia, chalazia and coloboma, and congenital blindness. All except the skeletal features increase with age, but there is considerable variability of expression of these features in different affected people (Gorlin, 1987; 1995). The condition is inherited as an autosomal dominant trait with almost complete penetrance but highly variable expression. Diagnostic features are described in Table 12.2.

A variety of other, less common, abnormalities have been noted in affected people, including milia, epidermoid cysts, chalazia and comedones of the skin, cleft lip and palate, pectus carinatum, and hypogonadotrophic hypogonadism in males. Hamartomatous upper GI polyposis has also been reported (Schwartz, 1978). There is a definite increase in incidence of non-dermatological malignancies, including squamous cell carcinoma and fibrosarcoma in the jaw cysts, and nasopharyngeal carcinomas. Mental retardation has been reported in about 3 per cent of cases, but its true incidence is unclear. Detailed CT and MRI have revealed a high incidence of asymmetric or dilated ventricles in 24 per cent, and one in ten individuals have dysgenesis or agenesis of the corpus callosum (Kimonis et al., 2004). Childhood medulloblastoma may occur in the first 2 years of life, and meningioma and craniopharyngioma have been described. Bilateral ovarian fibromas (which can be hormonally active) are common in affected women, and there is a risk of ovarian fibrosarcoma or other malignancy developing in these lesions (Ismail and Walker,

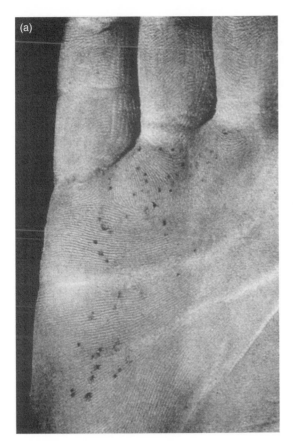

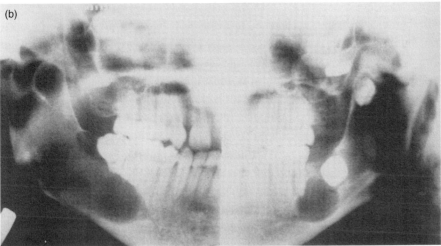

Fig. 12.5. Gorlin syndrome: (a) palmar pits, (b) odontogenic keratocysts and (c) calcified falx cerebri (courtesy of Robert Gorlin).

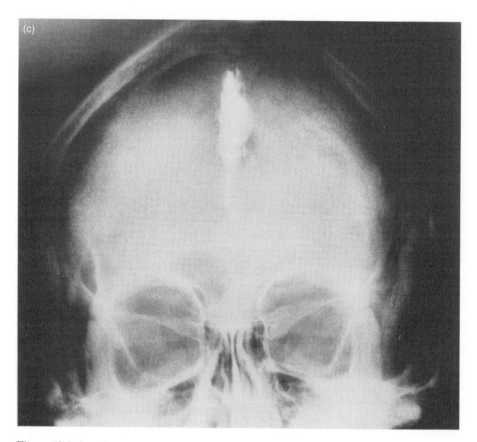

Figure 12.5. (cont.)

1990). Seminoma has been reported in males. Cardiac fibromas may occur from early childhood; these may remain static, or possibly regress or enlarge with age (Cotton et al., 1991). Other tumours that have been described in association with Gorlin syndrome include renal fibroma, melanoma, neurofibroma, leiomyoma and rhabdomyoma/sarcoma. Mesenteric lymphatic or chylous cysts may occur.

Surveillance of affected people should consist of yearly dermatological examinations and 6-monthly evaluation of the jaw cysts by means of an oropantogram, since odontogenic cysts can erode locally and be very destructive, and early enucleation of these cysts can prevent this. Infants should be kept under surveillance for signs of medulloblastoma, and some have recommended 6-monthly MRI until the age of 7 years (after which the risk declines significantly) (Kimonis et al., 2004). Cranial ultrasound may also be a useful investigation because care should be taken to restrict exposure to radiation to a minimum in view of the extreme radiation sensitivity in this condition. Pelvic ultrasound scanning may detect ovarian tumours, but in view of the low incidence of this complication, regular scanning is generally not advised.

Table 12.2. *Diagnostic criteria for Gorlin syndrome (Evans et al., 1993)*

Major criteria
More than two BCC or one BCC under 20 years at diagnosis
Histologically proven odontogenic keratocysts of the jaw
Three or more cutaneous palmar or plantar pits
Bifid, fused or markedly splayed ribs
First-degree relative with Gorlin syndrome

Minor criteria
Height-adjusted macrocephaly
One of the following orofacial characteristics: cleft lip or palate; frontal bossing; coarse face;
    moderate or severe hypertelorism
One of the following skeletal abnormalities: Sprengel, pectus excavatum (marked), severe
    syndactyly
One of the following radiological features: bridging of the sella turcica, hemi/fused/elongation
    of vertebral bodies, modelling defects and flame-shaped lucencies of the hands and feet
Ovarian fibroma
Medulloblastoma

The diagnosis requires the presence of two major, or one major and one minor features.

Genetic counselling should be facilitated by molecular genetic analysis. Affected children show few features. However, if at the age of 5 years an at-risk child has no abnormality on X-ray of spine or skull and has no osteomas or dermatological lesions, the risk of the child being a gene carrier is very small (Farndon et al., 1992).

Gorlin syndrome is caused by mutations in the human homologue (*PTCH*) of the *Drosophila* segment polarity gene *patched* which maps to chromosome 9q (Hahn et al., 1996; Johnson et al., 1996). There is no evidence of locus heterogeneity in Gorlin syndrome and most reported mutations are predicted to cause protein truncation. No genotype–phenotype relationships have been identified (Wicking et al., 1997). *PTCH* encodes a transmembrane glycoprotein that acts as an antagonist in the Hedgehog signalling pathway. PTCH inhibits smoothened (SMO), which in turn activates transcription factors in the Wnt and decapentaplegic pathways. It appears likely that some manifestations of Gorlin syndrome (e.g. symmetrical developmental defects, such as macrocephaly, etc.) result from haploinsufficiency, but that basal call carcinomas and other tumours require inactivation of both alleles in a two-step mechanism of tumourigenesis (Levanat et al., 1996). Interestingly, too much activity in the Hedgehog pathway leads to Gorlin syndrome with the associated cancer risk, whereas under-activity causes holoprosencephaly (Roessler et al., 1997; Odent et al., 1999).

Hemihypertrophy

Idiopathic asymmetrical overgrowth is usually a sporadic condition and is to be distinguished from that associated with Klippel–Trenaunay–Weber syndrome, neurofibromatosis type 1 (NF1) and Beckwith–Wiedemann syndrome. Idiopathic hemihypertrophy is associated with a significant risk of mental handicap, genito-urinary abnormalities and neoplasia (Viljeon et al., 1984). Wilms tumour occurs in approximately 3 per cent of patients with hemihypertrophy and there are also reported associations with adrenal cortical tumours and hepatoblastoma (Viljeon et al., 1984). Uniparental paternal isodisomy for chromosome 11 was described in a patient with hemihypertrophy, Wilms tumour and congenital adrenal carcinoma (Grundy et al., 1991), suggesting overlap between isolated hemipertrophy and BWS (see Section Beckwith–Wiedemann Syndrome, p. 170). There are now several reports of uniparental disomy for chromosome 11 in isolated hemihypertrophy so this diagnosis should be sought, although it may not be detected on blood analysis and require analysis of skin fibroblasts from the hypertrophied side. Children with idiopathic hemihypertrophy should be kept under surveillance for abdominal neoplasms using a similar protocol to that recommended for BWS (see p. 170).

Hereditary non-polyposis colorectal cancer

It is commonly abbreviated as HNPCC; and is also known as Lynch syndrome, or Lynch family cancer syndrome. Lynch syndrome is now the preferred term.

Background: history and epidemiology

Lynch et al. (1967; 1985) delineated two disorders characterised by an autosomal dominantly inherited predisposition to colon cancer without florid polyposis. These disorders, "Lynch syndromes I and II" (the latter reserved for families with extracolonic cancers, have been collectively referred to as HNPCC for some time, and are not truly distinct entities (Lynch et al., 1993; Menko, 1993). Paradoxically, in some HNPCC pedigrees, colorectal cancer is absent, and led to the re-introduction of the term "Lynch syndrome" to describe this syndrome (Umar et al., 2004a). The condition is due to inherited changes in the DNA mismatch repair (MMR) genes, most commonly *MLH1* and *MSH2*, but mutations have also been reported in *MSH6* and *PMS2*. In addition to a high risk of colon cancer (up to 80 per cent lifetime risk, but probably lower in females (40 per cent) than males) (Dunlop et al., 1997), HNPCC is characterised by an early age at diagnosis of colon cancer (40–50 years compared with 60–70 years in the general population), a preponderance of right-sided tumours (60–70 per cent versus 15 per cent), and susceptibility to multiple primary cancers (25 per cent versus 5 per cent) (Mecklin et al., 1986; Lanspa et al., 1990, Aarnio et al., 1999). The overall lifetime risk for metachronous colorectal cancer has been estimated at up to 30 per cent, but prospective data are lacking, and survival bias may be present. There is clear evidence that colorectal cancers exhibiting MSI have a better survival than those that do not (Bubb et al., 1996; Gryfe et al., 2000), and some early data suggested that this is also true for those with HNPCC (Sankila et al., 1996; Watson et al., 1998). However, more recent data have questioned the data obtained in those with germline mutations, particularly with respect to possible ascertainment bias (Farrington et al., 2002; Clark et al., 2004).

In individuals with HNPCC there is a predisposition to a variety of extra-colonic cancers, most commonly endometrial, but also ovarian, gastric, pancreatic, hepatobiliary tract, urothelial and small intestine (Watson and Lynch 2001). In one study from Finland, estimates of the cumulative lifetime risks of the various cancer types in gene carriers were 78 per cent for colorectal cancer, 43–60 per cent for endometrial cancer in women, 19 per cent for gastric cancer, 18 per cent for biliary tract cancer, 10 per cent for urinary tract cancer and 9 per cent for ovarian cancer in women, with a 1 per cent risk of small bowel and brain tumours, representing a significantly increased relative risk for these tumour types (Aarnio et al., 1995; 1999). In other studies women may have a lower risk of colorectal cancer than males: 61 per cent versus 91 per cent risk to age of 70 years (Dunlop et al., 1997). The estimated relative risks for extra-colonic cancer may vary with different germline mutations: those for small intestinal cancer are 291 for *MLH1* mutation carriers and 102 for *MSH2* mutation carriers, for gastric cancer 4 and 19 respectively, for ovarian cancer 6 and 8 respectively, and for urinary tract cancer 75 in *MSH2* mutation carriers only (Vasen et al., 1996; 2001). Overall, *MSH2* mutations appear to confer a higher risk of cancer than *MLH1* mutations, mainly due to an increased risk of urinary tract and endometrial cancers in *MSH2* mutation carriers. *MSH6* mutations are associated with less of a risk of colorectal cancer but an increased risk of endometrial and, to a lesser extent, urothelial cancer (Wijnen et al., 1999; Vasen et al., 2001).

Clinical features and pathology

Florid polyposis does not occur in HNPCC, but colonic adenomas (particularly right sided) have been reported to be more common than in controls: 30 per cent of HNPCC patients have at least one colonic adenoma, and 20 per cent have multiple lesions, compared with 11 per cent and 4 per cent in age-matched and sex-matched controls (Lanspa et al., 1990; Gaglia et al., 1995). Other studies have, however, suggested that the prevalence of adenomas, however, is not greatly increased, but they develop more rapidly through the adenoma-carcinoma sequence in this disease (Jass, 1995a). If multiple adenomas occur, it is very rare to find more than 50, which differentiates HNPCC syndrome from FAP, in which characteristically there are more than 100 polyps. A subgroup of patients with HNPCC develop flat adenomas (slightly elevated lesions with adenoma-tous changes confined to the colonic crypts) (Lynch et al., 1990c), although it is not clear that this subset can be distinguished by molecular means.

The mean age at diagnosis of colon cancer in this disease is about 44 years, compared to 65 years in the general population; 65 per cent of tumours occur in the right hemicolon, and 23 per cent have metachronous cancers (Mecklin, 1987, Lynch and de la Chapelle, 1999). About 5 per cent of colorectal cancers occur before 30 years of age (Vasen et al., 1989; 2001).

The pathology of colorectal cancers in HNPCC is notable for a slight over-representation of mucinous carcinomas, mainly well differentiated and rarely of the signet-ring cell type, with a medullary pattern in about 9 per cent of cases. Lymphocytic infiltration and tumour budding with de-differentiation are more common in HNPCC than in sporadic cancers, and in HNPCC there are char-acteristically more *APC*, *β-catenin* and *K-RAS* mutations than in sporadic can-cers, whereas DNA methylation and *BRAF* mutations are rare in HNPCC (Jass, 2004).

The dermatological features of Muir–Torre syndrome (Smyrk et al., 2001) with sebaceous adenomas and carcinomas, may occur occasionally in individuals with HNPCC, but genotype–phenotype correlations are not evident, beyond the interesting observation that mutations are much more common in *MSH2* than in *MLH1* (Lucci-Cordisco et al., 2003).

Turcot syndrome is the co-occurrence of colorectal polyps and brain tumours (see p. 250). This can be caused by germline mutations in the *APC* gene or one of the *HNPCC* genes. Some children have been described with adenomatous colonic polyps, primary brain tumours, leukaemia and café-au-lait skin patches, with an autosomal recessive inheritance pattern, and the condition has been shown to be due to homozygosity or compound heterozygosity for mutations in *MLH1*, *MSH2*, *MSH6* or PMS2 (Ricciardone et al., 1999; Whiteside et al., 2002; Menko et al. 2004 reviewed in Bandipalliam, 2005).

Diagnostic features

For practical purposes, and for research, criteria for the diagnosis of HNPCC known as the Amsterdam Criteria, were drawn up in 1991 (see Tables 12.3 and 12.3).

Table 12.3. *The original Amsterdam Criteria: AC1*

1. At least three relatives (all related to each other) affected by colorectal cancer, one a first-degree relative of the other two
2. At least two successive generations affected.
3. Colorectal cancer diagnosed before 50 years of age in one relative
4. Familial adenomatous polyposis excluded.

Vasen et al. (1991).

Table 12.4. *The revised Amsterdam Criteria: AC2*

1. At least three relatives (all related to each other) affected by an HNPCC-related cancer*, one a first-degree relative of the other two.
2. At least two successive generations affected.
3. HNPCC-related cancer diagnosed before 50 years of age in one relative
4. Familial adenomatous polyposis excluded.

Vasen et al. (1999).
*The only cancers permitted are colorectal carcinoma, endometrial adenocarcinoma, small intestinal adenocarcinoma, transitional cell carcinoma of the renal pelvis, and transitional cell carcinoma of the ureter.

Table 12.3 can easily be memorised as 3-2-1-0 (three cases, two generations, one case diagnosed under 50, no FAP).

Subsequently, because of the increased relative risk for the related tumours referred to above, the occurrence of an endometrial or upper GI carcinoma in a young individual in such a family was included to indicate affected status with regard to HNPCC (Amsterdam 2 (AC2) criteria; Vasen et al., 1999, see Table 12.4).

The seven-point Bethesda guidelines were introduced to increase the sensitivity of diagnosis, identifying 94 per cent of patients with a pathogenic mutation, but with low specificity (25 per cent) (Rodriguez-Bigas et al., 1997). These guidelines were introduced initially to indicate who might benefit from MSI analysis, not to replace the Amsterdam criteria, which was originally designed to identify families most likely to carry mutations in the causative genes. On the basis of further research into the sensitivity and specificity of the original guidelines, they have recently been changed, simplified, and in some ways made broader (Umar et al., 2004a). These guidelines differ from the original in that fulfilling the Amsterdam criteria is no longer included, the presence of colonic adenomas alone is not sufficient for inclusion, the age at diagnosis for inclusion has been

Table 12.5. *The revised Bethesda guidelines*

Tumours from individuals should be tested for MSI in the following situations

1. Colorectal cancer diagnosed in a patient who is less than 50 years of age.
2. Presence of synchronous, metachronous colorectal, or other HNPCC-associated tumours, regardless of age.
3. Colorectal cancer with the MSI-H histology (such as tumour infiltrating lymphocytes, Crohns-like lymphocytic reaction, mucinous/signet-ring differentiation, or medullary growth pattern) diagnosed in a patient who is less than 60 years of age.
4. Colorectal cancer diagnosed in one or more first-degree relatives with an HNPCC-related tumour, with one of the cancers being diagnosed under age 50 years.
5. Colorectal cancer diagnosed in two or more first- or second-degree relatives with HNPCC-related tumours, regardless of age.

Adapted from Umar et al. (2004).

increased to 50 or abolished altogether, and finally, the pathological features of colorectal cancers that are likely to carry *MMR* gene mutations have been refined (see Table 12.5).

Wijnen et al. (1998) proposed a logistic model that takes into account various clinical parameters of the family, to estimate the probability of a mutation being present in *MLH1* or *MSH2* (Wijnen et al., 1998). One study showed that in a high-risk clinic setting, virtually all *MLH1* and *MSH2* mutation carriers can be identified by applying only the first 3 of the original 7 Bethesda guidelines; on the other hand, the specificity is substantially reduced (Syngal et al., 2000). Studies in the population have indicated that identifying all mutation carriers using family history alone is not possible (Aaltonen et al., 1998). The most recent models (such as the so-called "Amsterdam-Plus" model) have tried to improve on previous models by including additional information such as the number of family members with one or more adenoma, or double primary cancers (Lipton et al., 2004). Further improvements, incorporating molecular markers found in the cancers may be possible. A series of recommendations have been established for the process of evaluation of at-risk patients, see below.

Recommendations for the process of molecular evaluation of patients identified as being at risk, based on meeting the Bethesda Guidelines (adapted from Umar et al., 2004a).

1. The optimal approach to evaluation is MSI or immunohistochemical (IHC) analysis of tumours, followed by germline *MMR* gene testing in

patients with MSI-H tumours or tumours with a loss of expression of one of the *MMR* genes.

2. After the mutation is identified, at-risk relatives should be referred for genetic counselling.

3. An alternative approach, if tissue testing is not feasible, is to proceed directly to germline analysis of the *MMR* genes.

4. If no *MMR* gene mutation is found in a proband with an MSI-H tumour and/ or a clinical history of HNPCC, the genetic test result is non-informative. The patients and the at-risk individuals should be counselled as if HNPCC was confirmed and high-risk surveillance should be undertaken.

Molecular genetics

The most common genes in which germline mutations may cause this disease are *MSH2* on chromosome 2p16, *MLH1* on chromosome 3p21, which account for approximately 90 per cent of cases of HNPCC; and *MSH6* on 2p15, and much less commonly, *PMS2* on chromosome 7p22, which interestingly, can be a rare cause childhood brain cancer, when mutations are present in the homozygous state (De Vos et al., 2004). Mutations in *MSH3* are very rarely reported in patients with colorectal cancer (Nicoliades et al., 1994; Akiyama et al., 1997; de la Chapelle 2004). Interpretation of reported mutations in *PMS2* is complicated by the presence of pseudogenes (Hayward et al., 2004). Studies suggest that nearly one half of individuals diagnosed with colorectal cancer before the age of 35 years may have such a germline mutation in one of these genes (Liu et al., 1995), but that only a minority of patients with colorectal cancer diagnosed between the ages of 35 and 45 years without a family history of colorectal cancer have such mutations. The overall contribution of HNPCC to colorectal cancer is probably 2–3 per cent (de la Chapelle, 2004), but only very extensive, multimodal mutation analysis can hope to find more than 75 per cent of all mutations. Exonic deletions are particularly common in *MSH2*.

All these genes are involved in the same pathway for repair of mismatches in DNA, and MSI may be demonstrated as DNA replication errors detectable in tumour relative to genomic DNA (Parsons et al., 1993; Liu et al., 1995). Frameshift mutations of the transforming growth factor β (TGF) type II receptor gene and other growth/apoptosis-related genes such as BAX are common, and are due to the runs of mono or dinucleotide repeats present in these target genes. Analysis of a series of families with HNPCC suggests that perhaps half of the cases are due to mutations in the *MSH2* gene, 30–40 per cent to mutations in the *MLH1* gene, less than 10 per cent are attributable to mutations in *MSH6* and only a handful are due to mutations in other genes. When multiple techniques are used, most families that fulfil the Amsterdam Criteria are found to have germline *HNPCC* mutations (Wagner et al., 2003; Difiore et al., 2004). Founder mutations in the genes causing HNPCC are known, for instance there is an *MLH1* deletion of exon 16 in the Finns (Nystrom-Lahti et al., 1995) and a founder mutation in *MSH2*, known as A636P, probably accounts for a third of all HNPCC in the Ashkenazi Jewish population (Foulkes et al., 2002). Attenuated forms of FAP may rarely masquerade as HNPCC, usually due to unusual mutations in the *APC* gene (Spirio et al., 1993). Other genes that may be involved in colorectal cancer predisposition, with single reports of germline mutations reported in cases, include *AXIN2* and *TGFβRII*. Subsequent data have suggested that the latter mutation is most likely to be a neutral polymorphism (Lu et al., 1998; de la Chapelle, 2004).

The molecular defect in HNPCC is repair of DNA mismatches (MMR defect). Heterozygous cells repair DNA normally (or at levels that generally do not have clinical consequences), but in cells where the second allele has been inactivated, for instance by deletion, in the colonic epithelium, a mutator phenotype is generated and MSI is seen. Genes with microsatellite sequences in their coding regions (such as *TGFβRII*) are prone to somatic mutation, which is thought to promote the carcinogenic progression (de la Chapelle, 2004).

Affected individuals from families fulfilling Amsterdam Criteria 2 are usually tested for germline mutations in the genes causing HNPCC without pre-testing (e.g. of pathology blocks), although IHC staining of tumour blocks will likely indicate (by lack of staining of *MSH2, MLH1, MSH6 or PMS2*) the gene likely to be involved (Shia et al., 2005). MSH6 staining is usually absent in cases due to a *MSH2* mutation, (although the reverse is not observed) and is not always abnormal in tumours arising in *MSH6* mutation carriers (Berends et al., 2002). Tumours in individuals with HNPCC characteristically demonstrate MSI, but this may also occur in 15 per cent of all colorectal cancers. Testing the tumour for MSI using a panel of microsatellites (BAT 25, BAT 26 and three others) helps to identify tumours from individuals with an increased likelihood of having HNPCC (Boland et al., 1998), but as more microsatellites are used, the numbers of MSI-high tumours increases and the test becomes less specific for HNPCC (Laiho et al., 2002; Reyes et al., 2002). MLH1 methylation is common (86 per cent) in MSI-high tumours from non-HNPCC subjects (de la Chapelle, 2004), so lack of such methylation makes HNPCC more likely. *BRAF* mutations are rarely seen in HNPCC-related cancers, and their presence in a colorectal cancer occurring in a hereditary colorectal cancer family makes a MMR gene mutation unlikely (Wang et al., 2003). Taken together, these observations suggest that pathological analysis of colorectal cancers can considerably simplify germline mutation analysis in hereditary colorectal cancer families.

Screening

First-degree relatives of individuals affected by HNPCC should be offered screening for colorectal cancer and possibly for other cancers seen in their family. Since colorectal adenomas are assumed to be the premalignant lesions (for colorectal cancer) and the majority of lesions are right sided, colonoscopy is the screening method of choice (Hodgson et al., 1995). Asymptomatic at-risk relatives (with an affected first-degree relative with HNPCC) should be offered biennial colonoscopy from the age of 25–40 years and yearly thereafter (Umar et al., 2004b). Interval cancers have been detected in individuals screened at 2-yearly intervals. Annual examinations are probably optimal but often not very practical, and therefore a "compromise" has been made by starting annual colonoscopies at an age when the annual risk begins to rise more sharply. The adenoma-carcinoma progression rate appears to be very much increased in HNPCC, above that in the general population (Jass, 1995b). If adenomas are found, they are removed, and colonoscopy should be repeated annually. There is good evidence that such screening does reduce cancer morbidity and mortality in screened individuals (Jarvinen et al., 1995; Vasen et al., 1995; Renkonen-Sinisalo et al., 2000). These data suggest that a 3-year screening interval is too long.

When colorectal cancer is detected in an affected individual many centres advocate subtotal or even total colectomy because of the significant risk of a second colorectal cancer, but the evidence for and against such management options is still lacking, and there is currently a European trial to evaluate this (Olschwang et al., 2005). Lifetime surveillance for rectal cancer should be continued after such surgery. The risk of rectal cancer has been assessed at 12 per cent over a 12-year follow-up period (Jarvinen et al., 2000). Such surgery could also be offered to *MMR* gene mutation carriers who have been found to have recurrent or dysplastic adenomas. Carrier women found to have colon cancer require careful preoperative assessment for ovarian and uterine cancer. Even if there is no evidence of current malignancy, prophylactic hysterectomy and bilateral oophorectomy at the time of colon surgery should be considered when there is a strong family history of these neoplasms.

There is some evidence that individuals with HNPCC may have a survival benefit from treatment with adjuvant chemotherapy (Elsaleh et al., 2001), although the evidence for this is conflicting, and other studies suggest that tumours demonstrating MMR deficiency are resistant to chemotherapeutic agents including 5-FU, methylating agents and antimetabolites (Bignami et al., 2003; Clark et al., 2004).

Because of the increased risk of gynaecological cancers in females with HNPCC (possibly up to a half of total cancer risk) women with this disease and those at high risk of inheriting it should be followed up with annual bimanual pelvic examination and transvaginal ultrasound scan for ovarian and uterine cancers from 30 years of age. Transvaginal ultrasound with Doppler examination may delineate ovarian lesions, and a serum CA125 is also suggested annually (Jacobs and Lancaster, 1996), but the efficacy of such surveillance is still unproven. Regular endometrial aspiration and biopsy (pipelle, or hysteroscopic biopsy) is more sensitive than ultrasound for the detection of endometrial cancer, but since endometrial cancer has a relatively good prognosis, and the efficacy of surveillance is as yet unknown, screening would be best performed in the setting of a prospective study (Vasen et al., 1996) (see section below on endometrial cancer). A high incidence of other HNPCC-associated cancers in particular families is an indication for screening for the specific cancer within that kindred showing an increased frequency of these extracolonic cancers. Thus dermatological surveillance may be offered in Muir-Torre families, and annual assessment for urological malignancy by abdominal ultrasound and cytological examination of an early-morning urine sample for red blood cells and cytology, from 30 to 35 years of age. Gastroscopies annually, with eradication of *Helicobacter pylori* infection, when present, could be considered from the age of 30 to 35 years in individuals with a strong family history of gastric cancer (Park et al., 2000), although the efficacy of such screening has not yet been established. (For more discussion see p. 63.)

Endometrial cancer in HNPCC

Endometrial cancer is the fifth most common cancer in women in the UK, accounting for 7 per cent of invasive cancers in women, occurring in 1 in 100 women by 75 years of age. The commonest histological type (90 per cent) is adenocarcinoma (see p. 87). Women with HNPCC have a very high lifetime risk of endometrial cancer. Tumours characteristically demonstrate MSI (due to impaired repair of mismatch DNA errors), and complex atypical endometrial hyperplasia appears to be the premalignant endometrial lesion (Lohse et al., 2002; Sutter et al., 2004). Carriers of *MSH6* mutations have the highest endometrial cancer risk (Wijnen et al., 1999), and the risk is higher in MSH2 than in MLH1 mutation carriers (Vasen et al., 2001; Huang et al., 2004). Women with HNPCC have a lifetime risk of endometrial cancer of up to 60 per cent, with the highest incidence between 40 and 60 years of age, average 49.3 years. There are characteristics of endometrial cancer in HNPCC which appear to be different from sporadic cancers, including more poorly differentiated histology (83 per cent versus 27 per cent in sporadic cancers) with Crohn-like lymphoid reaction (100 per cent versus 27 per cent), lymphangio-invasive growth (67 per cent versus 0 per cent) and tumour invasion by lymphocytes (100 per cent versus 36 per cent) (Van den Bos et al., 2004). It has been suggested that the DNA MMR defect in HNPCC generates increased numbers of novel and potentially immunogenic mutations, which result in an increased immunologic response to tumours in affected individuals. MSI can be demonstrated in hyperplastic endometrium in women without HNPCC, but not in normal endometrium, and is also detectable in about 20 per cent of endometrial cancers (Baldinu et al., 2002). Gynaecological surveillance has been advocated annually for women with HNPCC, by pelvic ultrasound and endometrial aspiration and/or biopsy, and preliminary results indicate that this allows the detection of premalignant lesions, including complex atypical hyperplasia and early cancers (Wood and Duffy, 2003).

Genetic counselling in HNPCC

Now that it is possible to delineate the mutation responsible for this disease in some families, it is possible to carry out predictive testing for the condition in families in which the pathogenic mutation has been detected in an affected individual. Such testing should only be offered with a full counselling protocol. Discussions should include providing information about the chances of developing cancer at a given age, and about the possible emotional effects of receiving a positive or a negative result, and the potential implications with regard to insurance and employment (Aktan-Collan et al., 2000). Before using such molecular tests, it is important to be confident of the pathogenicity of the mutation by for example, the demonstration that it segregates with the disease or has been shown to be pathogenic in other families, and that the nature of the mutation is likely to cause disruption of function.

The ascertainment and counselling of at-risk family members is of great importance and should be encouraged; there is often poor communication between different parts of a family. Genetic registers of families with this disease facilitate the follow-up of affected and at-risk individuals, and the ascertainment of other individuals within a family who may benefit from screening (see screening for colorectal cancer, p. 63).

Autosomal recessive childhood cancer predisposition syndrome

It has become appreciated that homozygous mutations in *MLH1*, *MSH2*, *MSH6* and *PMS2*) can be responsible for an autosomal recessive condition characterised by childhood malignancies, particularly haematological (lymphomas and leukaemias) and brain tumours, including medulloblastomas, glioblastomas and oligodendrogliomata), other cancers (GI or uterine cancer) and dermatological features of NF (café-au-lait patches) (De Vos et al., 2004; Menko et al., 2004). This has in the past been described as a variant of Turcot syndrome

(De Rosa et al., 2000; Bougeard et al., 2003; Trimbath et al 2001), and it is interesting to speculate what proportion of Turcot syndrome is attributable to mutations in *APC* and the *MMR* genes, particularly as both autosomal dominant and recessive forms of Turcot syndrome have been described.

Hyperparathyroidism–jaw tumour syndrome

Hyperparathyroidism–jaw tumour syndrome (HPT-JT) is an autosomal dominant disorder characterised by parathyroid adenoma or carcinoma, ossifying fibroma of the mandible and/or maxilla, and renal cysts, adenomas and carcinomas. Germline mutations in *HRPT2* are associated with HPT-JT (Carpten et al., 2002).

Typically, HPT-JT patients present with solitary parathyroid adenomas or carcinomas. Rarely, they present with double neoplasias. Parathyroid carcinomas are extremely rare and are not components of any other heritable syndrome. So its presence should raise the genetic differential diagnosis of HPT-JT. Approximately 80 per cent of these patients present with hyperparathyroidism (HPT). Parathyroid carcinoma occurs in approximately 10–15 per cent of affected individuals. A unique pathologic feature of parathyroid lesions in HPT-JT is the high frequency of cystic changes. About 30 per cent of patients also develop fibro-osseous lesions, primarily in the mandible and/or maxilla. Kidney lesions have been reported including bilateral cysts, renal adenoma, hamartomas and papillary RCC. It is important to be aware that in some families, only parathyroid lesions are present. As more families are currently being tested genetically, it is expected that the incidence and spectrum of its associated clinical features will become better defined.

Germline mutations in *HRPT2*, located on 1q25–q31, cause HPT-JT (Teh et al., 1996; Carpten et al., 2002). The *HRPT2* gene has 17 exons spanning 18.5 kb of genomic distance. HPT-JT-associated mutations are truncating, mainly frameshift and nonsense, with the majority occurring in exon 1 (Carpten et al., 2002). Because this gene was recently identified, it remains unknown whether a genotype–phenotype association exists. The penetrance for HPT is 80 per cent, which mainly will develop by the late teens. The *HRPT2* transcript is 2.7 kb and is predicted to encode a 531-amino acid protein. While the gene is ubiquitously expressed, its function remains unknown.

Individuals and families who have or are suspected of having HPT-JT should be offered clinical cancer genetic consultation, which includes genetic counselling. When HPT-JT is suspected in a family or individual, DNA-based testing may be offered to establish the diagnosis and for medical management. Because the *HRPT2* gene has now been identified, molecular-based differentiation of the various complex syndromes associated with hereditary primary HPT has become possible.

Clinical surveillance and prophylactic manoeuvers in HPT-JT are based on expert opinion. Annual blood-based biochemical tests for ionised calcium and intact parathyroid hormone levels beginning by the mid-teens have been advocated. Following the example of multiple endocrine neoplasia type 1 (MEN 1), some believe that surgical intervention should occur once serum levels confirm the presence of HPT. Parathyroid disease in HPT-JT is typically asynchronous adenomas although the potential for malignancy needs to be considered (Howell et al., 2003; Shattuck et al., 2003). While some groups advocate removal only of the enlarged parathyroid gland with continued regular monitoring, the alternative approach would be complete parathyroidectomy with fresh parathyroid auto-transplantation to the forearm (or sternocleidomastoid) (Marx et al., 2002; Chen et al., 2003). Because of the unclear frequencies of jaw manifestations and renal neoplasias, it is unknown if surveillance for these component features would prove useful. The more aggressive amongst HPT-JT exponents would suggest orthopentography of the jaw every 3 years as well as annual abdominal ultrasound or CT scan with and without contrast at least every other year to screen for polycystic disease, Wilms tumour or carcinoma, and renal hamartomas (Chen et al., 2003).

Juvenile polyposis syndrome

Solitary juvenile intestinal polyps are relatively common in the paediatric population, occurring in approximately 1–5 per cent. A clinical diagnosis of juvenile polyposis syndrome (JPS) is made when multiple (>5) juvenile polyps occur in any one individual (Waite and Eng, 2003). Despite its name, the age at diagnosis is bimodal, in childhood and in the mid-50s. JPS is an autosomal dominant hamartoma polyposis syndrome often clinically diagnosed when other inherited hamartoma polyposis syndromes, such as PJS (see below) and BRRS (see above, p. 169) have been excluded.

The prevalence of JPS is believed to be 1 in 100 000. The number of polyps varies between individuals, even in the same family, but can be anywhere from 5 to 200. They are most often found in the lower bowel (98 per cent) but can also develop in the stomach (15 per cent) and small intestine (7 per cent). Patients can become symptomatic from their polyps: haematochezia, melena, rectal prolapse, intussusception or abdominal pain. There is also an increased lifetime risk for malignancy of 10–60 per cent for GI (colorectal, gastric, duodenal) and pancreatic cancer (Jarvinen and Franssila, 1984; Jass et al., 1988).

Histopathology plays a critical role in the diagnosis of JPS. The typical JPS polyp is unilobulated and pedunculated, spherical in shape with a smooth outer surface. In contrast to other hamartomatous polyps, these lack a smooth muscle core but instead show an internal dense inflammatory response, with predominant mesenchymal stroma that entraps normal epithelial cells, often forming dilated cysts (Jass et al., 1988). Less typical (20 per cent) are JPS polyps that are multi-lobulated, with each lobe separated by well-defined clefts (Jass et al., 1988).

Congenital anomalies have been reported in 11–20 per cent of individuals with JPS, more often in the sporadic cases (Coburn et al., 1995). These can involve the GI tract (including malrotation of the gut), heart, CNS and genitourinary system. Clubbing of the fingertips is common, as is macrocephaly and congenital cardiac anomalies.

JPS is associated with mutations in one of at least two genes. Germline mutations in *MADH4* and *BMPR1A* have been found in approximately 40 per cent of familial and sporadic JPS probands (Howe et al., 1998b; 2001; Zhou et al., 2001a). Germline mutations in *MADH4* account for 15–25 per cent of JPS while mutations in *BMPR1A* account for another 15–25 per cent. Both *MADH4* and *BMPR1A* belong to the TGFβ superfamily. BMPR1A is phosphorylated by, and dimerises with, a specific type II BMP receptor. In turn, this activated complex signals through the intracellular SMAD1 or related SMAD5 and SMAD8 proteins, increasing their affinity for SMAD4, and gaining access to the nucleus for the transcriptional regulation of downstream target genes (Massague, 2000; Eng, 2001; Waite and Eng, 2003). The prominent role of the BMP pathway in cardiac development and in the development of the GI tract might explain the association of some JPS with congenital cardiac anomalies and malrotation of the gut (Waite and Eng, 2003). Further investigation might reveal cardiac anomalies predominating in those with *BMPR1A* mutations compared to those with *MADH4* mutations.

To date, the only genotype–phenotype correlation observed is the marked prevalence of giant gastric polyps in individuals with *MADH4* mutations as compared to families with germline *BMPR1A* alterations (Friedl et al., 2002). It is likely that there is at least one other JPS gene that has not been identified yet. While other members of the TGFβ-SMAD superfamily would be ideal candidates, no germline mutations in the genes encoding *SMAD1*, *SMAD2*, *SMAD3* and *SMAD5* have been identified to date (Bevan et al., 1999).

While there were early reports of germline *PTEN* mutations in "JPS" these were not confirmed as the individuals labelled as "JPS" either had features suggestive of Cowden syndrome or were too young for the manifestations of Cowden syndrome to be apparent. Indeed, when a single hospital series of individuals given the diagnosis of JPS were analysed for the presence of *PTEN* mutations, only one was found to harbour such a mutation (Kurose et al., 1999; Olsohwang et al 1998). This patient was asked to return for a meticulous physical examination and indeed, pathognomonic cutaneous features of CS were noted (Kurose et al., 1999). A second study now exists: 55 individuals in whom JPS has been diagnosed were examined and one was found to carry a germline *PTEN* mutation (Howe JR, personal communication) (Waite and Eng, 2003). In retrospective review of medical records, it became obvious that this person probably had Cowden syndrome. Thus, JPS individuals found to carry germline *PTEN* mutations should in fact be reclassified as Cowden syndrome or *PTEN* Hamartoma Tumour syndrome (PHTS).

Clinical cancer genetic consultation, which includes genetic counselling, should be offered to all probands and families with JPS or suspected to have JPS. As with most inherited cancer syndromes with known susceptibility genes, the known affected individual should be tested for mutations in *MADH4* and *BMPR1A*. Once the family-specific mutation is known, all first-degree relatives can be offered genetic testing in the setting of clinical cancer genetic consultation including genetic counselling. In such families, a mutation negative result in a family member offered predictive testing is a true negative. An individual believed to have JPS and found to have a germline *PTEN* mutation should be informed they have PHTS or Cowden syndrome and medically managed as in CS (see above, p. 179).

Clinical surveillance guidelines and intervention is based on expert opinion and based heavily on the experience of FAP and HNPCC. Individuals found to carry a germline mutation in *MADH4* or *BMPR1A* should undergo upper and lower endoscopy to determine whether they have polyps at that time, whether these require further medical attention and to decide upon the interval of further endoscopies. In asymptomatic at-risk individuals, screening endoscopies should begin in the second decade. Symptomatic individuals should have upper and lower endoscopies at the time of symptomatology. If no polyps are noted, then the screening interval may be every 2–3 years so long as the individuals remains asymptomatic. When polyps are found, they should be removed, followed by an endoscopy at 1 year. When the tract is polyp-free, then screening intervals of 2–3 years can occur. If a JPS individual presents with non-metastatic colorectal cancer, total colectomy should be advocated to remove all at-risk colonic epithelium at the time of surgery.

Probands or families with the clinical diagnosis of JPS but are mutation negative at both *BMPR1A* and *MADH4* should have all clinically at-risk individuals be managed as if they had mutation-proven JPS. Because large deletions and promoter mutations have not been systematically looked for in these 2 genes, it is possible that current "mutation negative" JPS patients might harbour deletions and promoter mutations.

Klinefelter syndrome

In men, the incidence of cancer of the breast is about 1 per cent of the frequency in females. It has been estimated that about 3.8 per cent of males with breast cancer have Klinefelter syndrome, giving an extrapolated risk of breast cancer in males with the 47XXY karyotype of about 7 per cent. This is almost equivalent to the population risk of the disease in females to age 70 (Nadel and Koss, 1967; Lynch et al., 1974). Studies vary in the extent of risk increase estimated: a risk 20 times the usual male breast cancer risk has been estimated (Jackson et al., 1965; Harnden et al., 1971). There is an increased risk of breast cancer in males carrying mutations in *BRCA2*, but no data are available on the breast cancer risk in individuals with Klinefelter syndrome who carry such mutations.

Extragonadal malignant germ cell tumours (teratomas, usually mediastinal, diagnosed before the age of 30 years) are significantly more prevalent in Klinefelter syndrome (relative risk 67), and any individual with early sexual development or testicular growth should be screened by measurement of germ cell tumour markers, including alphafetoprotein and human chorionic gonadotrophin-B (Evans and Critchlow, 1987; Scheike et al., 1973; Nichols, 1992; Derenoncourt et al., 1995; Hasle et al., 1995; Ganslandt et al., 2000; Yong et al., 2000).

Testicular tumours may be more common (perhaps secondary to cryptorchidism), and an association with AML and lymphoma has been proposed (Attard-Montalto et al., 1994), but this has not been substantiated (Machatschek et al., 2004) and may be due to the fact that cytogenetic studies are often performed in individuals with haematological malignancies (Hasle et al., 1995; Keung et al., 2002).

The overall risk of cancer in Klinefelter syndrome is not substantially increased, so that no routine cancer surveillance is recommended.

Kostmann syndrome (Kostmann infantile agranulocytosis)

This is a rare autosomal recessive disorder characterised by granulocytopenia and monocytosis in infancy. There is an increased risk of myelodysplastic syndrome and/or AML in the severe congenital neutropenia syndromes, such that in follow-up study (mean 6 years) malignant transformation occurred in ~10 per cent (Freedman et al., 2000). Neutropenia may respond to treatment with recombinant human granulocyte-colony stimulating factor. Germline mutations in the ELA2 (neutrophil elastase) account for many dominantly inherited and sporadic cases of severe congenital neutropenia, but not Kostmann syndrome (Ancliff et al., 2001).

Li–Fraumeni syndrome

Li–Fraumeni syndrome (LFS) is a rare autosomal dominant disorder characterised by sarcoma, breast cancer, brain tumour, leukaemia/lymphoma and adrenocortical carcinoma (ACC) (Li and Fraumeni, 1969; Li et al., 1988). Germline mutations in the *TP53* tumour suppressor gene on 17p13.1 have been found in 70 per cent of LFS (Malkin et al., 1990; Srivastava et al., 1990; Varley et al., 1997).

Clinical features

The major component malignancies in LFS include sarcomas, breast cancer, brain tumours, ACC and acute leukaemias (Li and Fraumeni, 1969; Garber et al., 1991; Li et al., 1991). Other associated cancers may include Wilms tumour, cancers of the colon, stomach, lung and pancreas, as well as melanoma and gonadal germ cell tumours (Garber et al., 1991; Varley et al., 1997; Birch et al., 2001), although some of these are isolated observations in a single family and so, their exact frequencies in mutation-positive individuals are unknown. The operational diagnostic criteria for LFS is as follows (Li and Fraumeni, 1969):

- An individual (index case) with a sarcoma diagnosed before age of 45 years.
- A first-degree relative with any cancer before age of 45 years.
- A third family member who is a first- or second-degree relative with either a sarcoma diagnosed at any age or any cancer diagnosed before age of 45 years.

There are several sets of operational criteria for the diagnosis of LFS-like (LFL) families. The two most commonly used include the so-called Manchester criteria (Varley, 2003) and Eeles criteria (Eeles, 1995).

- Manchester criteria:
  - A proband with any childhood cancer or sarcoma, brain tumour, or adrenal cortical tumour diagnosed under age of 45 years.
  - A first- or second-degree relative with a typical LFS cancer (sarcoma, breast cancer, brain tumour, adrenal cortical tumour, or acute leukaemia) at any age.
  - An additional first- or second-degree relative with any cancer under the age of 60 years.
- Eeles criteria:
  - Two first- or second-degree relatives with LFS-related malignancies (sarcoma, breast cancer, malignant brain tumour, adrenal cortical carcinoma, or acute leukaemia) at any age.

Genetics

Germline *TP53* mutations cause LFS, and at least 70 per cent of those who meet the diagnostic criteria have an identified mutation (Malkin et al., 1990;

Varley et al., 1997). Amongst these mutations, 70 per cent occur within exons 5 through 8 (Varley et al., 1997). In contrast to other cancer syndromes, missense mutations are the most common variety in LFS (Varley, 2003). The mutation frequency in families meeting the standard clinical criteria for LFS is 70–80 per cent in most clinical laboratories (Varley et al., 1997; Friedl et al., 1999; Frebourg et al., 1995; Varley, 2003). In families meeting the LFL criteria the frequency is lower: 8 per cent using the Eeles criteria and 22–40 per cent using the Manchester criteria (Eng et al., 1997; Varley et al., 1997; Varley, 2003; Birch et al., 1990; 1994).

Genotype–phenotype correlations have been observed in some studies but not in others. For example, in one, families with missense mutations in the DNA-binding domain trended towards an overall higher cancer incidence, particularly of those of the breast and CNS, with an earlier age at onset, when compared to families with protein truncating or inactivating mutations, or families with no mutation at all (Birch et al., 1998). Further, a systematic database study of all LFS families revealed that the mean age of breast cancer diagnosis in *TP53* mutation-positive families was a mean of 34.6 years in contrast to 42.5 years in mutation negative families ($P = 0.0035$) (Olivier et al., 2003). In mutation-positive families, brain tumours were over-represented in those families with missense mutations in the DNA-binding loop that contacts the minor groove of DNA. Development of ACCs were associated with missense mutations in the loops opposing the protein–DNA contact surface ($P = 0.0003$) (Olivier et al., 2003). In contrast, a study of 56 *TP53* mutation-positive individuals from 107 kindreds ascertained through cases of childhood soft tissue sarcoma reported no difference in phenotype between patients with missense mutations compared to those with truncating mutations (Hwang et al., 2003). Differences in patient accrual, study design, and mutation site classification may have contributed to these disparate findings, and thus more studies or a pooled analysis are needed to clarify this issue.

The frequency of germline *TP53* mutations in patients with multiple primary cancers unselected for family history and in those with apparently sporadic LFS component tumours has been extensively studied. While only 1 per cent of early-onset breast cancer cases will harbour a germline *TP53* mutation (Sidransky et al., 1992; Lalloo et al., 2003), the frequencies may be higher in sporadic osteosarcomas, 2–3 per cent (McIntyre et al., 1994), 9 per cent for rhabdomyosarcomas (Diller et al., 1995) and 2–10 per cent for brain tumours (Felix et al., 1995). Perhaps the most striking association occurs in cases of childhood ACC. In a series of 14 ACC patients unselected for family history, 11 (82 per cent) carried a germline *TP53* mutation. Interestingly, the same two mutations (at codons 152 and 158) were present in 9 of the 11 mutation-positive cases. In another series of

36 cases of childhood ACC in southern Brazil, 35 carried an identical *R337H* mutation. Initially, a founder effect was considered to be ruled-out (Ribeiro et al, 2001), but a subsequent study indicated that in fact a single common origin for all carriers of the Brazilian R337H mutation is likely (Pinto et al., 2004). The cancer family history in mutation-positive cases was not striking (there has been no evidence for Li-Fraumeni syndrome in the 30 mutation-positive kindred), suggesting a low-penetrance and possibly tissue-specific effect of this particular mutation (Figueiredo et al., 2006).

Genetic and medical management

The genetic-based management of LFS is not straightforward. It may be useful to view *TP53* mutation analysis as a molecular diagnostic test for LFS especially in the setting of LFL or apparently sporadic component neoplasias. However, it is less clear whether benefit derives from pre-morbid predictive testing, in particular when the predictive test is mutation positive. While breast cancer screening can be instituted, little effective surveillance is available for the other component tumours. Most clinical cancer geneticists will acknowledge that a predictive test that is negative in the setting of a known family-specific germline *TP53* mutation can be useful. Such an informative negative test will relieve that particular family member from LFS-directed clinical surveillance as his/her cancer risk would be no different from that of the general population.

Maffucci syndrome

Maffucci syndrome (MIM 166000) also known as Ollier disease is usually a sporadic condition, in which osteochondromatosis (mostly enchondromas) and haemangiomas occur. Cavernous or capillary haemangiomas, phlebectasia and lymphangiomas may develop and can be disfiguring. The dyschondroplasia may result in shortening of bones, fractures and deformities from enchondromas. Many mesenchymal neoplasias may occur, possibly in 15–30 per cent of cases (Harris, 1990; Albrechts and Rapini, 1995). Chondrosarcoma is the most common malignancy to develop in this condition (75 per cent), but fibrosarcoma, angiosarcoma, osteosarcoma, ovarian granulosa cell tumours or teratomas and gliomas have been reported (Sun et al., 1985; Schwartz et al., 1987; Christian and Ballon, 1990; Chang and Prados, 1994). Multiple primary tumours may develop (Loewinger et al., 1977). This syndrome may be the same as osteochondromatosis (Lewis and Ketcham, 1973; Tamimi and Bolen, 1984).

A germline variant in *PTHrP*, R150C, was found in one individual with enchondromatosis (Hopyan et al., 2002). Another individual had an enchondroma with a somatic or mosaic R150C variant (absent in normal adjacent bone) while another four such individuals neither had germline nor somatic *PTHrP* mutations. However another study failed to identify this mutation in 31 patients (Rozeman et al., 2004).

McCune–Albright syndrome

McCune–Albright syndrome (MAS, MIM 174800) is a non-heritable disorder classically characterised by the triad of polyostotic fibrous dysplasia (POFD), café-au-lait spots and sexual precocity. Somatic gain-of-function mutations in the *GNAS1* locus on 20q13.2–q13.3 have been described in affected tissues. Since these mutations arise post-zygotically, affected individuals are considered somatic mosaics.

POFD is characterised by fibrous tissue proliferation with destruction of bone, leading to pathological fractures and pseudoarthroses. The diagnosis of MAS is usually clinically obvious and is confirmed by excess circulating levels of one or more hormones (thyroid hormone, cortisol, growth hormone, or estrogen) in the absence of the respective stimulating hormones. Fibrous dysplasia is usually diagnosed by its characteristic ground glass (but occasionally sclerotic) appearance on X-ray, although it can be confused with osteofibrous dysplasia or HPT-JT (Hammami et al., 1997; Weinstein et al., 2002). Deafness and blindness may result from pressure within the cranial foramina. In addition, café-au-lait patches, with irregular borders, and multiple endocrinopathies occur. The most frequent endocrine disturbances are precocious puberty, especially in females (Albright et al., 1937), but thyroid dysfunction, HPT, acromegaly, Cushing syndrome or hyperprolactinaemia may occur. The condition is almost always sporadic, although some familial cases have been described, with affected individuals in several generations. However, there is dispute about whether these familial cases were really MAS (Alvarez-Arratia et al., 1983). Osteosarcomatous transformation in areas of fibrous dysplasia has been described as a complication of this condition (Taconis, 1988). It had been suggested that this disorder might be caused by somatic mutations in an autosomal dominant lethal gene, which would only be compatible with survival if present in mosaic form (Happle, 1989). Subsequently, mutations in the *GNAS1* gene that encodes a subunit of the stimulatory G protein, $G_s\alpha$, were identified (Weinstein et al., 1991). It has been postulated that somatic mutations of this type occur early in embryogenesis and result in a mosaic population of cells, which would explain the sporadic occurrence and variable abnormalities in this syndrome (Marie et al., 1997). Subsequent to the initial description of somatic mosaic *GNAS1* mutations in this syndrome, alternative exons with multiple transcripts and imprinting were described (Weinstein et al.,

2002; Rickard and Wilson, 2003). Loss of exon 1A imprinting causes pseudohy-poparathyroidism type Ib (Weinstein et al., 2002). $G_s\alpha$ is bi-allelically expressed in most human tissues, but shows exclusive or preferential expression from the maternal allele in some tissues, including pituitary, thyroid and ovary (Weinstein et al., 2002). In pituitary tumours that harbour an activating $G_s\alpha$ mutation, the mutation almost always occurs on the maternal allele (Weinstein et al., 2002). Therefore the clinical manifestations observed in each MAS patient might be affected by which parental allele harbours the $G_s\alpha$ gene mutation.

Since MAS and FD result from somatic mosaic mutations, and not germline mutations, in *GNAS1*, these syndromes are virtually never inherited. Patients with fibrous dysplasia should not be treated with radiation, as it is ineffective and may increase the risk for malignant transformation. It would be prudent for all POFD patients to be screened for endocrine manifestations of MAS.

Mosaic variegated aneuploidy

This term was first used by Warburton and colleagues to describe a rare clinical entity associated with specific cytogenetic findings in cell lines (Warburton et al., 1991). The clinical picture is severe microcephaly, growth deficiency, mild physical abnormalities and mental retardation. Many other features have been reported. Malignancies have also, been found, with myelodysplasia, rhab-domyosarcoma, leukaemia and Wilms tumour reported. Cytogenetically, the main features are aneuploidy for different chromosomes occurring mosaically; the proportion of cells showing aneuploidy varies considerably, but often more than a quarter of all cells show aneuploidy. Based on these findings, it was postulated that the underlying molecular defect was homozygosity for an auto-somal recessive gene that predisposed to mitotic instability. Other cases of affected children whose parents were consanguineous supported this conjecture (Tolmie et al., 1988; Papi et al., 1989). It has been noted that in mosaic varie-gated aneuploidy 3 of 14 reported cases developed a malignancy (Jacquemont et al., 2002). The finding of homozygous mutations in *BUB1B* (Hanks et al., 2004) confirmed the earlier prediction, and are of particular interest because of the associated cancer predisposition. *BUB1B* encodes BUBR1, a protein that is essential for mitosis. BUBR1 regulates the mitotic spindle. Somatic muta-tions in *BUB1B* are rare in most cancers studied thus far, but have been identi-fied (Cahill et al., 1998) and genes that regulate mitosis are likely to have an important role in cancer (Lengauer et al., 1997). The question of whether cancers can arise solely from chromosomal instability has been debated (Rajagopalan et al., 2003; Sieber et al., 2003). The recent findings in mosaic variegated aneuploidy supports the notion that aneuploidy is a sufficient cause of carcinogenesis.

Multiple endocrine neoplasia type 1

Multiple endocrine neoplasia type 1 (MEN 1, MIM 131100), also known as Wermer syndrome, is an autosomal dominant inherited cancer syndrome occurring in 1–2/100 000 live births and characterised by the classic triad of pituitary tumours, parathyroid neoplasia and pancreatic endocrine neoplasia (Thakker, 2000). Germline mutations in *MEN1*, encoding MENIN, on 11q13, are associated with MEN 1 (Larsson et al., 1988; Larsson and Friedman, 1994; Chandrasekharappa et al., 1997).

Clinical features

The major endocrine features of MEN 1 are parathyroid adenomas, entero-pancreatic endocrine tumours, and pituitary tumours. As defined by the consensus diagnostic criteria, a diagnosis of MEN 1 is made in a person with 2 of the 3 major endocrine tumours. Familial MEN 1 is defined as at least one MEN 1 case plus at least one first-degree relative with 1 of these 3 tumours (Brandi et al., 1987; Thakker, 2000). Primary HPT is the most common manifestation and usually the first sign of MEN 1, occurring in 80–100 per cent of all such patients (Thakker, 2000). These tumours are typically multiglandular and often hyperplastic. The mean age at onset of MEN 1-related HPT is 30 years earlier in patients with MEN 1 than in the general population (20–25 years versus 50 years). Parathyroid carcinoma is not known to be associated with MEN 1 unlike in HPT-JT, caused by mutations in the *HRPT2* gene.

Pancreatic islet cell tumours, now referred to as neuroendocrine carcinomas of the pancreas, usually gastrinomas and insulinomas, and less commonly VIPomas (vasoactive intestinal peptide), glucagonomas and somatostatinomas, are the second most common endocrine manifestation, occurring in up to 30–80 per cent of patients by age of 40 years (Thakker, 2000). These are usually multifocal and can arise in the pancreas or more commonly, as small (<0.5 cm) foci throughout the duodenum. Gastrinomas represent over half of the pancreatic islet cell tumours in MEN 1 and are the major cause of morbidity and mortality in these patients (Skogseid et al., 1994; Trump et al., 1996; Norton et al., 1999; Brandi et al., 2001). Most result in peptic ulcer disease (Zollinger–Ellison syndrome) and half are malignant at the time of diagnosis (Skogseid et al., 1994; Weber et al., 1995; Norton et al., 1999). Non-functional tumours of the entero-pancreas, some of which produce pancreatic polypeptide, are seen in 20 per cent of patients (Skogseid et al., 1994, p. 351).

Approximately 15–50 per cent of individuals with MEN 1 develop a pituitary tumour (Skogseid, 1994; Thakker, 2000). Two-thirds are microadenomas (<1.0 cm in diameter) and the majority are prolactin-secreting (Corbetta et al., 1997). Other manifestations include carcinoids of the foregut (typically bronchial or thymic), skin tumours including lipomas (30 per cent), facial angiomas (85 per cent), and collagenomas (70 per cent) (Thakker, 2000; Skogseid et al., 1994) and adrenal cortical lesions, including cortical adenomas, diffuse or nodular hyperplasia or rarely carcinoma. These adrenal lesions do not show loss of heterozygosity for the *MEN1* locus and might represent a secondary phenomenon (Skogseid et al., 1992; Burgess et al., 1996a). Thyroid adenomas, phaeochromocytoma (PC) (usually unilateral), spinal ependymoma, leiomyoma and melanoma have also been reported but their frequency is not known.

Genetics

Germline loss-of-function mutations in *MEN1*, on 11q13 and encoding MENIN, have been found in 60–70 per cent of MEN 1 probands (Larsson et al., 1988; Larsson and Friedman, 1994; Chandrasekharappa et al., 1997). Loss of the wild-type allele in many familial and sporadic MEN 1-associated tumours, as well as the fact that most mutations result in protein truncation, suggests that *MEN1* is a tumour suppressor gene. The exact role of MENIN is not currently known, but its localisation to the nucleus and its interactions with proteins chief of which is JUN-D suggest that it may play a role in transcriptional regulation (Agarwal et al., 1999; 2003; Kim et al., 2003). While other MENIN partners such as NF-kappa-B, SMAD3 and REL-A have been described in vitro, it remains unclear whether these relationships hold in vivo. It is also possible that it plays a role in other regulatory pathways that lead to the control of cell growth and/ or genomic integrity, but this remains to be seen.

Over 300 *MEN1* mutations have been reported to date and like most tumour suppressor gene-associated loss-of-function mutations, they are nonsense, frameshift and missense, and are scattered throughout the gene. There is currently no evidence of genotype–phenotype correlations and inter- and intra-familial variability is the rule (Giraud et al., 1998; Wautot et al., 2002).

Genetic and medical management

Individuals or families with MEN 1 or suspected or having MEN 1 should be referred for clinical cancer genetic consultation which includes genetic counselling. The frequency of MEN 1 among patients with apparently sporadic component tumours varies but can be high for some tumour types. For instance, approximately one-third of patients with Zollinger–Ellison syndrome will have a clinical diagnosis of MEN 1 (Bardram and Stage, 1985; Roy et al., 2001). Only 2–3 per cent of patients presenting with primary HPT have MEN 1 (Uchino et al., 2000), although, familial isolated hyperparathyroidism (FIHP) is allelic to MEN 1, with 20 per cent of probands harbouring a germline *MEN1*

Table 12.6. *Sanple surveillance programme for patients with MEN 1 and asymptomatic* MEN1 *mutation carriers (from Dreijerink and Lips, 2005)*

From age of 5 years
2-yearly clinical examination and biochemical measurement of ionised calcium, phosphate, parathyroid hormone, glucose, insulin, C-peptide, glucagon, gastrin, pancreatic polypeptide, prolactin, IGF1, platelet serotonin and chromogranin A.

Every 2 years from age of 15 years
Upper abdominal MRI scan
MRI scan of the pituitary with gadolinium contrast
MRI scan of the mediastinum in males

mutation (see below) (Pannett et al., 2003). Among patients with pituitary tumours, the prevalence of MEN 1 is 2.5–5 per cent (Scheithauer et al., 1987; Corbetta et al., 1997), but is as high as 14 per cent in patients with prolactinoma (Corbetta et al., 1997). These results underscore the importance of carefully taking a thorough medical and family history in patients with a diagnosis of an MEN 1-associated endocrine tumour, even seemingly in isolation.

Germline *MEN1* mutation analysis can be a useful molecular diagnostic in the setting of apparently sporadic presentations of MEN 1-component neoplasias. Finding a mutation is diagnostic of MEN 1. Not finding a mutation is non-diagnostic. Mutation analysis for *MEN1* and other genes, such as *HRPT2* can help differentiate MEN 1 from HPT-JT in the setting of HPT presentation. HPT-JT also carries a risk for parathyroid carcinoma.

The precise strategy for clinical surveillance of individuals with or at risk for MEN 1 remains controversial and based, for the most part, on region-specific expert opinion but a sample surveillance protocol is shown in Table 12.6 (Dreijerink and Lips, 2005).

Multiple endocrine neoplasia type 2

MEN 2 (MIM 171400), also known as Sipple syndrome, is an autosomal dominant inherited cancer syndrome occurring in 1 in 300 000 live births and comprises three subtypes depending on the combination of clinical features (Schimke, 1984). MEN 2A, the most common clinical subtype, is characterised by medullary thyroid carcinoma (MTC), PC and HPT. MEN 2B, the least common subtype, is similar to MEN 2A except that component neoplasias occur an average of 10 years earlier than that in MEN 2A, clinically apparent HPT is rarely, if ever, seen, and other features such as marfanoid habitus, ganglioneuromatosis of the mucosae and medullated corneal nerve fibres are present (Gorlin et al., 1968). Familial MTC (FMTC) is characterised by MTC only in any given family (Farndon et al., 1986). Germline mutations in the *RET* proto-oncogene, on 10q11.2, have been found in >95 per cent of all MEN 2 probands (Eng et al., 1996a).

Multiple endocrine neoplasia type 2A

MTC is the most frequent complication of MEN 2A and occurs in more than 95 per cent of clinically affected patients. PC develops in about 50 per cent of patients, but there are interfamilial variations in predisposition, and the variations in frequency of PC have been correlated with specific *RET* mutations (Eng et al., 1996a) (see below). Similarly, the incidence of HPT, which occurs in 15–30 per cent of patients, is also correlated with allelic variation (Eng et al., 1996b; Schuffenecker et al., 1998).

MTC is almost always the first manifestation of MEN 2A. Clinical epidemiologic studies suggested that about 25 per cent of all MTC presentations are MEN 2 and are characterised by C-cell hyperplasia. MTC arise from these parafollicular C-cells, which derive from the neural crest, and secrete calcitonin. Other hormones may also be secreted, including adrenocorticotropic hormone (ACTH), melanocyte-stimulating hormone (MSH), prolactin, serotonin, VIP, somatostatin, prostaglandins and gastrin, so the symptomatology may be complex. About one-third of patients with MTC develop diarrhoea, which resolves on removal of the thyroid gland. MEN 2A-related MTCs often present clinically between 20 and 40 years of age, and up to a quarter present with cervical lymphadenopathy. They may metastasise to liver, lungs and bone. Over 90 per cent are bilateral and multifocal.

MEN 2A-related PC occurs, on average, about 8 years after MTC, with a mean age at diagnosis of 37 years (Howe et al., 1993), and is bilateral in approximately 50 per cent of affected patients. However, extra-adrenal or malignant tumours are infrequent. Up to 50 per cent of patients with PC are asymptomatic, and a rise in urinary catecholamines and vanillyl mandelic acid (VMA) may be a late feature. Hypertension may develop but paroxysmal hypertension, especially related to postural changes, is typical of PC. An increase in the adrenaline:noradrenaline ratio in the urine may be noted earlier, as would serum chromogranin-A levels.

Although clinical penetrance for MEN 2A is incomplete (approximately 45 per cent at age of 50 years, and 60–75 per cent at age of 70 years), hyperplasia of thyroid C-cells, which is the precursor of MTC, has a much earlier age at onset. C-cell hyperplasia may be detected in asymptomatic gene carriers by measuring serum calcitonin levels following pentagastrin administration. Using such biochemical screening tests increases the apparent penetrance of MEN 2A to 93 per cent at age of 31 years (Easton et al., 1989).

Multiple endocrine neoplasia type 2B

MEN 2B is similar to MEN 2A except that the mean age of tumour development in the former is an average 10 years earlier than the latter (Schimke, 1984; Eng et al., 2001). Interestingly, clinically apparent HPT is rarely, if ever, observed in individuals with MEN 2B. Instead, they have characteristic stigmata including multiple mucosal neuromas and intestinal ganglioneuromatosis. There is a thin, asthenic marfanoid build, with some muscle wasting and possibly weakness. Joint laxity, kyphoscoliosis, pectus excavatum, pes cavus and genu valgum are common. The face is elongated, the eyebrows are large and prominent, and the lips enlarged and nodular secondary to the neuromata – "blubbery" (Gorlin et al., 1968; Schimke, 1984) (see Fig. 12.6). There may be multiple mucosal neuromas, which can be plexiform and are visible on the eyelids, conjunctivae and corneas. Enlarged corneal nerves (medullated corneal nerve fibres) may be seen. Cutaneous neuromas may also occur, and rarely, there may be café-au-lait patches and facial lentigenes. The skin features may resemble those of NF 1, from which MEN 2B must be distinguished. Bowel malfunction, usually presenting with constipation or even obstipation, may result from ganglioneuromatosis of the gut (Carney et al., 1976). This must be distinguished from Hirschsprung disease (see below).

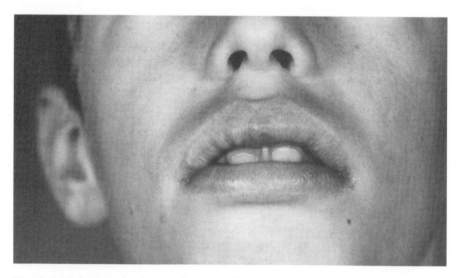

Fig. 12.6. Multiple endocrine neoplasia type 2B.

MTC and PC develop in virtually all patients with MEN 2B. The tumours are bilateral and multicentric, and metastasise locally and distantly, often before the disease is recognised. MEN 2B-related MTC develop at a younger age (mean age at diagnosis, 20 years) than MEN 2A and has been observed to be metastatic by the age of 4 years (Wells et al., 1978; Eng et al., 2001). While it is widely believed that the prognosis for MEN 2B-related MTC is worse than that in MEN 2A, well-controlled studies suggest that this is largely due to lead time bias.

Familial medullary thyroid carcinoma

This is a relatively infrequent clinical subtype of MEN 2, believed to represent 5–10 per cent of all MEN 2 cases. FMTC is characterised by familial later-onset MTC with objective evidence against the presence of PC or HPT (Farndon et al., 1986). Given our current knowledge of the genetics of MEN 2, it is believed that FMTC and MEN 2A are artificially divided subtypes and may be on a continuum but represent phenotypes resulting from different penetrance.

Molecular genetics of MEN 2

The *MEN2* locus was mapped to 10q11.2 and subsequently, germline gain-of-function mutations in the *RET* proto-oncogene were found in probands with MEN 2A, MEN 2B and FMTC (Mathew et al., 1987; Gardner et al., 1993; Mulligan et al., 1993; Eng et al., 1994b; 1995d; Hofstra et al., 1994; Bolino et al., 1995; Santoro et al., 1995).

Before identification of *RET* as the *MEN2* susceptibility gene, the clinical penetrance of MEN 2A was said to be 70 per cent by the age of 70 years (Ponder et al., 1988). After the putative susceptibility locus was found, the biochemically induced penetrance of MEN 2A was found to be 100 per cent by the age of 70 years (Easton et al., 1989). Similarly, original epidemiologic studies suggested that approximately 25 per cent of all MTC presentations were due to MEN 2. After *RET* was identified, several series examined the frequency of unexpected germline *RET* mutations in apparently sporadic MTC. When individuals with MTC were tested without taking a good family history or excluding syndromic features, the mutation frequency was approximately 25 per cent (Decker et al., 1995). However, several other series accruing MTC cases with no family history and no syndromic features reveal that the unexpected germline *RET* mutation frequency ranges from 5 to 10 per cent (Eng et al., 1995c; Wohlik et al., 1996; Schuffenecker et al., 1997; Wiench et al., 2001). A population-based series of apparently sporadic PC, defined as no family history and no syndromic features, suggests a ~5 per cent occult germline *RET* mutation frequency (Neumann et al., 2002).

Germline *RET* mutations have been identified in >95 per cent of all MEN 2, with 98 per cent of MEN 2A probands found to have a mutation, 97 per cent in

MEN 2B and 85 per cent in FMTC (Eng et al., 1996b; Gimm et al., 1997; Smith D.P. et al., 1997). The characteristic mutational spectrum found in MEN 2A includes missense mutations in one of cysteine codons 609, 611, 618, 620 (exon 10) or 634 (exon 11) (Mulligan et al., 1994; Eng et al., 1996). Approximately 85 per cent of MEN 2A individuals carry a codon 634 mutation (Eng et al., 1996a). Genotype–phenotype analyses reveal that codon 634 mutations are associated with the presence of PC and HPT (Eng et al., 1996b). In particular, the *C634R* mutation is likely associated with the development of HPT (Mulligan et al., 1994; Eng et al., 1996a; Schuffenecker et al., 1998). Rare "one-off" missense mutations seen in MEN 2A include those involving codons 630 and 790 (Eng et al., 1996b; Eng, 1999). FMTC-associated mutations occur at the same cysteine codons as those in MEN 2A although mutations at codons 609–620 are more proportionately frequent in FMTC than MEN 2A. Consistent with the C634R-HPT association, FMTC families have not been found to have C634R mutations, but C634Y and other 634 mutations (Eng et al., 1996a). Germline mutations probably unique to FMTC include E768D (exon 13), V804L and V804M (exon 14), although one family segregating V804L has been described with older-onset unilateral PC in 2 members (Eng et al., 1996a; Nilsson et al., 1999).

Germline M918T and A883F mutations occur in 95 per cent and ~2 per cent, respectively, of MEN 2B patients (Eng et al., 1996b; Gimm et al., 1997; Smith D.P. et al., 1997). These two mutations are unique to MEN2B and have never been observed in MEN 2A or FMTC. Interestingly, at least one MEN 2B family appears to carry a *V804M* mutation in the presence of a *RET* variant of unknown significance (Miyauchi et al., 1999).

Discovering that *RET* is the susceptibility gene for MEN 2 also led to the realisation that variable penetrance characterised various genotypes. For example, it has now become obvious that *RET* codons 918, 883 and 634 mutations have the highest penetrance, predisposing to MEN 2B and MEN 2A with MTC, PC and HPT involvement (Eng et al., 1996a; Eng, 2000b). In contrast, germline *V804M* mutations and perhaps cysteine codon 609 mutations have the lowest penetrance and the older ages of onset (Eng et al., 1996a; Shannon et al., 1999). Mutations at codons 611–620 have a broad range of penetrance and expressivity. Taken together, these data suggest that each of the component organs has a different threshold for transformation to neoplasia, with the highest threshold in the parathyroid glands and the lowest in the C-cells of the thyroid, the precursor cells of MTC.

RET and the practice of molecular-based medical management in MEN 2

RET testing in MEN 2 is considered the paradigm for the practice of clinical cancer genetics. Since *RET* mutations have been identified in >95 per cent of individuals with MEN 2, *RET* gene testing as a molecular diagnostic test and as a predictive test is considered the standard of medical care around the world (Eng et al., 1996a; 2001). In addition, because of the frequency of germline *RET* mutation in apparently sporadic cases of MTC, all presentations of MTC, irrespective of syndromic features or family history should be offered *RET* gene testing in the setting of clinical cancer genetics consultation which includes genetic counselling.

In an MEN 2 family without a known mutation, *RET* testing should begin with an affected individual. Once a family-specific mutation is found, all at-risk family members should be offered testing, before the age of 5 years in MEN 2A/ FMTC and before the age of 2 years, preferably within the first year, in MEN 2B. For those individuals found to have a mutation, a prophylactic total thyroidectomy is recommended for all MEN 2 subtypes. This should be completed before the age of 5–6 years for MEN 2A/FMTC and before the age of 2 years, some believe 6 months, for MEN 2B (Wells et al., 1994). The precise timing of prophylactic surgery remains controversial for FMTC and in particular those with codon 609, 768 and 804 mutations who seem to have a lower penetrance and perhaps later onset of MTC (Eng et al., 1996a; Shannon et al., 1999). Clinical surveillance following thyroidectomy is dictated by what is found during the surgery. If the patient is found to have invasive MTC at the time of surgery, screening should include calcium-stimulated calcitonin testing every 3–6 months for the first 2 years, every 6 months from 3 to 5 years after surgery, and then annually. If only a small focus of MTC is found at the time of surgery, follow-up screening should involve annual basal (unstimulated) calcitonin for 5–10 years. If no cancer is present in the thyroid at the time of prophylactive surgery, no follow-up screening is indicated, even if C-cell hyperplasia is present. All individuals who have undergone thyroidectomy need thyroid hormone replacement therapy and monitoring.

MEN 2-related PC almost always occur after MTC. All mutation-positive individuals should undergo annual screening for PC beginning at the age of 6 years. This usually consists of 24-h urine studies for VMA, metanephrines and catecholamines. Most centres also advocate annual serum measurements for catecholamine levels and chromogranin-A. Abdominal ultrasound or CT/MRI scans for routine surveillance remain controversial.

In MEN 2, HPT is usually later onset and has age-related penetrance (Schuffenecker et al., 1998). Clinical surveillance in MEN 2A includes annual measurement of serum ionised calcium and intact parathyroid hormone levels beginning at the time of MEN 2 diagnosis. Once HPT is detected, removal of all four parathyroid glands is necessary. At that time or at the time of thyroidectomy, whichever occurs first, all glands and the thymus are removed. Half of a parathyroid gland should be pulverised and autografted into an easily accessible muscle of the arm or neck to control the body's calcium levels and can be easily removed should HPT recur (Wells et al., 1994). Since clinically evident HPT is rare, or even non-existent, in MEN 2B, parathyroid screening is not generally recommended for this subtype.

In the era of routine clinical *RET* mutation testing, the clinician may find it uncomfortable to manage *RET* mutation negative MEN 2 families. If there are sufficient clinically affected members in such families, linkage analysis using 10q11 markers within and around *RET* should be performed. In the event that the family is not large enough or not informative for linkage, then management should follow that in the pre-*RET* testing era. For *RET* mutation negative families, at-risk individuals should undergo annual screening for MTC (stimulated calcitonin screening), PC and HPT from the age of 6–35 years. Prophylactic thyroidectomy is usually not routinely offered to this subgroup.

Muir–Torre syndrome

Muir–Torre syndrome is a rare autosomal dominant condition, first described in 1967 in an individual who had multiple benign sebaceous adenomas and kera-toacanthomas of the skin, and multiple internal malignancies (large bowel, duodenum and larynx) (Muir et al., 1967; Schwartz et al., 1989). The skin stigmata of this condition include sebaceous hyperplasia, adenoma and carcinoma, with keratoacanthoma and BCC. The internal neoplasias include tumours of the colon, stomach and oesophagus, breast, uterus, ovaries, bladder, larynx, and squamous cell carcinomas of the mucous membranes (Grignon et al., 1987). The syndrome is defined by dermatologists as a combination of at least one sebaceous gland tumour and a minimum of one internal malignancy (Cohen et al., 1991). The condition usually becomes manifest from the fifth decade of life, and multiple skin lesions develop.

It has become apparent that the only known hereditary cause of Muir–Torre syndrome is mutations in the *MMR* genes *MLH1* and *MSH2*. No mutations have been reported in *MSH6* in this syndrome. The presence of identical mutations in families with HNPCC and Muir–Torre syndrome confirms that this syndrome is essentially a variant of HNPCC (Kolodner et al., 1994). The implication of this conclusion is that individuals with sebaceous carcinoma and a mutation in a *MMR* gene should be considered to be at an elevated lifetime risk of all the cancers that are known to occur in HNPCC. In a large, single-institution study, 27 of 41 patients with Muir–Torre syndrome had mutations in *MLH1* or *MSH2* (Mangold et al., 2004). Interestingly, 25 of the 27 mutations were in *MSH2*, confirming multiple earlier observations that found far more mutations in *MSH2* than in *MLH1* (Lucci-Cordisco et al., 2003). Because the ascertainment criteria in the recent study of Mangold et al. were a sebaceous gland neoplasm and at least one internal neoplasm in the same patient (regardless of site of cancer or family history), it is not surprising that not all individuals with germline MMR gene mutations fell within the Bethesda guidelines for gene testing. Probably all sebaceous neoplasms occurring in the context of Muir–Torre syndrome are associated with MSI (Kruse et al., 2003), or loss of expression of MSH2 (or rarely MLH1) (Fiorentino et al., 2004), so all patients with sebaceous neoplasms, should be offered either or both of these tests. If either test suggests a MMR gene mutation, analysis should be carried out, even in the absence of an internal malignancy or a positive family history. The situation may be particularly challenging on the rare occasion when a child is diagnosed with a sebaceous neoplasm (which are usually peri-ocular) (Omura et al., 2002), as in the absence of family history, testing of a minor may be warranted. From a laboratory standpoint, the spectrum of mutations in *MSH2* is similar to that seen in non-Muir–Torre-associated HNPCC, no genotype–phenotype associations within *MSH2* are seen (Mangold et al., 2004) and a search for genomic deletions is indicated if sequenced-based analysis is negative (Barana et al., 2004).

Screening for cancer in relatives of individuals with this disorder is obviously important, and should be similar to that outlined for HNPCC, with extra-colonic surveillance, particularly of the skin. It is interesting to note that in many families with Muir–Torre syndrome, only one person is affected by a sebaceous cancer, suggesting that other modifying factors may be present. In one Quebec family, which was later identified to carry a germline deletion in *MLH1*, the one person who developed sebaceous carcinoma only did so after receiving a heart transplant and subsequent immunosuppression (Paraf et al., 1995). The generality of this finding has been confirmed in a more recent study (Harwood et al., 2003).

Although no other genes have been implicated in Muir–Torre syndrome, when exposed to N-nitrosomethylbenzylamine, mice heterozygous for the gene encoding the fragile histidine triad gene, *Fhit* developed a syndrome akin to human Muir–Torre syndrome (Fong et al., 2000). In human sebaceous carcinomas, FHIT protein was absent only from those tumours that were microsatellite stable, suggesting an alternative pathway to skin tumours in this syndrome (Holbach et al., 2002). No germline mutations in *FHIT* have been identified in Muir-Torre (or any other human cancer) syndrome.

MYH-associated polyposis (MAP)

Bi-allelic mutations in the *MYH* gene (now known as MUTYH) have been shown to be responsible for an autosomal recessive form of adenomatous polyposis. The product of the *MYH* gene is involved in repair of oxidative DNA damage, and adenomas from affected patients show characteristic DNA repair errors. The number of colonic polyps in this condition tends to be between 15 and 200, significantly fewer than in classical FAP, although approximately 8 per cent of cases of polyposis with no detectable germline *APC* mutation, particularly cases with relatively few (100–500) polyps, have been found to carry bi-allelic mutations in *MYH*. The disorder accounts for approximately 30 per cent of cases of attenuated polyposis, with 15–100 colonic adenomas (Al-Tassan et al., 2002; Sampson et al., 2003, Sieber et al., 2003).

Management of patients with *MYH* polyposis should be along the lines of FAP management, with upper GI surveillance, since affected individuals do have a risk of upper GI neoplasia. Heterozygotes do not appear to have a significantly increased risk of GI polyps and do not require surveillance, but it is important to be certain that close relatives of affected individuals are offered genetic testing for the familial *MYH* mutations identified.

N syndrome

This rare, X-linked recessive disorder was described in a single family (two affected brothers) and was characterised by mental retardation, chromosome breakage and a predisposition to T-cell leukaemia. It is suggested to be caused by a mutation of DNA polymerase alpha (Floy et al., 1990).

NAME syndrome

See Carney Complex (above).

Neurofibromatosis type 1 (NF1, von Recklinghausen disease, peripheral NF)

NF1 is the most common form of NF, with a prevalence of about 1 per 3000 persons. Inheritance is autosomal dominant with variable expression, but approximately 50 per cent of cases represent new mutations. Characteristic clinical features are listed in Table 12.7. Conventional diagnostic criteria require two or more of the following features: (i) six or more café-au-lait lesions (more than 5 mm greatest diameter in children and more than 15 mm greatest diameter in adults); (ii) two or more neurofibromas (Fig. 12.7) or one plexiform neurofibroma; (iii) axillary or inguinal freckling; (iv) two or more Lisch nodules; (v) optic glioma; (vi) characteristic osseous lesion (sphenoid dysplasia or cortical thinning of long bone, with or without pseudoarthrosis); (vi) a first-degree relative (parent, sibling or child) with NF1 according to the above criteria.

The diagnosis of NF1 among at-risk relatives can usually be made early. Huson et al. (1989) found that all gene carriers have developed six or more café-au-lait

Table 12.7. *Clinical features of NF1*

Neurofibromas
Café-au-lait spots
Axillary freckling
Lisch nodules
Intellectual impairment
Epilepsy
Macrocephaly
Short stature
Kyphoscoliosis
Pseudoarthrosis
Renal artery stenosis
Cerebrovascular disease

Neoplasia
CNS
Optic glioma, astrocytoma and glioma, neurilemomas
Neurofibrosarcoma or malignant schwannoma

Endocrine
PC, carcinoid

Other
Rhabdomyosarcoma, leukaemia, neuroblastoma, Wilms tumour

spots by the age of 5 years, and 90 per cent of affected subjects have Lisch nodules by this age. Huson et al. (1989) and Lubs et al. (1991) found, respectively, that Lisch nodules were present in 93 per cent and 100 per cent of adults (aged over 20 years) with NF1. Unlike café-au-lait spots and neurofibromas, multiple Lisch nodules are specific for NF1, and have only been reported rarely in NF2. In addition, Lisch nodules frequently develop before neurofibromas (Lubs et al., 1991), which is very useful in the differentiation between minimally affected and unaffected individuals. In children with possible NF and no Lisch nodules, the ophthalmological assessment should be repeated periodically. Slit-lamp examination allows Lisch nodules to be distinguished from common iris naevi.

The approximate frequencies of disabling non-neoplastic complications of NF1 were estimated by Huson et al. (1989) to be 33 per cent for intellectual handicap (3 per cent moderate–severe retardation, 30 per cent minimal retardation or learning difficulties), 5 per cent for scoliosis requiring surgery, 4 per cent for epilepsy, 2 per cent for severe pseudoarthrosis, and 2 per cent for renal artery stenosis. Café-au-lait spots occur in more than 99 per cent of patients with NF1 but are not specific and may fade in older patients.

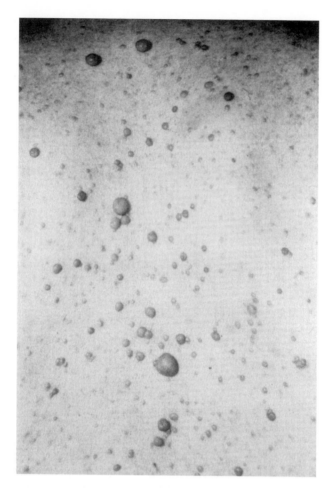

Fig. 12.7. Neurofibromatosis type 1. Dermal neurofibromata. Courtesy of Susan Huson.

Individuals with NF1 are at increased risk of a variety of neoplastic lesions, including optic glioma, neurofibrosarcoma, brain gliomas, PC and leukaemia. Estimates of the increased risk of neoplasia are variable because of differences in the methods of ascertainment, and some older studies have not distinguished between NF1 and NF2. Sorensen et al. (1986) found that the common perception of NF as a severe disorder with greatly increased risk of cancer is not true. Although probands in a hospital-based study had a fourfold increase in the incidence of malignant neoplasms or benign CNS tumours, the relative risk among affected relatives was only 1.5 (0.9 in males, 1.9 in females). There was a significant excess of glioma, and although the relative risk of PC was greatly increased (because it is rare in the general population), the absolute risk was small. In a population-based study, Huson et al. (1989) estimated the overall risk of malignant or CNS tumours to be approximately 5 per cent (0.7 per cent for optic glioma, 0.7–1.5 per cent for other CNS tumours, 1.5 per cent for rhabdomyosarcoma, and 1.5 per cent for peripheral nerve malignancy). Endocrine tumours (PCs, pancreatic apudomas) may occur in 3.1 per cent and spinal and visceral neurofibromas each occur in about 2.1 per cent of patients. Stiller et al. (1994) reported a relative risk of chronic myelomonocytic leukaemia of 221 in NF1, whereas the relative risks for acute lymphoblastic leukaemia (ALL) and non-Hodgkin lymphoma were 5.4 and 10 respectively.

Specific tumour types in NF1

Neurofibromas are benign tumours that usually involve the skin, although they can be subcutaneous or, rarely, visceral. Solitary neurofibromas may occur in an individual without a germline *NF1* mutation. The number of cutaneous neurofibromas increases with advancing age but shows wide variation (Huson et al., 1989). Two types of neurofibroma are distinguished: the common discrete variety in which the lesion arises from a single site along a peripheral nerve and has well-defined margins. Cutaneous neurofibromas are usually present in adults with NF1 and are most common on the trunk. About 20 per cent have head and neck lesions and more than 100 neurofibromas are found in most older patients. Neurofibromas often appear during puberty and may increase in size and number in pregnancy. Plexiform neurofibromas are peripheral nerve tumours that extend along the nerve and can involve multiple nerve branches. Plexiform neurofibromas are often associated with local soft tissue overgrowth and, when the cranial nerves are involved, cause marked disfigurement. Plexiform neurofibromas appear as large, soft, subcutaneous swellings with ill-defined margins and may be present in about 25 per cent of NF1 patients (usually on the trunk), but facial involvement is rare (Huson et al., 1988). The principal complication of neurofibromas is cosmetic disfigurement, but there is also the risk of malignant change (malignant peripheral nerve sheath tumour, MPNST). When malignancy does occur, it is often in a plexiform neurofibroma (Huson et al., 1989). Malignant change is usually signalled by pain and rapid increase in size, and all patients should be alerted to the significance of these events. Plexiform neurofibroma is locally aggressive and may grow along the nerve of origin to involve the spinal cord or brain. The risk of malignant change was estimated to be 2–4 per cent (Huson et al., 1988), but a population-based longitudinal study reported a lifetime risk of 8–13 per cent (median age at diagnosis 26 years) (Evans et al., 2002).

Optic glioma is the most frequently reported CNS lesion in NF1 and about a third of children with optic glioma have NF1. Estimates of the incidence of optic glioma in NF1 patients vary: Huson et al. (1988) found in a population-based study that less than 2 per cent of patients with NF1 had a symptomatic glioma, but Lewis et al. (1984) observed a frequency of up to 15 per cent with routine cranial magnetic resonance imaging. Histologically, optic gliomas are pilocytic astrocytomas and these are generally non-progressive tumours and are usually treated conservatively.

Other CNS gliomas reported in NF1 include brainstem gliomas, pilocytic astrocytomas of the hypothalamus and third ventricle, and, infrequently, diffuse gliomas of the cerebral hemispheres, cerebellum or spinal cord. Although brainstem glioma may produce aqueduct stenosis and hydrocephalus, NF1 patients are also at risk for non-neoplastic lesions, such as dural ectasia and aqueduct stenosis without mass lesions.

NF1 is a well-recognised, but infrequent, cause of PC. The most frequent age at diagnosis of PC in NF1 patients is in the fifth decade (Walther et al., 1999b). Onset before the age of 20 years is uncommon, and this tumour is virtually unknown in childhood (Knudson and Strong, 1972). Multiple tumours are seen in 12 per cent of patients.

The other endocrine tumour that has been associated with *NF1* is duodenal carcinoid. Typically, this is somatostatinoma with distinctive histological appearance (psammoma bodies) and somatostatin immunoreactivity (Griffiths et al., 1987; Swinburn et al., 1988).

A variety of embryonal tumours have been reported in children with NF1, including rhabdomyosarcoma, Wilms tumour and neuroblastoma (McKeen et al., 1978; Hartley et al., 1988). In addition, children with NF1 are predisposed to myeloid malignancies (200–500 times the normal risk), particularly juvenile myelomonocytic leukaemia (Bader and Miller, 1978; Clark and Hutter, 1982).

The *NF1* gene was mapped to chromosome 17 by genetic linkage studies in 1987 (Barker et al., 1987; Seizinger et al., 1987) and was cloned 3 years later (Wallace et al., 1990; Viskochil et al., 1990). The isolation of the *NF1* gene was facilitated by the identification of two patients with constitutional chromosome 17 translocations involving band 17q11.2. The arrangement of the *NF1* gene is unusual in that it appears to span at least three active genes within an intron (Wallace et al., 1990; Cawthon et al., 1990; Viskochil et al., 1990). The *NF1* gene encodes an mRNA of approximately 11 kb and both deletions and point mutations have been described in the germline of affected patients. The cloning of the *NF1* gene provides an opportunity to define the relationship between the molecular pathology and the clinical phenotype, but progress was delayed by the large size of the gene (>60 exons and several alternatively spliced isoforms) and the difficulty in identifying germline mutations. A wide variety of loss-of-function mutations, including germline deletions, have been described. Generally, no clear genotype–phenotype relationship has been defined, and there is evidence that the phenotype of *NF1* is influenced by modifier effects (Easton et al., 1993b). However, individuals with an NF1 microdeletion have, on average, an earlier onset of, and a greater number of neurofibromas and an increased lifetime risk of MPNSTs (De Raedt et al., 2003).

NF1 gene product (neurofibromin) contains a domain homologous to GTPase activating protein (GAP) and the *NF1* gene appears to function as a classical tumour suppressor gene and NF1 allele loss has been detected in both malignant neurofibroma.

Patients with NF1 should be kept under surveillance, with annual clinical examination (every 2 years in children), but routine biochemical or radiological screening is probably not indicated in a service setting (Huson et al., 1988). The affectation status for most at-risk relatives can be reliably established on clinical criteria because penetrance is close to 100 per cent for offspring of unequivocal cases (Riccardi and Lewis, 1988). Although presymptomatic and prenatal diagnoses of NF1 by mutation analysis or linked DNA markers are available, uptake is limited by the fact that many NF1 patients are isolated cases and do not have a suitable family structure for linkage-based diagnosis. Direct mutation analysis is technically challenging but is becoming more widely available. Although mutation analysis might allow prenatal diagnosis to be considered, molecular genetic testing is of limited value because the severity of the disorder cannot be predicted. NF1 characteristically has a very wide variation in expression. Parents of apparently sporadic cases should undergo careful assessment for subclinical signs of NF1 (e.g. detailed skin examination with Wood's light and ophthalmological testing for Lisch nodules). If these investigations are normal, the recurrence risk is very small, but the possibility of gonosomal mosaicism should be borne in mind.

Neurofibromatosis type 2 (central neurofibromatosis and bilateral acoustic neuroma neurofibromatosis)

NF2 is an autosomal dominantly inherited disorder estimated to have an incidence of 1 in 40 000 persons per year and a prevalence of 1 in 210 000 (Evans et al., 1992a), although recent data suggests that NF2 may be more common (birth incidence 1 in 25 000) and account for 7 per cent of the patients with vestibular schwannoma (Evans et al., 2005). The hallmark of NF2 is bilateral vestibular schwannomas (acoustic neuromas), but there is also a predisposition to other CNS tumours, such as meningioma, astrocytoma, ependymoma and schwannoma of the dorsal spinal roots. NF1 and NF2 are distinct disorders, with the *NF1* and *NF2* genes mapping to chromosomes 17 and 22 respectively.

The clinical features of NF2 as reported by Evans et al. (1992b) in a large UK study are shown in Table 12.8. Although peripheral neurofibromas may occur

Table 12.8. *Clinical features of NF2*

Clinical features	Frequency (%)
Vestibular schwannoma	85
Meningioma	45
Spinal tumours	26
Skin tumours	68
Café-au-lait patch	43
Cataracts	38
Ependymoma	3
Astrocytoma	4
Optic sheath meningioma	4

Source: Adapted from Evans et al. (1992b).

in NF2 they are rarely numerous, and Lisch nodules (iris hamartomas), axillary or groin freckling and multiple (six or more) café-au-lait spots are not features of NF2. However, café-au-lait patches do occur in excess: Kanter et al. (1980) found that 61 per cent of NF2 patients had at least one café-au-lait spot or neurofibroma but that none had more than five, and Evans et al. (1992b) found only one out of 97 patients had six café-au-lait patches. Glial tumours are less common than meningiomas or schwannomas, and astrocytomas and ependymomas are usually low grade, affecting the lower brain stem or upper spinal cord. A generalised peripheral neuropathy occurs in some cases (Evans et al., 1992b).

Several sets of diagnostic criteria for NF2 are available. The most accurate appear to be the Manchester and the National Neurofibromatosis Foundation (NNFF) Criteria (see Table 12.9), but all current criteria have a low sensitivity for diagnosing people who present without bilateral vestibular schwannomas, particularly if there is no family history of NF2 (Baser et al., 2002b).

The age of onset of NF2 is variable. Symptoms of vestibular schwannoma (usually hearing loss, which may be unilateral, sometimes vestibular disturbance or tinnitus) typically begin in the second or third decade (mean age of 23 years), but NF2 can present in the first or seventh decade (Kanter et al., 1980; Martuza and Eldridge, 1988; Evans et al., 1992b). Penetrance is more than 95 per cent at the age of 50 years and the mean age at diagnosis is 28 years. The first manifestation of NF2 in some cases may be a congenital cataract. Some studies have suggested that there is an earlier age at onset in familial cases with maternal transmission (Kanter et al., 1980; Evans et al., 1992b); however, there is no evidence of imprinting of the *NF2* gene and this observation may result from a tendency for severely affected men not to have children. About 50 per cent of

Table 12.9 *Diagnostic criteria for NF2*

Manchester criteria[a]

A. Bilateral vestibular schwannomas
B. First-degree family relative with NF2 *and* unilateral vestibular schwannoma *or* any two
   of: meningioma, schwannoma, glioma, neurofibroma, posterior subcapsular lenticular
   opacities
C. Unilateral vestibular schwannoma *and* any two of: meningioma, schwannoma, glioma,
   neurofibroma, posterior subcapsular lenticular opacities
D. Multiple meningiomas (two or more) *and* unilateral vestibular schwannoma *or* any two
   of: schwannoma, glioma, neurofibroma, cataract

National Neurofibromatosis Foundation (NNFF) Criteria[b]

A. Confirmed or definite NF2
   1. Bilateral vestibular schwannomas
   2. First-degree family relative with NF2 *and* unilateral vestibular schwannoma at less
      than 30 years of age *or* any two of: meningioma, schwannoma, glioma, juvenile lens
      opacity (posterior subcapsular cataract or cortical cataract)
B. Presumptive or probable NF2
   1. Unilateral vestibular schwannoma at less than 30 years of age *and* at least one of:
      meningioma, schwannoma, glioma, juvenile lens opacity (posterior subcapsular
      cataract or cortical cataract)
   2. Multiple meningiomas (two or more) *and* unilateral vestibular schwannoma at less
      than 30 years of age *or* at least one of: schwannoma, glioma, juvenile lens opacity
      (posterior subcapsular cataract or cortical cataract)

[a] In the Manchester criteria, "any two of" refers to two individual tumours or cataract, whereas
in the other sets of criteria, it refers to two tumour types or cataract.
[b] For the purposes of this study, the NNFF criteria for confirmed or definite NF2 and for
presumptive or probable criteria were considered to be equivalent.
Source: (Adapted from Baser et al., 2002a)

patients with NF2 represent new mutations and the mutation rate is approximately 6×10^{-6}.

The proportion of NF2 patients reported to have other non-acoustic CNS tumours is variable. Kanter et al. (1980) estimated it at 18 per cent and Evans et al. (1992b) at 45 per cent, but studies of single families have shown a higher incidence. Wertelecki et al. (1988) reported that in a single large family 16 out of 23 affected individuals had non-acoustic CNS tumours (9 meningiomas, 4 ependymomas, 2 spinal neurofibromas, 1 pontine glioma). These higher frequencies probably reflect more complete ascertainment through diagnosis of asymptomatic tumours and also interfamilial variations in predisposition to other non-acoustic CNS tumours. Meningiomas in NF2 are frequently multiple and may be intracranial or spinal. NF2 has been subdivided into two forms, according to a mild phenotype (Gardner type) with late onset (above 25 years) and a more severe form (Wishart) with early onset and multiple meningiomas and spinal tumours. However, many cases do not fit neatly into either category.

Individuals in the following categories should be evaluated for evidence of NF2 (Martuza and Eldridge, 1988): (i) acoustic neuroma at age less than 30 years, (ii) child with meningeal or Schwann-cell tumour; (iii) multiple CNS tumours with no diagnosed cause; and (iv) adolescent or adult with one or more neurofibromas but no family history of NF1, no Lisch nodules and only a few café-au-lait spots. A careful skin examination, ophthalmological assessment and audiometry with brainstem auditory-evoked response should be performed initially, and an MRI brain scan (to detect acoustic neuroma and other intracranial tumours) should be arranged for those individuals with any abnormalities suggestive of NF2. Skin neurofibromas occur less commonly in NF2 than in NF1, but skin tumours should be carefully sought. The most common types of skin tumours are: (i) discrete subcutaneous swellings appearing to arise from peripheral nerves; and (ii) well-circumscribed, slightly raised lesions with a roughened appearance and prominent hairs (Evans et al., 1992b).

Relatives of affected people should be investigated for stigmata of NF2. Congenital cataracts should be sought by detailed ophthalmoscopy and annual clinical examination (for evidence of cutaneous stigmata) should be performed during childhood. From the age of 10 years, annual audiometry and brainstem auditory-evoked potential should be performed (Evans et al., 1992b). Skin and eye examinations are also indicated. A gandolinium-enhanced MRI scan is a sensitive but expensive investigation. Although an MRI scan every 3 years could be advocated, when scan access is limited these intervals may be extended. In many cases, surveillance will be continued until the age of 40 years, but the decision about when to discontinue screening will depend on the individual family. Although early diagnosis and surgery will prevent progressive neurological impairment, often hearing cannot be preserved. Affected patients should be prepared for the possibility of progressive hearing loss and warned to avoid heights and swimming alone. At-risk individuals demonstrated not to be gene carriers by molecular genetic analysis can be excluded from further surveillance.

A notable feature of NF2 is a high prevalence of somatic mosaicism such that up to 30 per cent of people with new mutations are mosaic (Kluwe et al., 2003, Moyhuddin et al., 2003). Mosaicism should be suspected in individuals with mild disease and no detectable NF2 mutation in blood. In cases with bilateral tumours and no detectable mutation in blood, the identification of an identical

NF2 mutation in both vestibular schwannomas is an indicator of mosaicism. The risk of disease transmission from mosaic parents to offspring is low when the constitutional *NF2* mutation cannot be identified in the parent blood using standard techniques and somatic mosaicism can cause misleading results in linkage analysis for the second generation (such that individual predicted to be at high risk on linkage analysis may have inherited a wild-type allele (Moyhuddin et al., 2003). Conversely children who inherit a *NF2* mutation from a mosaic parent will generally be more severely affected.

The gene for NF2 maps to chromosome 22 and was cloned in 1993 (Rouleau et al., 1993). No evidence of significant locus heterogeneity has been reported, and molecular genetic diagnosis is usually possible by direct mutation analysis. Inactivation of both alleles of the *NF2* gene has been demonstrated in familial and sporadic vestibular schwannomas, compatible with a classical tumour suppressor gene model (Irving et al., 1994). Identification of germline *NF2* mutations has provided genotype–phenotype correlations such that patients with nonsense or frameshift mutations appear generally to have more severe disease (Wishart type) than those with missense or splice site mutations (Parry et al., 1996; Ruttledge et al., 1996). However, some missense mutations may be associated with a severe phenotype. For non-VIII nerve NF2-associated tumours (e.g. intracranial meningiomas, spinal tumours, and peripheral nerve tumours), people with constitutional *NF2* missense mutations, splice-site mutations, large deletions, or somatic mosaicism had significantly fewer tumours than patients with nonsense or frameshift mutations (Baser et al., 2004). The prognosis of patients with NF2 is influenced not only by genotype–phenotype correlations, but also by surgical management with lower mortality in specialist centres (Baser et al., 2002a).

Evans et al. (1997a) described families segregating multiple spinal and cutaneous schwannomas (schwannomatosis) as a dominant trait. In most cases, vestibular schwannomas did not appear, but linkage to the *NF2* gene was established, suggesting that this disorder represented a variant of NF2 and it has been suggested that this may represent an attenuated form of NF2. However, in two kindreds with schwannomatosis, MacCollin et al. (2003) found linkage to chromosome 22, but not to the *NF2* gene suggesting that, at least in some cases, the pathogenesis is distinct from NF2.

Neurofibromatosis: atypical

This group comprises forms of NF that do not neatly fall into the NF1 or NF2 categories. For example, in NF3 there are features of NF1 (café-au-lait spots, cutaneous neurofibromas characteristically on the palms of the hand), and of NF2 (bilateral vestibular schwannomas, meningiomas and spinal neurofibromas).

Molecular genetic analysis of the *NF1* and *NF2* can be used to clarify the relationship of atypical forms of NF to NF1 and NF2. Schwannomatosis, a variant of NF2, has been linked with the *NF2* gene on chromosome 22 but may have a distinct pathogenesis (see above).

Nijmegen breakage syndrome (including Semanova syndrome)

This rare autosomal recessive disorder is characterised by microcephaly, growth retardation, "bird-like" face and humoral and cellular immunodeficiency. A characteristic feature is the marked discrepancy between the (usually) normal intelligence and severe microcephaly. There is an increased risk of lymphoreticular malignancy. Laboratory findings include chromosome instability in cultured lymphocytes with frequent rearrangements involving chromosomes 7 and 14, cellular and chromosomal hypersensitivity to X-irradiation, and radioresistance of DNA replication (Taalman et al., 1989). Most reported cases are of eastern European origin where a NBS1 founder mutation (657del5 in exon 6) is common. The cellular phenotype, chromosome breakage and immunodeficiency features of Nijmegen breakage syndrome and AT are similar, but the clinical phenotypes are distinct. The gene for Nijmegen breakage syndrome (*NBS1*) maps to 8q21 and encodes a protein (nibrin) (Varon et al., 1998) that is phosphorylated by the ATM protein. *NBS1* heterozygotes may have an increased risk of cancer including prostate (Cybulski et al., 2004). There is evidence for locus heterogeneity in Nijmegen breakage syndrome (Maraschio et al., 2003).

Perlman syndrome

This rare disorder is characterised by macrosomia, visceromegaly, renal hamartomas with or without nephroblastomatosis, dysmorphic features (enophthalmos, broad depressed nasal bridge and everted upper lip), neurodevelopmental delay and cryptorchidism in males (Greenberg et al., 1986). The disease should be distinguished from Beckwith–Wiedemann and Simson–Golabi–Behmel syndromes, but inheritance appears to be autosomal recessive (Henneveld et al., 1999). There is a very high risk of Wilms tumour, which is frequently bilateral.

Peutz–Jegher syndrome

PJS (MIM 175200) is a rare autosomal dominant inherited hamartoma-cancer syndrome characterised by tiny pigmented mucocutaneous macules and GI hamartomatous polyps and a high risk of GI, breast and pancreatic carcinomas (Hemminki et al., 1997; Eng et al., 2001). Germline mutations in *LKB1/STK11* are associated with PJS.

Clinical features

The presence of melanin spots on the lips, perioral region and buccal mucosa is pathognomonic for PJS and likely occurs in 95 per cent of such individuals (Peutz, 1921; Jeghers et al., 1949). These tiny macules can also occur as black or bluish spots on the hands (especially the palms), arms, feet (especially plantar areas), legs, genitalia and anus. The skin pigmentation is present from early childhood and may fade after the age of 25 years. The absence of the pigmented spots, however, does not exclude the diagnosis of PJS (Lampe et al., 2003).

Most patients present because of symptomatology related to their GI hamartomatous polyps, although polyps can occur in the nasal mucosa, bladder, uterus and gallbladder as well. They can present with episodes of colicky abdominal pain from childhood (usually the second decade). Intussusception and obstruction are not uncommon complications, and rectal bleeding, severe enough to present with anaemia, may occur. The distribution of polyps is most commonly in the small intestine (64 per cent), but also in the colon (53 per cent), stomach (49 per cent) and rectum (32 per cent) (Jeghers et al., 1949). The polyps are broad-based hamartomas of the smooth muscle that extend into the lamina propria. Many show histological features of "pseudoinvasion" (Giardiello et al., 1987). Nevertheless, adenomatous change may develop within the polyps and there is an increased risk of malignancy (relative risk 13), and mortality from cancer may be as high as 40 per cent by 50 years of age has been quoted for this condition (Linos et al., 1981; Giardiello et al., 1987; Boardman et al., 1998).

In the absence of the characteristic melanin spots, histopathology of the polyps is critical in making the diagnosis of PJS, as the PJS polyp has a diagnostically useful central core of smooth muscle that extends, in a tree-like manner ("arborisation") into the superficial epithelial layer. Invagination of the epithelial layer occurs, essentially trapping these cells within the smooth muscle component, and causing "pseudoinvasion" of the bowel wall that can be misdiagnosed as cancer. This involvement of the three tissue layers predisposes to intussusception and the formation of the distinctive lobulated PJS polyp. Nonetheless, the operational clinical diagnostic criteria for PJS is as follows:

1. Three or more histologically confirmed PJS polyps
2. Any number of PJS polyps or characteristic mucocutaneous pigmentation, with a positive family history of PJS
3. Any number of PJS polyps with characteristic mucocutaneous pigmentation

In addition to an increased risk of GI cancer (Linos et al., 1981), extra-intestinal cancers are over-represented in PJS as well (Giardiello et al., 1987; Boardman et al., 1998). Invasive ductal carcinomas of the breast and pancreatic adenocarcinomas are significantly associated with PJS (Giardiello et al., 1987;

Boardman et al., 1998). Non-malignant tumours associated with this syndrome include ovarian sex cord tumours and testicular (Sertoli cell) tumours. The histology of these tumours is intermediate between granulosa cell tumours and Sertoli cell tumours. They are common in this syndrome, and rarely malignant, although at least one such malignancy has been described. The clinical effects are mainly due to the hyperoestrogenisation in females, and can give rise to adenoma malignum of the cervix. Many of these tumours occur in young adults, and the Sertoli and sex cord tumours may occur in prepubertal boys, causing sexual precocity and gynaecomastia. Sertoli cell tumours of the ovary may occur, and ovarian sex cord tumours are common, bilateral and multifocal.

The relative risks of all cancers in PJS are high, assessed as 3 per cent by age of 30 years, 19 per cent by 40 years, 32 per cent by 50 years, 63 per cent by 60 years and 81 per cent by age of 70 years. The respective risks of GI cancer (oesophagus, stomach, small bowel, colorectum and pancreas) are 1, 10, 18, 42 and 66 per cent; of gynaecological cancer 3, 6, 13 and 13 per cent overall; and the breast cancer risks are 8 per cent by 40 years of age, 11 per cent by 50 years and 32 per cent by 60 years of age. The risk of pancreatic cancer was 5 per cent by age 40 years and 8 per cent by 60 years (Lim et al., 2003; 2004).

Genetics

Germline loss-of-function mutations in *LKB1/STK11*, on19p13.3, encoding a multifunctional nuclear serine–threonine kinase, were found in a proportion of PJS individuals and kindreds (Hemminki A et al., 1997; 1998; Jenne et al., 1998). *LKB1/STK11* mutations have been found in only 40–50 per cent of cases, leading to the suggestion of either locus heterogeneity or the presence of large deletions and promoter mutations, which have not been systematically analysed. *LKB1/STK11* has nine exons, and the normal protein product acts as a tumour suppressor, a notable role for a protein kinase. Studies show that bi-allelic inactivation of *LKB1/STK11*, either through germline mutation plus somatic mutation, or more commonly promoter hypermethylation of the wild-type allele, cause hamartomatous polyps to develop.

Genetic and medical management

As with other inherited cancer syndromes, patients with or suspected to have PJS should be referred to clinical cancer genetics consultation. The presence of a germline *LKB1/STK11* mutation is diagnostic of PJS. However, failure to find a mutation in an individual who meets the clinical diagnostic criteria for PJS does not exclude the diagnosis and such individuals should be managed like anyone with PJS and/or germline *LKB1/STK11* mutation.

Patients with PJS require careful follow-up, although the precise follow-up is based on expert opinion due to the rarity of this syndrome. Since the risk of cancer is high, regular (2 yearly from early adulthood) upper and lower bowel endoscopy and 2-yearly small bowel follow-through have been recommended. Laparotomy may be required for suspicious symptoms. Polypectomy should be as complete as possible, and can be performed at endoscopy. Surveillance for extra-intestinal malignancy includes mammography, yearly gynaecological evaluation and pelvic ultrasound, and 3-yearly cervical smears. Testicular ultrasound is suggested for males with feminising features because of the risk of feminising sertoli cell tumours of the testis.

Porphyria

There are several forms of porphyria – inborn errors of porphyrin metabolism with sunlight-sensitive dermatological eruptions and abnormal porphyrin excretion patterns – most of which are inherited as autosomal dominant traits. Congenital erythropoietic porphyria is an autosomal recessive trait. Clinical and molecular aspects of the different porphyrias are reviewed by Kauppinen (2005). Siderosis of the liver develops in the hepatic porphyrias and can lead to inflammation and fibrosis, with the risk of hepatoma developing, particularly in porphyria cutanea tarda and variegate porphyria (Gilbert et al., 2004). The dermatological features of these two types are bullae and fragile skin in sun-exposed areas, with hyperpigmentation, hypertrichosis, photosensitivity, erosions, milia and sclerodermoid areas. Treatment is by phlebotomy and chloroquine. Many of the genes underlying the porphyrias – notably coproporphyria, acute intermittent, erythropoietic and variegate porphyria (Martasek et al., 1994; Kauppinen et al., 1995; Ostasiewicz et al., 1995; Meissner et al., 1996) have been delineated, and it is possible to detect germline mutations in these in affected probands. In a study of 650 patients with acute hepatic porphyria followed up for 7 years, 7 were diagnosed with hepatocellular cancer (3 asymptomatic), with an overall standardised rate ratio of 36 (95 per cent CI: 14–74). The occurrence of cancer was not related to the specific haeme biosynthetic abnormality, but haeme precursors were significantly increased and melatonin decreased in cancer cases (Andant et al., 2000). From a follow-up study of 39 patients with porphyria cutanea tarda on surveillance with 6-monthly ultrasound and CA125 measurements, on treatment with phlebotomies resulting in clinical remission, only one patient developed hepatocellular cancer (cumulative incidence 0.26 per cent) and this patient was an alcoholic with hepatitis C virus (HCV) infection (Gisbert et al., 2004) The authors concluded that the risk of hepatocellular carcinoma was relatively low in such patients, but that the risk increased with HCV infection and advanced fibrosis/cirrhosis. They recommended that PCT patients should have liver biopsies to determine the presence of such factors, and surveillance if they were present. The percentage of hepatocellular cancer attributable to HCV infection may be 25 per cent, and most develop in cirrhotic livers; surveillance should be by 6-monthly screening in such high-risk patients (Montalto et al., 2002). Other risk factors for hepatocellular cancer are haemochromatosis, tyrosinaemia and alpha-1 antitrypsin deficiency (see p. 48). Patients with porphyria should be checked for their hepatitis and haemochromatosis status as these may increase the risk of neoplasia.

Rothmund–Thomson syndrome (poikiloderma congenitale)

This rare autosomal recessive disorder is characterised by atrophy, pigmentation and telangiectasia of the skin associated with juvenile zonular cataracts and short stature. The dermal erythematous lesions may be present at birth and have usually appeared by the first 6 months of life. They begin on the face and spread to involve the whole of the body. The skin atrophy, pigmentation and telangiectasia develop from the 3rd to the 6th month of life, particularly on extensor surfaces of the hands, arms, legs and buttocks, and are worst over exposed surfaces. This inflammatory stage is followed by skin atrophy with pigmentation anomalies. Bilateral cataracts develop at 4–7 years, and there may be alopecia. Warty dyskeratosis is seen, and squamous cell carcinoma may develop in the skin in adulthood; multiple Bowen disease has been described (Haneke and Gutschmidt, 1979). There are two case reports of oral squamous cell carcinoma (Dahele et al., 2004). Associated abnormalities that may occur include sparse hair or alopecia, atrophic nails, microdontia or other dental malformations, hypogonadism, small saddle nose, hypoplastic thumbs, forearm reduction defects, small hands and feet, and osteoporosis or sclerosis. Osteogenic sarcoma has been described in a proportion of patients (32 per cent in one series) and skin malignancy may also occur (Starr et al., 1985; Wang et al., 2001). Myelodysplasia and fibrosarcoma have also been described in this condition (Naryan et al., 2001). In-vitro chromosomal instability has been described in cultured fibroblasts from such patients (Der Kaloustian et al., 1990; Lindor et al., 1996). A subset of cases are due to bi-allelic mutations in the *RECQL4* helicase, and these may have an increased osteosarcoma risk (Kitao et al., 1999; Wang et al., 2003). In a large 25-year retrospective study of 938 individuals with osteosarcoma, 66 had multiple primary cancers. One of these cases had Rothmund–Thompson syndrome, illustrating the rarity of this condition in patients ascertained by a diagnosis of osteosarcoma (Hauben et al., 2003). Mutations in *RECQL4* are rare in sporadic osteosarcoma (Nishijo et al., 2004).

A similar condition, Kindler syndrome (characterised by poikiloderma congenitale with trauma-induced blister formation, especially in childhood, and photosensitivity), also predisposes to solar-induced malignancies of skin and mucous membranes. Histologically, tonofilament clumping is seen (Haber and Hanna,

1996). Protection against sunlight may help to prevent complications developing. Mutations in kindlin-1, a novel keratinocyte focal contact protein, have been found to cause this autosomal recessive mutation, and recurrent mutations occur (Ashton et al., 2004).

Severe combined immunodeficiency disease

This comprises a heterogeneous group of disorders characterised by severe cell-mediated and humoral immunodeficiency. Autosomal recessive and X-linked forms (the most common form in males) occur. Although infection is the most common cause of death, there is also an increased risk of lymphoma (see p. 126). Following the mapping of X-linked severe combined immunodeficiency disease to Xq13.1, mutations in the interleukin-2 receptor γ chain gene were identified (Noguchi et al., 1993; Puck et al., 1993). Mutations are heterogeneous and molecular genetic analysis is technically demanding (Puck et al., 1997). At least eight autosomal genes are implicated in recessive SCID including adenosine deaminase, CD3 delta and CD3 epsilon chain, CD45, IL-7 receptor alpha chain, Jak3 and RAG1/RAG2 deficiencies and *Artemis* mutations (Buckley, 2004a,b). There is no evidence that heterozygotes for autosomal recessive causes of the disease (including adenosine deaminase deficiency) are at increased risk for cancer (Morrell et al., 1987).

Shwachman–Diamond syndrome

This is a rare autosomal recessive disease characterised by exocrine pancreatic insufficiency, skeletal abnormalities (e.g. metaphyseal dysostosis), growth retardation, recurrent infections, and haematological abnormalities (neutropenia, hypoplastic anaemia, thrombocytopenia, or pancytopenia) (Dror and Freedman, 1999). The risk of leukaemia in Shwachman–Diamond syndrome was calculated to be increased 27-fold (Woods et al., 1981). A range of leukaemic types have been described in this condition including ALL, AML, chronic myeloid leukaemia (CML) and erythroleukaemia. Although the risk of leukaemic transformation had been considered to be 5–10 per cent, Smith et al. (1996) suggested that this was an underestimate. The Shwachman–Diamond syndrome gene maps to 7q11 and encodes a protein of 250 amino acids (Boocock et al., 2003). Most mutations appeared to result from gene conversion events with a pseudogene.

Simpson–Golabi–Behmel syndrome

An X-linked congenital overgrowth syndrome with some expression in carrier females, Simpson–Golabi–Behmel syndrome is characterised by prenatal and postnatal overgrowth, coarse facies with hypertelorism and a midline groove of the lower lip, and a variety of developmental defects including cleft lip and palate, polydactyly, supernumerary nipples, congenital heart disease and cryptorchidism. Mental retardation is not usually a feature, but has been reported in some cases. Simpson–Golabi–Behmel syndrome must be distinguished from other overgrowth syndromes, in particular BWS (p. 170). There is an increased risk of embryonal tumours, and screening for Wilms tumour may be offered as described for BWS.

Simpson–Golabi–Behmel syndrome is caused by mutations in the glypican 3 (*GPC3*) gene, which maps to Xq26 (Pilia et al., 1996; Hughes-Benzie et al., 1996). The GPC3 protein is proposed to modulate the action of *IGF2* by binding extracellular IGF2 protein. In addition, a second locus (SGBS2), maps to Xp22 (Brzustowicz et al., 1999). Li et al. (2001) suggested that hepatoblastoma and nephroblastomatosis are part of the Simpson–Golabi–Behmel syndrome phenotype and identified GPC3 deletion in two patients previously diagnosed as Sotos syndrome and Perlman syndrome.

Tuberous sclerosis (tuberose sclerosis)

This autosomal dominant hamartomatous disorder with an incidence of approximately 1 per 12 000 live births. New mutations account for 70 per cent of cases, and the mutation rate is 2.5×10^{-5}/haploid genome. Most serious morbidity is caused by the CNS lesions, which produce mental retardation and epilepsy, but renal angiomyolipomas can occasionally be life threatening, and RCC may occur at an increased rate, albeit infrequently (Washecka and Hanna, 1991).

Tuberous sclerosis is a multisystem disorder and the clinical features are diverse (Lendvay and Marshall, 2003):

Skin: Hypopigmented oval or "ash leaf" patches (80–90 per cent), facial angiofibromas (adenoma sebaceum; 40–90 per cent), Shagreen patches (20–40 per cent), forehead fibrous plaque (25 per cent), periungual fibromas (Koenen tumours) (15–50 per cent), molluscum fibrosum pendulum (23 per cent).

Eyes: Hamartomas of the retina or optic nerve occur in about 50 per cent of patients with tuberous sclerosis. Just under half of these are calcified. Most retinal lesions do not grow and although visual impairment from retinal or optic nerve astrocytoma is recorded, it is a rare complication (Robertson, 1988).

CNS: Epilepsy (approximately 80 per cent of patients), mental retardation (50 per cent) and giant-cell astrocytomas (5–10 per cent) are important features (Webb et al., 1996). Although MRI scanning demonstrates cortical tubers more easily than CT scanning, the latter is more sensitive in detecting small areas of intracranial calcification. Intracranial tumours are usually benign astrocytomas (subependymal nodules), which often calcify and are typically situated around the lateral aspects of the lateral ventricles. Infrequently, malignant giant-cell astrocytomas develop from these subependymal nodules, most commonly near the foramen of Monro and resulting in bilateral (but often asymmetric) obstructive hydrocephalus. Less often, the tumour occurs at the frontal or temporal horns of the lateral ventricle or in the third ventricle. On CT scan, giant-cell astrocytomas have a mixed pattern with foci of calcification and areas of vascularity showing enhancement with intravenous contrast. Most tumours are slow growing and distant metastases have not been reported. Subependymal giant-cell astrocytomas can be demonstrated in about 8 per cent of patients, and although the proportion of tuberous sclerosis patients who develop intracranial hypertension is not accurately defined, it is estimated to be less than 3 per cent (Gomez, 1988).

Teeth: Enamel "pits" due to enamel hypoplasia (70 per cent). However these are very common in the general population and are not of any diagnostic value.

Kidney: Renal lesions occur in up to 75 per cent of cases and are a major cause of morbidity and mortality in older patients and their importance has increased with the advent of more effective seizure control. The most frequent renal complications of tuberous sclerosis are angiomyolipomas (49 per cent) and renal cysts (32 per cent) (Cook et al., 1996). Angiomyolipomas are frequently multiple and bilateral. Most patients with a single angiomyolipoma do not have tuberous sclerosis and patients with non-tuberous sclerosis-associated angiomyolipomas are usually middle-aged or elderly women (Robbins and Bernstein, 1988). Angiomyolipomas in tuberous sclerosis patients present earlier (mean 32 versus 54 years) in non-tuberous sclerosis cases (Steiner et al., 1993). Most angiomyolipomas are asymptomatic and although severe haemorrhage may occur, there is no indication to treat asymptomatic tumours. There is no convincing evidence for malignant transformation occurring in an angiomyolipoma (Robbins and Bernstein, 1988). Angiomyolipomas consist of disorganised smooth muscle cells, adipose tissue and aberrant blood vessels which do not have an internal elastic lamina and are prone to rupture. Larger tumours tend to be symptomatic and whereas small asymptomatic lesions may be kept under surveillance, it has been recommended that symptomatic angiomyolipomas >4 cm are investigated (angiography) and treated (embolisation or renal sparing surgery). Renal cystic disease is the second most common renal manifestation and renal cysts tend to occur at a younger age than angiomyolipomas. Severe renal cystic disease may result from a contiguous deletion of the *TSC2* (see below) and *PKD1* (autosomal dominant adult-onset polycystic kidney disease) genes (Brook-Carter et al., 1994, Sampson et al., 1997).

The risk of RCC in tuberous sclerosis is controversial (Tello et al., 1998), but although it appears to affect only a minority of cases (~2 per cent), those cases reported were frequently bilateral (43 per cent), with an early age at onset (median 28 years) (Washecka and Hanna, 1991).

GI: Benign, small, adenomatous rectal polyps.

Bones: Cysts (60 per cent), areas of periosteal new bone/sclerosis (60 per cent). However, these findings are of no diagnostic value.

Cardiac: Rhabdomyomas are present in most infants with tuberous sclerosis. Thereafter many regress and echocardiographically demonstrable lesions occur in only about 30 per cent of adult patients. Obstructive symptoms or rhabdomyoma-induced arrhythmias are rare, and the likelihood of spontaneous regression favours conservative management in most cases.

Lungs: A specific feature of tuberous sclerosis is lymphangioleiomyomatosis (LAM) caused by an overgrowth of atypical smooth muscle cells. It is nearly always restricted to women, and is very rare in the general population (1 per million) (Johnson and Tattersfield, 2002) Honeycomb fibrosis also occurs, but is rare.

Conventional diagnostic criteria for tuberous sclerosis are shown in Table 12.10. The manifestations of tuberous sclerosis can be mild and easily overlooked, so that the assessment of at-risk relatives must be performed assiduously. In addition to careful examination of the skin (including Wood's lamp examination) and nails, further examinations usually indicated include brain CT or MRI scan, renal ultrasound, specialist eye examination and echocardiogram (in children). Dental pits are more common in patients with tuberous sclerosis, but their usefulness as a diagnostic feature is limited because many normal persons have small numbers of these. Truly non-penetrant gene carriers are extremely unusual, so that the risk to individuals with negative investigations as outlined above will be small. A frequent diagnostic problem occurs in assessing the significance of a single ambiguous lesion (e.g. ashleaf patch or equivocal CT scan finding) in an at-risk individual. Parents of a child with tuberous sclerosis who have been fully investigated with negative results should be given a 2 per cent recurrence risk for tuberous sclerosis in further children, because of the possibility of germline mosaicism or non-penetrance.

The presence of locus heterogeneity in tuberous sclerosis is firmly established, with two genes (*TSC1* and *TSC2* respectively) mapped at 9q34 and 16p13.3 adjacent to the autosomal dominant polycystic kidney locus (APKD1). The *TSC2* gene was isolated first (The European Chromosome 16 Tuberous Sclerosis Consortium, 1993; Wienecke et al., 1995) and the *TSC1* gene was cloned 10 years after the initial mapping to chromosome 9 (van Slegtenhorst et al., 1997). Loss of heterozygosity at *TSC1* or *TSC2* is observed in hamartomas

Table 12.10. *Diagnostic criteria for tuberous sclerosis. A diagnosis of tuberous sclerosis is suggested if a single primary or two secondary diagnostic features are present*

Primary features	Secondary features
Classical shagreen patch	Ashleaf patch (hypomelanotic macules)
Ungual fibroma	Gingival fibroma
Retinal hamartoma	Bilateral polycystic kidney
Facial angiofibromas	Cardiac rhabdomyoma
Subependymal glial nodule (on	Cortical tuber
CT scan)	Radiographic "honeycomb" lungs
Renal angiomyolipoma	Infantile spasms
Lymphangioleiomyomatosis (lung)	Myoclonic, tonic or atonic seizures
	First-degree relative with tuberous sclerosis
	Forehead fibrous plaque
	Giant-cell astrocytoma

Source: After Gomez (1988).

from tuberous sclerosis patients, consistent with both genes having a tumour suppressor function (Sepp et al., 1996). Half of familial cases are linked to *TSC1* and half to *TSC2*, but >80 per cent of sporadic cases have *TSC2* mutations (Jones et al., 1999). The proteins specified by the *TSC1* and *TSC2* genes (hamartin and tuberin respectively) interact directly with each other and mutations affecting either gene result in the tuberous sclerosis phenotype (Hodges et al., 2001). Hamartin or tuberin inactivation leads to dysregulation of the mammalian target of rapamycin (mTOR) and abnormal cell growth (Inoki et al., 2005). This finding suggests that inhibitors of mTOR (e.g. rapamycin) have a potential role in tuberous sclerosis therapy.

Large kindreds with tuberous sclerosis are unusual and in most cases reliable presymptomatic or prenatal diagnosis using linked DNA markers is not usually feasible. Molecular diagnosis by direct mutation analysis is possible, but the *TSC2* gene is very large and mutations are heterogeneous and so molecular diagnosis may not be available. All parents of apparently isolated cases of tuberous sclerosis should undergo detailed clinical examination (including examination of nails and Wood's light), a CT or MRI brain scan, and renal and liver ultrasound examination. If these investigations are negative, the recurrence risk is reduced to approximately 2 per cent.

The clinical features of germline mutations in *TSC1* and *TSC2* appear similar, except that the presence of severe renal cystic disease is strongly correlated with deletions of both *TSC2* and *APKD1* genes (Brook-Carter et al., 1994) and intellectual disability is more frequent in sporadic cases which are mostly caused by *TSC2* mutations. Renal carcinoma has been described in families linked to *TSC1* and to *TSC2*, and although RCC is uncommon in tuberous sclerosis, a germline mutation in rat *TSC2* gene is responsible for the Eker rat model of hereditary renal carcinoma *TSC2* (Kobayashi et al., 1995).

The investigation of asymptomatic at-risk relatives has been described. For unequivocally affected individuals, management is directed towards the active clinical problems, however regular surveillance of asymptomatic angiomyolipomas may be undertaken, particularly if large (>4 cm). Symptomatic angiomyolipomas may be investigated by angiography and, particularly if >4 cm, embolisation or renal sparing surgery performed.

Turcot syndrome

The association of multiple polyps of the colon with malignant tumours of the CNS is known as Turcot syndrome (Turcot et al., 1959). The condition seems to be rare. The colorectal polyps are characteristically not as numerous as in FAP (fewer than 100), and are larger, developing in the second decade of life, but the brain tumours may occur in childhood. Medulloblastomas and glioblastomas predominate. Café-au-lait spots and pigmented spots have been noted (Itoh and Ohsato, 1985), and sebaceous cysts and BCC may occur (Michels and Stevens, 1982).

Despite original suggestions that the condition was only an autosomal recessive trait, it is clearly autosomal dominant in some families (Costa et al., 1987; Kumar et al., 1989). Current evidence suggests that in the majority of families, Turcot syndrome is allelic with FAP, especially where medulloblastomas predominate, and truncating germline *APC* mutations have been found in about two-thirds of families with Turcot syndrome (Hamilton et al., 1995). In a minority of Turcot families (particularly those with glioblastomas) germline mismatch repair gene mutations have been reported (Tops et al., 1992; Liu et al., 1995). In these families, genomic instability was demonstrated in the brain and colonic tumours of affected individuals (Paraf et al., 1997). This has even been seen in normal tissue from patients with Turcot syndrome, perhaps suggesting that the single mutation in *PMS2* identified in this report was actually accompanied by another, hidden mutation (Miyaki et al., 1997). Clear evidence for autosomal recessive Turcot syndrome was provided by the report of two siblings who were diagnosed with a brain tumour and a colorectal cancer respectively at very young ages (De Rosa et al., 2000). The authors identified two germline mutations in *PMS2* in the two children: 1221delG and 2361delCTTC, both of which were inherited from the patient's unaffected parents. A literature review of individuals with café-au-lait spots and early-onset colorectal cancer revealed excesses of early-onset brain tumours (mean age of diagnosis of 16.5 ± 1.2) and lymphoma and/or leukaemia. Several could be accounted for by homozygous mutations in *PMS2* or heterozygous mutations in *MLH1* (Trimbath et al., 2001).

Interestingly, homozygous *PMS2* mutations occur in some children with brain tumours, but these cases are not strictly Turcot syndrome, as the supratentorial primitive neuroectodermal tumours (PNETs) that occur (along with café-au-lait lesions and susceptibility to haematological malignancies) (De Vos et al., 2004) are not usually associated with a personal or family history of colorectal cancer. However, De Vos et al. identified a two germline *PMS2* mutations in the two siblings who were described by Turcot in 1959. Previously, a single *PMS2* mutation R134X had been identified in the two affected sibs and their father (Hamilton et al., 1995), and although the parents were unaffected, it was assumed to be a dominantly inherited disorder in that family. The identification of another mutation, 2184delTC, and its presence in the mother, confirms the original Turcot pedigree as an example of autosomal recessive Turcot syndrome. This stresses the need for genomic analysis of *PMS2* in families with childhood supratentorial PNETs and/or other brain tumours, particularly if café-au-lait spots are present. Surveillance of first-degree relatives at risk for Turcot syndrome should include regular colonoscopies from age of 25 years in cases associated with HNPCC, or surveillance appropriate for FAP if this is the underlying condition.

Tylosis (keratosis palmaris et plantaris)

This autosomal dominant condition is characterised by a diffuse keratoderma of the palms and soles developing from the age of 5 years (typically around puberty). It is associated with a very high risk of developing cancer of the oesophagus (95 per cent risk by the age of 60 years) (Harper et al., 1970). Oral leucoplakia also occurs and there is a risk of squamous carcinoma of the lip and mouth. The differential diagnosis from the more common diffuse palmoplantar keratoderma, which carries no increased risk of carcinoma of the oesophagus, is that in the latter condition, lesions develop in infancy and are well established by 6–12 months of life.

The incidence of oesophageal cancer in gene carriers (heterozygotes) reaches 95 per cent by the age of 63 years, and the mean age at onset of the cancer is 45 years (Shine and Allison, 1966). Prophylactic oesophagectomy with interposition of a segment of colon has been suggested for affected individuals. If prophylactic oesophagectomy has not been performed, then annual oesophagoscopy is recommended and immediate oesophagectomy is advisable if dysplasia is detected.

The gene for this condition has been mapped to chromosome 17q, but distal to the keratin gene cluster on 17q (Hennies et al., 1995; Kelsell et al., 1996).

Von Hippel–Lindau disease

This is an autosomal dominant disorder with a minimal birth incidence of 1 per 35 000 (Maher et al., 1991). A wide variety of tumours have been reported in von Hippel–Lindau (VHL) disease (Horton et al., 1976), but the most frequent manifestations are retinal angioma (60 per cent of patients), cerebellar (60 per cent), spinal (13–44 per cent) and brainstem haemangioblastomas (18 per cent), RCC (28 per cent) and PC (7–20 per cent) (Maher et al., 1990b). Renal, pancreatic and epididymal cysts are also frequent findings. Other less frequent complications include pancreatic tumours (usually non-secretory endocrine tumours), endolymphatic sac tumours (ELST) and broad ligament cystadenoma (Kaelin and Maher, 1998). Clinical penetrance is age dependent and almost complete by the age of 60 years (0.19 at age of 15 years, 0.52 at 25 years and 0.91 at 45 years). The mean age at clinical diagnosis is 26 years (but rarely, affected patients can present in infancy) and age at diagnosis will be earlier if at-risk relatives are under routine surveillance (see later). There is a high probability of a patient with VHL disease developing a major complication (at age of 60 years, the risk of cerebellar haemangioblastoma, retinal angioma and of RCC is 0.7 or more. However the frequency of PC is more variable and shows marked interfamilial variability.

Conventional diagnostic criteria for VHL disease are: (i) *for isolated cases*, two or more haemangioblastomas (retinal or CNS) or a single haemangioblastoma in association with a visceral tumour or ELST; or (ii) *if there is a family history of retinal or CNS haemangioblastoma*, only one haemangioblastoma, ELST or visceral tumour is required for the diagnosis. Small numbers of visceral cysts do not provide a reliable basis for the diagnosis of the disease in familial cases. The mutation rate for VHL disease (4.4×10^{-6}/gene per generation) is significant (Maher et al., 1991), but isolated cases are underdiagnosed because they can only be recognised when they have developed two complications, whereas familial cases can be diagnosed after a single manifestation. Increasingly diagnosis of VHL disease is by molecular genetic analysis, so that isolated cases can be recognised after the first manifestation of the disease.

Cerebellar haemangioblastoma (see p. 15)

This is the joint most frequent complication (with retinal angiomatosis) of VHL disease. Approximately 30 per cent of cerebellar haemangioblastomas occur as part of VHL disease and evidence of the disease should be sought in all patients with apparently sporadic cerebellar haemangioblastoma. Tumours complicating VHL disease occur, on average, at a younger age than sporadic cerebellar haemangioblastoma (see p. 15) and in about 20 per cent of cases the tumours are multiple or recurrent. CT scanning demonstrates a contrast-enhancing mass, but MRI scanning is more sensitive and is preferred when available. These tumours are benign, may be cystic or solid, and the histological appearance is identical to that of a retinal angioma (haemangioblastoma). Approximately 4 per cent of patients with apparently sporadic cerebellar haemangioblastoma have a germline *VHL* gene mutation (Hes et al., 2000). In view of the risk of false negative mutation analysis and somatic mosaicism, apparently sporadic early-onset cases may be kept under review in case evidence of VHL disease develops. Surgery is usually performed when a haemangioblastoma becomes symptomatic. Stereotaxic radiotherapy may be an option for small non-cystic hemangioblastomas that are not amenable to standard surgery (Patrice et al., 1996).

Spinal cord haemangioblastoma

This is the second most frequent site for CNS haemangioblastomas. Pain is the most common symptom and may be followed by sensory loss and signs of cord compression. MRI scanning is the preferred method of investigation. Symptomatic lesions should be excised, and although the prognosis can be good, if diagnosis is delayed or surgery difficult, paraplegia may result. Medical treatment with anti-angiogenic agents should be considered if conventional surgery is not possible.

Brain stem haemangioblastoma

This occurs in 18 per cent of patients, most often in the dorsal medulla and craniocervical junction (Filling-Katz et al., 1991). Supratentorial haemangioblastomas are rare. Many CNS haemangioblastomas detected by MRI scanning are asymptomatic. The detection of such tumours is helpful in determining carrier status, but surgery is usually only performed for symptomatic tumours.

Retinal angiomatosis (see Fig. 12.8)

This is often the earliest manifestation of VHL disease. Retinal angiomas are frequently asymptomatic and most occur in the peripheral retina. They have been reported in infancy and in the ninth decade (Ridley et al., 1986), but the risk of retinal angioma before the age of 5 years is less than 1 per cent and mean age at diagnosis is 25 years. Early detection of retinal angiomas facilitates treatment and prevents blindness. Direct and indirect ophthalmoscopy should be performed on all patients and at-risk relatives (see Table 12.10). Fluoroscein angioscopy can improve the detection of small lesions.

Renal cell carcinoma

In cross-sectional studies 25–30 per cent of VHL patients have had clear cell RCC (Maher et al., 1990a). The risk of RCC in VHL disease was under-estimated for many years because the mean age at diagnosis (44 years) is significantly older than for retinal angioma (25 years) and cerebellar haemangioblastoma (29 years) and although the risk of RCC is influenced by allelic heterogeneity, in most cases lifetime risk of RCC is high (more than 70 per cent). The clinical presentation and risk of metastasis in RCC complicating VHL disease are similar to those of sporadic non-familial tumours. However, tumours in VHL disease occur at an earlier age and are often multiple and bilateral. Renal cysts may be detected in the second decade, and RCC has been detected at age of 16 years, but is rare in patients aged less than 20 years. RCC may arise from the wall of renal cysts, and complex cysts require careful follow-up. Renal tumours and cysts may be demonstrated by ultrasonography, but in the presence of multiple cysts, identification of tumours by ultrasonography is less reliable. Although CT scanning is most sensitive, MRI scanning avoids repeated radiation exposure and is preferred for routine screening. The management of renal cancer in VHL disease has moved towards a conservative nephron-sparing approach. It is usual to follow small asymptomatic tumours by serial imaging until they reach about 3 cm in size. At that stage, conservative renal surgery is performed with the aim of conserving functioning renal tissue for as long as possible. Follow-up of VHL patients treated by nephron-sparing surgery reveals a high incidence of local recurrence from new primary tumours, but a low risk of distant metastasis (Steinbach et al., 1995). In contrast, 25 per cent of VHL patients with more advanced RCC (>3 cm) develop metastatic disease (Walther et al., 1999a). Repeated partial nephrectomies may eventually compromise renal function. In such cases dialysis is instigated, although renal transplantation is also an option. To date it appears that immunosuppression does not affect adversely the underlying course of VHL disease and the prognosis of VHL patients after transplantation appears similar to that of other comparable groups (Goldfarb et al., 1998).

Phaeochromocytoma

There are clear interfamilial differences in predisposition to PC in VHL disease. In a minority of families, PC is the most frequent complication of this disease but in other families it is rare (Green et al., 1986). VHL disease has been subclassified according to the presence (type 2) or absence (type 1) of PC. In most cases, PC-positive VHL families also have a high incidence of renal cancer (type 2B), but in some families PC is common and renal carcinoma is rare (type 2A). In addition about 40 per cent of familial PC-only cases have a germline *VHL* gene mutation (type 2C) (Woodward et al., 1997). In one series, 11 per cent

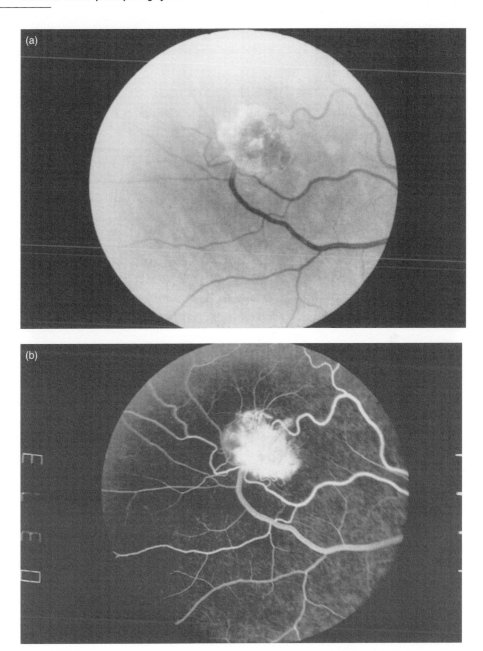

Fig. 12.8. VHL disease: (a) moderate-sized retinal angioma and (b) fluoroscein angiogram of the same lesion.

Table 12.11. *Typical screening protocol for VHL disease in affected patients and at-risk relatives*

Affected patient or gene carrier
Annual physical examination and urine testing
Annual direct and indirect ophthalmoscopy
MRI brain scan every 3 years to age of 50 years and every 5 years thereafter
Annual abdominal MRI or ultrasound scan (CT scan may be required periodically if
    following by ultrasound and multiple renal cysts are present)
Annual 24-h urine collection for catecholamines and VMAs

At-risk relative
Annual physical examination and urine testing
Annual direct and indirect ophthalmoscopy from age of 5 years until age of 60 years
MRI brain scan every 3 years from age 15 to 40 years and then every 5 years until age of
    60 years
Annual renal MRI or ultrasound scan from age 16 to 65 years
Annual 24-h urine collection for catecholamines and VMAs

of patients with apparently sporadic PC had a germline *VHL* mutation (Neumann et al., 2002), although the frequency in a UK series is approximately half of this (unpublished observations). Both adrenal and extra-adrenal PCs can occur in VHL disease. VHL patients with PC usually have missense mutations (see below) and although the overall risk of malignancy in PCs is generally considered to be ~10 per cent, the rate in VHL disease appears to be less than this (~5 per cent).

Pancreas

Pancreas cysts and tumours are relatively common features of VHL disease. Multiple cysts are the most frequent pancreatic manifestation and are present in most older patients. However pancreatic cysts rarely impair pancreatic function. Pancreatic tumours occur in 5–10 per cent of cases. A high frequency of that malignancy has been reported in VHL associated islet cell tumours and surgery is indicated in tumours >3 cm while tumours <1 cm may be monitored (Libutti et al., 1998).

Endolymphatic sac tumours

ELSTs have only been recognised as a specific component of VHL disease in the last decade. In a large survey of VHL patients using MRI and CT scans, Manski et al. (1997) found that 11 per cent of patients with VHL disease had an ELST. Hearing loss is the most common symptom of an ELST, but tinnitus and vertigo also occur in many cases. Hence an ELST should be considered in all VHL patients who complain of hearing loss. However ELSTs are frequently asymptomatic and surgical intervention is not always indicated.

Molecular genetics

The VHL disease gene maps to chromosome 3p25 and was isolated in 1993 (Latif et al., 1993). Germline mutations may be detected in 95–100 per cent of patients, and a genotype–phenotype correlation has been described such that large deletions and protein-truncating mutations are associated with a low risk of PC and specific missense mutations may produce a high risk of PC (type 2 families). Families with a high frequency of PC (types 2A, 2B and 2C) usually have a surface missense mutation whereas type 1 families have mostly germline deletions or truncating mutations. Regular screening of patients affected by VHL disease and of at-risk relatives is important to detect tumours at an early stage and to establish the carrier status for at-risk individuals (see Table 12.11). Molecular genetic analysis enables the screening protocols to be modified according to an individual's risk so that screening frequency may be reduced or discontinued as appropriate.

Werner syndrome

This is a rare autosomal recessive disorder characterised by features of premature senescence and short stature with loss of subcutaneous fat and muscle, stocky trunk and slender limbs, a thin face with beaked nose, and a high-pitched and hoarse voice. The clinical features of senescence develop from the second decade, with premature greying of the hair from the third decade, generalised hair loss, juvenile cataracts from the third decade, premature arteriosclerosis and calcification of blood vessels with coronary heart disease, osteoporosis, metastatic calcification, and scleropoikiloderma of the skin giving an aged appearance. Diabetes mellitus and hypogonadism may be associated. There may be osteoporosis with ankylosis and destruction of joints and muscle atrophy, and hyperkeratosis over bony prominences and on the soles of the feet, which may ulcerate. There may be areas of hyperpigmentation and hypopigmentation of the skin, with lentigenes. About 10 per cent of affected individuals develop tumours, predominantly of types uncommon in the general population, notably of connective tissue or mesenchymal origin, such as soft tissue sarcomas, osteosarcomas, uterine myosarcomas, meningiomas and adenomas of the thyroid, parathyroid, adrenal cortex, breast and liver (Epstein et al., 1966; Goto et al., 1996). Thyroid carcinomas and melanomas have been reported more frequently in Japanese than in Caucasian Werner syndrome patients. Cultured cells from Werner Syndrome patients show chromosome instability and hyper sensitivity to DNA cross-linking agents (Moser et al., 2000).

Werner syndrome is caused by loss-of-function mutations in a gene (*WRN*) at chromosome 8p12 that encodes a predicted protein with homology to DNA and RNA helicases (Yu et al., 1996). However Chen et al., 2003 found that 20 per cent of patients referred to an international registry for molecular diagnosis of Werner syndrome had wild-type *WRN* mutation analysis. Sequence analysis of the *LMNA* gene (which is mutated in a rare childhood syndrome of premature ageing, Hutchinson–Gilford syndrome, and other disorders) in this subset revealed a heterozygous LMNA missense mutation in ~15 per cent of cases.

Wiscott–Aldrich syndrome

This X-linked recessive disorder is characterised by immunodeficiency, eczema and thrombocytopenia. Complications include susceptibility to pyogenic infection, bloody diarrhoea, arthritis, autoimmune disease and lymphoma. Death in childhood may occur from overwhelming bacterial or viral infections. Mucocutaneous petechiae, ecchymoses, purpuric rash and atopic-like dermatosis may develop, and there may be hepatosplenomegaly. There is progressive loss of lymphoid elements normally found in the thymus, spleen, lymph nodes, etc. There appears to be a lack of the 115-kDa glycoprotein sialophorin on lymphocyte surface membranes. Malignancy of the reticuloendothelial system, lymphomas and lymphomatoid granulomatosis are common, being the cause of death in about 10 per cent of cases (ten Bensel et al., 1964). However, by the age of 30 years the risk of non-Hodgkin lymphoma approaches 100 per cent. Patients have small platelets, and the immunodeficiency involves both T-cell and B-cell function. There is low antigen-induced lymphocyte proliferation, with low IgM and defective antibody production.

Linkage between DXS255 on the proximal short arm of the X chromosome (at Xp11.4–11.21) and Wiscott–Aldrich syndrome (Peackocke and Siminowitch, 1987) paved the way for the isolation of the *WASP* gene in 1994 (Derry et al., 1994). Since then, numerous *WASP* mutations have been characterised, a small number of hot spot mutations identified and genotype–phenotype correlations characterised. *WASP* mutations may result in three distinct phenotypes: the classic Wiscott–Aldrich syndrome triad of thrombocytopenia/small platelets, recurrent infections as a result of immunodeficiency, and eczema; the milder X-linked thrombocytopenia variant; and congenital neutropenia without features of Wiscott–Aldrich syndrome or X-linked thromobocytopenia. Patients with a normal sized, but mutated protein, associated with a missense mutation generally have a milder X-linked thrombocytopenia phenotype, whereas those with mutations leading to loss of protein expression or expression of only truncated protein have a more severe classical Wiscott–Aldrich syndrome phenotype and a higher risk of malignancy (Imai et al., 2004, Jin et al., 2004). Prior to the availability of mutation analysis, prenatal diagnosis was achieved by finding small platelets in a male fetus, and with the use of linkage analysis where possible (Arvelier et al., 1990).

X-linked lymphoproliferative disorder (Duncan disease)

This condition affects about 3 per million males and the gene has been mapped to Xq25. Affected males are susceptible to severe infectious mononucleosis infections (fatal in 50 per cent, often in childhood), and 25 per cent develop malignant lymphoma, typically Burkitt-type non-Hodgkin lymphoma in the ileocaecal region, but CNS, hepatic and renal lymphomas are also common. Systemic vasculitis is a rare complication (Dutz et al., 2001). X-linked lympho-proliferative disorder is caused by mutations in the SH2 domain protein 1A (*SH2D1A*) gene (Sumegi et al., 2000). At least one quarter of all mutations are missed by direct sequencing, so there may be a role for other, function-based assays in definite cases, or in possible heterozygotes (Tabata et al., 2005).

Xeroderma pigmentosum

This is a heterogeneous group of autosomal recessive disorders with a preva-lence of about 1 in 70 000 of the population. It is characterised by hypersensitivity to UV light and a high incidence of UV-induced skin cancers (Cohen and Levy, 1989). Clinical onset is before the age of 18 months in 50 per cent. Freckle-like skin lesions with erythema develop in sun-exposed skin in the first few years of life, and there may be extreme sunlight sensitivity (see Fig. 12.9). Macules of increased pigmentation develop on the skin and mucous membranes, and achromic areas may also occur. Subsequently, there is an atrophic and telan-giectatic stage in which the skin becomes dry and scaly, with atrophy and spotted dyschromia. Hyperkeratotic plaques, keratomas, keratoacanthomas, fibromas, angiomyomas, cutaneous horns and other benign tumours ensue, and there may be facial ulcerations. Multiple malignant basal and squamous cell carcin-omas and malignant melanoma develop in sun-exposed areas; the risk for malig-nancy is up to 2000-fold increased above normal. The median age at onset for skin cancer in XP has been estimated to be 8 years, compared with 60 years in the general population. Squamous cell carcinomas, sarcomas, melanomas and epitheliomas may develop in the eyes and mucous membranes, and squamous cell carcinomas of the tongue and oropharynx may occur, with a relative risk of 10 000 times normal. Other malignant tumours may develop, including neuri-nomas, sarcomas and adenocarcinomas. It has been suggested that there is also a 10–20-fold increased incidence of internal neoplasms, such as lung, uterine,

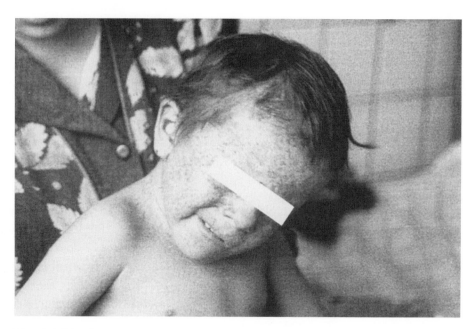

Fig. 12.9. Xeroderma pigmentosum.

brain, breast or testicular tumours in XP. Actinic damage to the eyes may cause keratitis and conjunctivitis, which can lead to symblepharon and neoplasia, particularly at the corneo-scleral junction. Entropion and ectropion may occur. Death results from disseminated tumours, usually by the second or third decade (Giannelli, 1986; Kraemer and Slor, 1985).

De Sanctis–Caccione syndrome emphasised neurological involvement in a subgroup of XP patients. Neurological complications are variable and include progressive mental deficiency, microcephaly, ataxia, choreoathetosis, spasticity, sensorineural deafness, lower motor neuron and cranial nerve damage. Onset of these neurological abnormalities may be in infancy or later in childhood, and may be mild or severe. They develop in about 18 per cent of cases of XP (Kraemer and Slor, 1985). They can occur in any subgroup of XP but do so most commonly in complementation group D (XPD) (see below). Loss or absence of neurons may be demonstrated in the cerebrum or cerebellum at autopsy in these cases.

The karyotype is normal, but there is hypersensitivity to chromosomal damage after exposure to UV light.

Different subgroups (complementation groups) of XP are described, each with a different type of mutation reducing the capacity for excision repair of UV-induced DNA damage (Giannelli, 1986). These subgroups are associated with different clinical severity. Complementation group A (XPA) includes cases of all degrees of clinical severity, with and without neurological complications; group C (XPC) is the most commonly described; and most are neurologically normal. Cockayne syndrome with XP has been described in single cases. The molecular bases for these conditions have been delineated, and are due to various defects in solar-induced DNA damage. These defects comprise lack of a functional helicase, endonuclease or lesion-recognising protein involved in the initial steps of nucleotide excision repair. Different enzyme defects are found in the different complementation groups. They include proteins involved in recognition of photoproducts (XPE), and of other DNA defects such as pyrimidine dimers (XPA), DNA helicases (XPB, XPD), and endonucleases that perform two incisions (XPG), and single-strand-binding proteins (XPC) (Boulikas, 1996; Chu and Mayne, 1996). Prenatal diagnosis by chorionic villus sampling is becoming available in those families in which the mutation can be defined at the DNA level.

Mutations in eight genes may cause XP. The genes for group A and group C xeroderma pigmentosum (*XPA* and *XPC*) are involved solely in nucleotide excision repair whereas the XPB and XPD proteins are both components of transcription factor TFIIH, which is involved in nucleotide excision repair, in basal transcription and in activated transcription (Lehmann, 2003). All bona fide patients with XPE have a mutation in the *DDB2* gene that encodes the smaller subunit of the heterodimeric damaged DNA-binding protein. XP group F (XPF) is caused by mutations in the *ERCC4* gene and group G (XPG) by mutations in *ERCC5*.

XP variant (XP-V) is indistinguishable from XP clinically, except the neurological features do not develop. Unlike other XP cells belonging to XPA to XPG, XP-V cells have normal nucleotide-excision repair processes but defective replication of UV-damaged DNA. This form of XP is caused by a mutation in the DNA polymerase eta gene (POLH) (Masutani et al., 1999).

Suggestions of an increased risk of lung cancer in heterozygote carriers (for all relatives: relative risk: 1.93) (Swift and Chase, 1979) have prompted association studies of XP gene variants and lung cancer risk with mixed results (Marin et al., 2004, Benhamou and Sarasin, 2005).

Treatment is by protection from sunlight and careful surveillance, with early excision of tumours. Avoidance of UV light should be instigated in childhood, when the apparent health of young children makes this difficult. The use of an UV light metre can be helpful. It is interesting that spontaneous regression of malignant melanoma has been described to occur in XP, although the mechanism for this is not understood (Lynch et al., 1978). There is a registry for cases of XP, which can help with their management (c/o Department of Pathology, Room C520, Medical Science Building, 100 Bergen Street, Newark, NJ 07103, USA).

Prenatal diagnosis of XP has been accomplished by demonstrating abnormal levels of DNA repair capacity on measurement of unscheduled DNA synthesis in UV-irradiated fetal amniocytes (Aras et al., 1985), or by mutation analysis.

A separate disorder of increased UV-A sensitivity has been described, in which there is an autosomal dominant predisposition to the development of cutaneous pigmented keratoses in sun-exposed skin associated with the development of carcinoma of the uterus and other internal malignancies (clinically more apparent in females) (Atherton et al., 1989). Fibroblasts from affected individuals demonstrated an increased frequency of single-strand breaks in DNA following exposure to long-wave UV-A.

Appendix: Genetic differential diagnoses by organ system neoplasms

Examples of conditions associated with specific cancers. Superscript numbers in this table refer to pages in this volume.

Organ or neoplasia type	Histologic type	Genetic differential diagnosis	Gene (if known)
Adrenal	Adrenocortical neoplasia	Li–Fraumeni syndrome[215]	TP53
		Beckwith–Wiedemann syndrome[170]	CDKN1C (p57KIP2), NSD1
		Carney complex[176]	PRKAR1A
		Multiple endocrine neoplasia type 1[220]	MEN1
		McCune–Albright syndrome[218]	GNAS1 (not germline)
	Adrenocortical carcinoma	Li–Fraumeni syndrome[215]	TP53
	Medulla – phaeochromocytoma	von Hippel–Lindau disease[252]	VHL
		Phaeochromocytoma–Paraganglioma syndrome[40]	SDHB, SDHC, SDHD
		Multiple endocrine neoplasia (MEN) type 2[222]	RET
		Neurofibromatosis type 1[230]	NF1
Bladder		Werner syndrome[257]	WRN
Brain	Glioma/glioblastoma	Li–Fraumeni syndrome[215]	TP53
		Turcot syndrome (autosomal dominant hereditary non-polyposis colorectal cancer syndrome) and biallelic (autosomal recessive) predisposition[250]	MLH1, MSH2, PMS2
	Optic glioma	Neurofibromatosis type 1[230]	NF1

(*Continued*)

Organ or neoplasia type	Histologic type	Genetic differential diagnosis	Gene (if known)
	Pinealoblastoma	Hereditary retinoblastoma[20]	*RB1*
	Astrocytoma	Neurofibromatosis type 1[230]	*NF1*
		Tuberous sclerosis complex[246]	*TSC1, TSC2*
		Melanoma–astrocytoma syndrome[139]	*CDKN2A/p16, p14ARF*
	Medulloblastoma/NET	Turcot syndrome (familial adenomatous polyposis)[250]	*APC*
		Nevoid basal cell carcinoma syndrome[196]	*PTC*
		Rhabdoid predisposition syndrome	*SNF5/INI1*
		Biallelic central PNET predisposition, with or without colorectal cancer	*PMS2*
	Neurofibromas	Neurofibromatosis type 1[230]	*NF1*
	Vestibular schwannomas	Neurofibromatosis type 2[235]	*NF2*
	Meningioma	Neurofibromatosis type 2[235]	*NF2*
		Neurofibromatosis type 1[230]	*NF1*
		Cowden syndrome[179]	*PTEN*
		Werner syndrome[257]	*WRN*
	Ependymoma	Neurofibromatosis type 2[230]	*NF2*
	Hemangioma, hemangioblastoma	Von Hippel–Lindau syndrome[252]	*VHL*
	Rhabdoid tumour/ atypical teratoid tumour	Rhabdoid predisposition syndrome	*SNF5/INI1*
	Cerebellum, dysplastic gangliocytoma (Lhermitte–Duclos disease)	Cowden syndrome[179]	*PTEN*
	Choroid plexus tumours	Li–Fraumeni syndrome[215]	*TP53*
Breast, female	Carcinoma	Hereditary breast-ovarian cancer syndrome[67]	*BRCA1, BRCA2*

Organ or neoplasia type	Histologic type	Genetic differential diagnosis	Gene (if known)
		Cowden syndrome/ Bannayan–Riley–Ruvalcaba syndrome[179]	PTEN
		Li–Fraumeni syndrome[215]	TP53
		Peutz–Jeghers syndrome[241]	LKB1/STK11
		Ataxiatelangiectasia heterozygotes[167]	ATM
		Werner syndrome[257]	WRN
		Hereditary lobular breast cancer with diffuse gastric cancer[45]	CDHI
Breast, male	Carcinoma	Hereditary breast–ovarian cancer syndrome[67]	BRCA2 (BRCA1)
		Cowden syndrome[179]	PTEN
		Reifenstein syndrome[214]	AR
		Klinefelter syndrome[200]	XXY
Colorectum	Adenocarcinoma	Hereditary non-polyposis colorectal cancer syndrome[200]	MLH1, MSH2, MSH6, PMS1, PMS2
		Familial adenomatous polyposis syndrome[184]	APC
		Juvenile polyposis syndrome SMAD4[211] BMPR1A	MADH4, BMPR1A
		Peutz–Jegher syndrome[241]	LKB1/STK11
		Hereditary mixed polyposis syndrome(s)	
		MAP; MUTYH-associated polyposis[230]	MYH
		Birt–Hogg–Dubé syndrome[173]	BHD
	Polyp – adenoma	Hereditary non-polyposis colorectal cancer syndrome[200]	MLH1, MSH2, MSH6, PMS1, PMS2
		Familial adenomatous polyposis syndrome[154]	APC

(Continued)

Organ or neoplasia type	Histologic type	Genetic differential diagnosis	Gene (if known)
Polyp – hamartoma		Hereditary mixed polyposis syndrome(s)	
		MAP; MUTYH-associated polyposis[230]	MYH
		Juvenile polyposis syndrome[211]	MADH4, BMPR1A
		Peutz–Jegher syndrome[241]	LKB1/STK11
		Cowden syndrome/Bannayan–Riley–Ruvalcaba syndrome[179]	PTEN
		Hereditary mixed polyposis syndrome(s)	—
		Hereditary hypoplastic polyposis	—
		Tuberous sclerosis complex[246]	TSC1, TSC2
Oesophagus	Adenocarcinoma	Familial Barrett oesophagus-adenocarcinoma[42]	
	Squamous cell carcinoma	Familial oesophageal squamous cell cancer[42]	
		Fanconi anaemia[193]	FANC-X
		Tylosis and oesophageal cancer[42]	
Eye	Retinoblastoma, retinoma	Hereditary retinoblastoma[20]	RB1
	Angioma, hemangioblastoma	von Hippel–Lindau syndrome[252]	VHL
	Melanoma	Li–Fraumeni syndrome[215]	TP53
		Ocular melanocytosis	
		Familial atypical multiple-mole melanoma/P16[139]	CDKN2A
		Hereditary breast-ovarian cancer syndrome[67]	BRCA2
	Squamous cell carcinoma, anterior eye	Xeroderma pigmentosum[259]	XP
	Hamartoma	Tuberous sclerosis complex[246]	TSC1, TSC2
		Familial adenomatous polyposis syndrome (CHRPE)[184]	APC
Head and neck	Squamous cell carcinomas	Fanconi anaemia[193]	FANC-X
		Bloom syndrome[174]	BLM

Organ or neoplasia type	Histologic type	Genetic differential diagnosis	Gene (if known)
		Dyskeratosis congenita[152]	TERC (AD), DKC1 (X-linked)
		Xeroderma pigmentosum[259]	XP
	Melanoma: nasal mucosa	Werner syndrome[258]	WRN
	Sebaceous carcinoma	Muir–Torre syndrome (40% eyelid)[228]	MSH2, MLH1
Heart	Myxoma	Carney complex[159]	PRKAR1A
	Rhabdomyoma	Tuberous sclerosis complex[246]	TSC1, TSC2
Haematologic	Leukemia, acute	Li–Fraumeni syndrome[215]	TP53
		Bloom syndrome[174]	BLM
	Leukemia, acute myeloid	Fanconi anaemia[193]	FANC-X
		Familial thrombocytopenia and predisposition to acute myeloid leukaemia[120]	RUNX1/AML1
		Amegakaryocytic thrombocytopenia[120]	C-MPL
		Diamond–Blackfan anaemia[120]	RPS19
		Shwachman–Diamond syndrome[120]	SBDS
		Severe congenital neutropenia/ Kostmann syndrome[120]	ELA2, GFI1
		Werner syndrome[257]	WRN
	Leukemia, acute lymphoid	Ataxiatelangiectasia[167]	ATM
		Nijmegen breakage syndrome[240]	NBS1
	Leukemia, juvenile chronic myeloid	Neurofibromatosis type 1[230]	NF1
	Lymphoma, non-Hodgkin	Ataxiatelangiectasia[167]	ATM
		Nijmegen breakage syndrome[240]	NBS1
		Bloom syndrome[174]	BLM

(Continued)

Organ or neoplasia type	Histologic type	Genetic differential diagnosis	Gene (if known)
		Autoimmune lymphoproliferative syndrome/Canale–Smith syndrome	FAS, FASL, CASP10
		Chediak–Higashi syndrome	LYST
		Wiskott–Aldrich syndrome[258]	WAS
		Duncan disease (X-linked lymphoproliferative disease)	SH2D1A
	Hodgkin disease	Autoimmune lymphoproliferative syndrome/Canale–Smith syndrome	FAS, FASL, CASP10
		Ataxia-telangiectasia[167]	ATM
		Wiskott–Aldrich syndrome[258]	WAS
		Nijmegen breakage syndrome[240]	NBS
Intestine, small	Carcinoma (ampullary)	Familial adenomatous polyposis syndrome[184]	APC
		MUTYH-associated polyposis	MUTYH (MYH)
	Carcinoma (any location)	Hereditary non-polyposis colorectal cancer syndrome[200]	MLH1, MSH2, MSH6, PMS2
		Peutz–Jegher syndrome[241]	LKB1/STK11
		Juvenile polyposis syndrome[211]	MADH4, BMPR1A
		Non-Hodgkin lymphoma (ileum) lymphoproliferative disorder[176]	SH2DIA
	Stromal tumour (gastrointestinal stromal tumours)	Hereditary gastrointestinal stromal tumour[230]	KIT
	Carcinoid tumour	Neurofibromatosis type 1[230]	NF1
		MEN 1[220]	MEN1
Kidney	Renal cell carcinoma, clear cell	von Hippel–Lindau syndrome[252]	VHL
		Birt–Hogg–Dubé syndrome[173]	BHD
		Cowden syndrome[179]	PTEN
		Hereditary clear cell renal carcinoma	
		Werner syndrome[257]	WRN

Organ or neoplasia type	Histologic type	Genetic differential diagnosis	Gene (if known)
	Renal cell carcinoma, papillary	Familial papillary renal cell cancer, type 1	MET
		Familial papillary renal cell cancer, type 2, with multiple leiomyomatosis syndrome[157]	FH
		Tuberous sclerosis complex[246]	TSC1, TSC2
		Hyperparathyroidism-jaw tumour syndrome[210]	HRPT2
		Birt–Hogg–Dubé syndrome[173]	BHD
	Renal pelvis, transitional cell	Hereditary non-polyposis colorectal cancer syndrome (Muir–Torre syndrome)[200]	MSH2, MLH1
	Angiomyolipoma	Tuberous sclerosis complex[246]	TSC1, TSC2
	Oncocytoma	Tuberous sclerosis complex[246]	TSC1, TSC2
		Birt–Hogg–Dubé[173]	BHD
	Wilms tumour	Hereditary Wilms tumour syndrome[112]	WT1
		Wilms tumour–aniridia–genital abnormality–mental retardation[112]	WT1, contiguous gene deletions
		Beckwith–Wiedemann syndrome[170]	CDKN1C (KIP2), NSD1
		Hyperparathyrodism-jaw tumour syndrome[210]	HRPT2
		Denys–Drash syndrome[183]	WT1
	Rhabdoid tumour/ atypical Teratoid tumour	Rhabdoid predisposition syndrome	SNF5/INI1
Liver	Hepatoblastoma	Familial adenomatous polyposis syndrome[184]	APC
		Beckwith–Wiedemann syndrome[170]	CDKN1C (KIP2), NSD1

(*Continued*)

Organ or neoplasia type	Histologic type	Genetic differential diagnosis	Gene (if known)
		Werner syndrome[257]	WRN
	Adenoma/carcinoma	Fanconi anaemia[193]	FANC-X
		Beckwith–Wiedemann syndrome[170]	CDKN1C (KIP2), NSD1
Ovary	Carcinoma	Hereditary breast-ovarian cancer syndrome[67]	BRCA1, BRCA2
		Hereditary non-polyposis colorectal cancer syndrome[200]	MLH1, MSH2, MSH6, PMS2
	Germ cell	Dysgenetic gonads (XY karyotype)	DHH
	Granulosa cell	Peutz–Jegher syndrome[241]	LKB1/STK11
		Ollier disease	PTHR1?
		Mafucci syndrome[217]	PTHR1?
Pancreas	Carcinoma	Hereditary non-polyposis colorectal cancer syndrome[200]	MLH1, MSH2, MSH6, PMS2
		Familial site specific pancreatic cancer	BRCA2
		Hereditary pancreatitis[52]	CFTR, SPINK, PRSS1
		Hereditary breast-ovarian cancer syndrome	BRCA2
		Familial melanoma[139]	CDKN2A
		von Hippel–Lindau syndrome[252]	VHL
		Peutz–Jegher syndrome[241]	LKB1/STK11
	Islet cell neoplasias	MEN 1[220]	MEN1
		von Hippel–Lindau syndrome[252]	VHL
		Neurofibromatosis type 1[230]	NF1
Paraganglia	Paraganglioma	Hereditary phaeochromocytoma–paraganglioma syndrome[40]	SDHB, SDHC, SDHD
		von Hippel–Lindau syndrome[252]	VHL
		MEN type 2[222]	RET
		Neurofibromatosis type 1[230]	NF1
		MEN 1[220]	MEN1

Organ or neoplasia type	Histologic type	Genetic differential diagnosis	Gene (if known)
Parathyroid	Adenoma/hyperplasia	MEN 1[220]	MEN1
		MEN 2[222]	RET
		Hyperparathyroidism-jaw tumour syndrome[210]	HRPT2
	Carcinoma	Hyperparathyroidism-jaw tumour syndrome[210]	HRPT2
Pituitary	Adenoma	MEN 1[220]	MEN1
		Carney complex[176]	PRKAR1A
Prostate	Carcinoma	Hereditary prostate cancer syndromes	—
		Hereditary breast-ovarian cancer syndrome[67]	BRCA1, BRCA2
Sarcoma	Osteosarcoma, soft tissue sarcoma	Li–Fraumeni syndrome[215]	TP53
		Werner syndrome[257]	WRN
		Hereditary retinoblastoma[20]	RB1
		Neurofibromatosis type 1[230]	NF1
		Rothmund–Thomson syndrome[244]	RECQL4
		Werner syndrome[257]	WRN
	Malignant peripheral nerve sheath tumour (neurofibrosarcoma, malignant schwannoma)	Neurofibromatosis type 1[230]	NF1
	Gastrointestinal	Paraganglioma and gastric sarcoma[40] Carney's triad	
	Gastrointestinal stromal tumours	Gastrointestinal stromal tumours	KIT
Skin	Melanoma	Familial melanoma[139]	CDKN2A/ CDK4
		Familial breast ovarian cancer[67]	BRCA2
		Xeroderma pigmentosum[259]	XP-X
		Werner syndrome[257]	WRN
		Hereditary retinoblastoma[20]	RB1
		Melanoma–astrocytoma syndrome[139]	CDKN2A/p16, p14ARF

(*Continued*)

Organ or neoplasia type	Histologic type	Genetic differential diagnosis	Gene (if known)
	Non-melanoma carcinoma	Nevoid basal cell carcinoma (Gorlin) syndrome[196]	PTCH
		Xeroderma pigmentosum[259]	XP-X
		Werner syndrome[257]	WRN
		Fanconi anaemia[193]	FANC-X
		Bazex–Christol–Dupré syndrome[150]	
		Ferguson–Smith syndrome[155]	
	Squamous cell carcinoma	Dyskeratosis congenita[152]	TERC (AD), DKC1 (X-linked)
	Sebaceous carcinoma	Muir–Torre syndrome[228]	MSH2, MLH1
	Leiomyoma	Multiple leiomyomatosis syndrome[157]	FH
	Angiofibromas (facial)	Tuberous sclerosis complex[246]	TSC1, TSC2
		MEN 1[220]	MEN1
	Neurofibroma	Neurofibromatosis type 1[230]	NF1
	Trichilemmomas/ trichodiscomas/ folliculomas	Cowden syndrome[179]	PTEN
		Birt–Hogg–Dubé syndrome[173]	BHD
Stomach	Carcinoma	Hereditary non-polyposis colorectal cancer syndrome[200]	MLH1, MSH2, MSH6, PMS2
		Hereditary diffuse gastric cancer syndrome	CDH1
		Ataxia-telangiectasia[167]	ATM
		Li–Fraumeni syndrome[215]	TP53
		Juvenile polyposis syndrome[211]	MADH4, BMPR1A
		Familial adenomatous polyposis syndrome[184]	APC
		Werner syndrome[257]	WRN
	Stromal tumours (gastrointestinal stromal tumours)	Hereditary gastrointestinal stromal tumour syndrome	KIT

Organ or neoplasia type	Histologic type	Genetic differential diagnosis	Gene (if known)
Testis		Klinefelter syndrome[214]	XXY
		Familial testicular cancer[176]	
		Carney complex	PRKAR1A
		Androgen insensitivity	AR
		Russell–Silver syndrome[112]	
	Gonadoblastoma	Wilms tumour–aniridia–genital abnormality–mental retardation	WT1, contiguous gene syndrome
Thyroid	Papillary	Familial adenomatous polyposis syndrome[184]	APC
		Cowden syndrome[179]	PTEN
		Carney complex[176]	PRKAR1A
		Familial non-medullary thyroid cancer syndromes	—
		Familial papillary thyroid carcinoma	—
	Follicular	Cowden syndrome[179]	PTEN
		Werner syndrome[257]	WRN
	Medullary	MEN 2[223]	RET
Uterus	Endometrial carcinoma	Hereditary non-polyposis colorectal cancer syndrome[200]	MLH1, MSH2, MSH6, PMS2
		Cowden syndrome[179]	PTEN
	Myometrial leiomyoma	Cowden syndrome[179]	PTEN
		Multiple leiomyomatosis papillary renal cell cancer[157]	FH
Vulva	Squamous cell	Fanconi anaemia[193]	FANC-X

References

Aaltonen, L.A., Salovaara, R., Kristo, P., Canzian, F., Hemminki, A., Peltomaki, P., Chadwick, R.B., Kaariainen, H., Eskelinen, M., Jarvinen, H., Mecklin, J.P., Delachapelle, A., Percesepe, A., Ahtola, H., Harkonen, N., Julkunen, R., Kangas, E., Ojala, S., Tulikoura, J. & Valkamo, E. (1998). Incidence of hereditary nonpolyposis colorectal cancer and the feasibility of molecular screening for the disease. *New Engl. J. Med.*, **338**(21), 1481–7.

Aarnio, M., Mecklin, J.-P., Aaltonen, L.A. et al. (1995). Life-time risk of different cancers in hereditary non-polyposis colorectal cancer (HNPCC) syndrome. *Int. J. Cancer*, **64**, 430–3.

Aarnio, M., Sanikala, R., Pukkala, E. et al. (1999). Cancer risk in mutation carriers of DNA-mismatch repair genes. *Int. J. Cancer*, **81**, 214–8.

Abeliovich, D., Kaduri, L., Lerer, I., Weinberg, N., Amir, G., Sagi, M., Zlotogora, J., Heching, N. & Peretz, T. (1997). The founder mutations 185delAG and 5382insC in BRCA1 and 6174delT in BRCA2 appear in 60-percent of ovarian cancer and 30-percent of early-onset breast cancer patients among Ashkenazi women. *Am. J. Hum. Genet.*, **60**, 505–14.

Aben, K.K. et al. (2001). Absence of karyotype abnormalities in patients with familial urothelial cell carcinoma. *Urology*, **57**(2), 266–9.

Abraham, S.C., Wu, T.T., Klimstra, D.S., Finn, L.S., Lee, J.H., Yeo, C.J., Cameron, J.L. & Hruban, R.H. (2001). Distinctive molecular genetic alterations in sporadic and familial adenomatous polyposis-associated pancreatoblastomas: frequent alterations in the APC/beta-catenin pathway and chromosome 11p. *Am. J. Pathol.*, **159**, 1619–27.

Agarwal, S.K., Guru, S.C., Heppner, C. et al. (1999). Menin interacts with the AP1 transcription factor JunD and represses JunD-activated transcription. *Cell*, **96**, 143–52.

Agarwal, S.K., Novotny, E.A., Crabtree, J.S. et al. (2003). Transcription factor JunD, deprived of menin, switches from growth suppressor to growth promoter. *Proc. Natl. Acad. Sci. USA*, **100**, 10770–5.

Ahlbom, A., Lichtenstein, P., Malmstrom, H., Feychting, M., Hemminki, K. & Pedersen, N.L. (1997). Cancer in twins: genetic and nongenetic familial risk factors. *J. Natl. Cancer Inst.*, **89**, 287–93.

Ahn, J., Ludecke, H.J., Lindow, S. et al. (1995). Cloning of he putative tumour supporssor gene for hereditary multiple exostoses (EXT1). *Nat. Genet.*, **11**, 137–43.

Ahonen, P. (1985). Autoimmune polyendocrinopathy-candidosis-ectodermal dystrophy (APECED): autosomal recessive inheritance. *Clin. Genet.*, **27**, 535–42.

Aida, H., Takakuwa, K., Nagata, H., Tsuneki, I., Takano, M., Tsuji, S. et al. (1998). Clinical features of ovarian cancer in Japanese women with germ-line mutations of BRCA1. *Clin. Cancer Res.*, **4**, 235–40.

Aitken, J., Welch, J., Duffy, D., Milligan, A., Green, A., Martin, N. & Hayward, N. (1999). CDKN2A variants in a population-based sample of Queensland families with melanoma. *J. Natl. Cancer Inst.*, **91**(5), 446–52.

Akiyama, Y., Satoh, H., Yamada, T. et al. (1997). Germline mutations of the HMSH6/9 TBP gene in an atypical hereditary nonpolyposis colorectal cancer kindred. *Cancer*, **57**, 3920–3.

Aktan-Collan, K., Mecklin, J.-P., Jarvinen, H. et al. (2000). Predictive genetic testing for hereitary non-polyposis colorectal cancer: uptake and long-term satisfaction. *Int. J. Cancer*, **89**, 44–50.

Aktas, D., Koc, A., Boduroglu, K., Hicsonmez, G. & Tuncbilek, E. (2000). Myelodysplastic syndrome associated with monosomy 7 in a child with Bloom syndrome. *Cancer Genet. Cytogenet.*, **116**(1), 44–6.

Alam, N.A., Bevan, S., Churchman, M. et al. (2001). Localization of a gene (*MCUL1*) for multiple cutaneous leiomyomata and uterine fibroids to chromosome 1q42.3–q42. *Am. J. Hum. Genet.*, **68**, 1264–9.

Alam, N.A., Rowan, A.J., Wortham, N. et al. (2003). Genetic and functional analyses of FH mutations in multiple cutaneous and uterine leiomatosis, hereditary leiomatosis and renal cancer, and fumarate hydratase deficiency. *Hum. Mol. Genet.*, **12**, 1–12.

Albeck, H. et al. (1993). Familial clusters of nasopharyngeal carcinoma and salivary gland carcinomas in Greenland natives. *Cancer*, **72**(1), 196–200.

Albrechts, A.E. & Rapini, R.P. (1995). Malignancy in Maffucci's syndrome. *Dermatol. Clin.*, **13**, 73–8.

Albright, F., Butler, A.M., Hampton, A.O. et al. (1937). Syndrome characterised by osteitis fibrosa disseminata, areas of pigmentation and endocrine dysfunction, with precocious puberty in females: report of 5 cases. *New Engl. J. Med.*, **216**, 727–46.

Aldred, M.A., Ginn-Pease, M.E., Morrison, C.D. et al. (2003a). Caveolin-1 and *caveolin-2*, together with three bone morphogenetic protein-related genes, may encode novel tumor suppressors downregulated in sporadic thyroid carcinogenesis. *Cancer Res.*, **63**, 2864–71.

Aldred, M.A., Morrison, C.D., Gimm, O. et al. (2003b). Peroxisome proliferator-activated receptor gamma is frequently downregulated in a diversity of sporadic non-medullary thyroid carcinomas. *Oncogene*, **22**, 3412–6.

Alexander, F.E., Jarrett, R.F., Cartwright, R.A., Armstrong, A.A., Gokhale, D.A., Kane, E., Gray, D., Lawrence, D.J. & Taylor, G.M. (2001). Epstein-Barr Virus and HLA-DPB1-*0301 in young adult Hodgkin's disease: evidence for inherited susceptibility to Epstein-Barr Virus in cases that are EBV(+ ve). *Cancer Epidemiol. Biomark. Prev.*, **10**(6), 705–9.

Alm, T. & Licznerski, G. (1973). The intestinal polyposes. *Clin. Gastroenterol.*, **2**, 577–602.

Alman, B.A., Greel, D.A. & Wolfe, H.J. (1996). Activating mutations of Gs protein in monostatic fibrous lesions of bone. *J. Orthop. Res.*, **14**, 311–15.

Alter, B.P. (1987). The bone marrow failure syndromes. In *Haematology of Infancy and Childhood*, 3rd edn, eds. Nathan, D.G. & Oski, F.S. W.B. Saunders, Philadelphia, PA.

Alter, B.P. (1996). Fanconi anaemia and malignancies. *Am. J. Hematol.*, **53**, 99–110.

Alter, B.P. (2003). Cancer in Fanconi anemia, 1927–2001. *Cancer*, **97**, 425–40.

Alter, B.P., Greene, M.H., Velazquez, I. & Rosenberg, P.S. (2003). Cancer in Fanconi anemia. *Blood*, **101**, 2072.

Altieri, A., Bermejo, J.L. & Hemminki, K. (2005). Familial risk for non-Hodgkin lymphoma and other lymphoproliferative malignancies by histopathologic subtype: the Swedish Family-Cancer Database. *Blood*, **106**, 668–72.

Al Saffar, M. & Foulkes, W.D. (2002). Hereditary ovarian cancer resulting from a non-ovarian cancer cluster region (OCCR) BRCA2 mutation: is the OCCR useful clinically? *J. Med. Genet.*, **39**, e68.

Al-Tassan, N., Chmiel, N.H., Maynard, J. et al. (2002). Inherited variants of MYH associated with somatic G:C-->T:A mutations in colorectal tumors. *Nat. Genet.*, **30**(2), 227–32.

Alvarez-Arratia, M.C., Rivas, F., Avia-Abundis, A., et al. (1983). A probable monogenic form of polyostotic fibrous dysplasia. *Clin. Genet.*, **24**, 132–9.

Ancliff, P.J., Gale, R.E., Liesner, R., Hann, I.M. & Linch, D.C. (2001). Mutations in the ELA2 gene encoding neutrophil elastase are present in most patients with sporadic severe congenital neutropenia but only in some patients with the familial form of the disease. *Blood*, **98**, 2645–50.

Andant, C., Puy, H., Bogard, C. et al. (2000). Hepatocellular carcinoma in patients with acute hepatic porphyria: frequency of occurrence and related factors. *J. Hepatol.*, **32**, 933–9.

Andersen, T.I., Borresen, A.L. & Moller, P. (1996). A common BRCA1 mutation in Norwegian breast and ovarian cancer families? [letter]. *Am. J. Hum. Genet.*, **59**, 486–7.

Anderson, D.E. & Badzioch, M.D. (1991). Hereditary cutaneous malignant melanoma: a 20-year family update. *Anticancer Res.*, **11**, 433–8.

Anderson, M.L., Pasha, T.M. & Leighton, J.A. (2000). Endoscopic perforation of the colon: lessons from a 10-year study. *Am. J. Gastroenterol.*, **95**, 3418–22.

Ang, S.O., Chen, H., Hirota, K., Gordeuk, V.R., Jelinek, J., Guan, Y., Liu, E., Sergueeva, A.I., Miasnikova, G.Y., Mole, D., Maxwell, P.H., Stockton, D.W., Semenza, G.L. & Prchal, J.T. (2002). Disruption of oxygen homeostasis underlies congenital Chuvash polycythemia. *Nat. Genet.*, **32**, 614–21.

Angelo, C., Groeso, M.G., Stella, P. et al. (2001). Becker's naevus syndrome. *Cutis*, **68**, 123–4.

Anthony, P.E., Morris, L.S. & Vowles, K.D.J. (1984). Multiple and recurrent inflammatory fibroid polyps in three generations of a Devon family. *Gut*, **25**, 854–62.

Antoniou, A., Pharoah, P.D., Narod, S., Risch, H.A., Eyfjord, J.E., Hopper, J.L., Loman, N., Olsson, H., Johannsson, O., Borg, A., Pasini, B., Radice, P., Manoukian, S., Eccles, D.M., Tang, N., Olah, E., Anton-Culver, H., Warner, E., Lubinski, J., Gronwald, J., Gorski, B., Tulinius, H., Thorlacius, S., Eerola, H., Nevanlinna, H., Syrjakoski, K., Kallioniemi, O.P., Thompson, D., Evans, C., Peto, J., Lalloo, F., Evans, D.G. & Easton, D.F. (2003). Average risks of breast and ovarian cancer associated with BRCA1 or BRCA2 mutations detected in case series unselected for family history: a combined analysis of 22 studies. *Am. J. Hum. Genet.*, **72**, 1117–30.

Antoniou, A.C., Gayther, S.A., Stratton, J.F., Ponder, B.A. & Easton, D.F. (2000). Risk models for familial ovarian and breast cancer. *Genet. Epidemiol.*, **18**, 173–90.

Antoniou, A.C., Pharoah, P.P., Smith, P. & Easton, D.F. (2004). The BOADICEA model of genetic susceptibility to breast and ovarian cancer. *Br. J. Cancer*, **91**, 1580–90.

Aoki, Y., Niihori, T., Kawame, H., Kurosawa, K., Ohashi, H., Tanaka, Y., Filocamo, M., Kato, K., Suzuki, Y., Kure, S. & Matsubara, Y. (2005). Germline mutations in HRAS proto-oncogene cause Costello syndrome. *Nat. Genet.*, **37**, 1038–40.

Apicella, C., Andrews, L., Hodgson, S.V., Fisher, S.A., Lewis, C.M., Solomon, E., Tucker, K., Friedlander, M., Bankier, A., Southey, M.C., Venter, D.J. & Hopper, J.L. (2003). Log odds of carrying an ancestral mutation in BRCA1 or BRCA2 for a defined personal and family history in an Ashkenazi Jewish woman (LAMBDA). *Breast Cancer Res.*, **5**, R206–16.

Apple, R.J., Becker, T.M., Wheeler, C.M. & Erlich, H.A. (1995). Comparison of human leukocyte antigen DR-DQ disease associations found with cervical dysplasia and invasive cervical carcinoma. *J. Natl. Cancer Inst.*, **87**, 427–36.

Araim, M., Nosaka, K., Koshiara, K. et al. (2004). Neurocutaneous melanosis associated with Dandy Walker malformation and a meningohydroencephalocoele. *J. Neurosurg. Spine*, **100**, 501–5.

Aras, S., Bohnert, E., Fischer, E. & Jung, E.G. (1985). Prenatal exclusion of xeroderma pigmentosa (XP-D) by amniotic cell analysis. *Photodermatology*, **2**, 181–3.

Arico, M., Nichols, K., Whitlock, J.A., Arceci, R., Haupt, R., Mittler, U., Kuhne, T., Lombardi, A., Ishii, E., Egeler, R.M. & Danesino, C. (1999). Familial clustering of Langerhans cell histiocytosis. *Br. J. Haematol.*, **107**, 883–8.

Arinami, T., Kondo, I., Hamaguchi, H. & Nakajima, S. (1986). Multifocal meningiomas in a patient with a constitutional ring chromosome 22. *J. Med. Genet.*, **23**, 178–80.

Armstrong, J.G., Davies, D.R., Guy, S.P. et al. (1997). APC mutations in familial adenomatous polyposis families in the Northwest of England. *Hum. Mutat.*, **10**, 376–80.

Armstrong, R.M. & Hanson, C.W. (1969). Familial gliomas. *Neurology*, **19**, 1061–3.

Arngrimsson, R., Dokal, I., Luzzato, L. & Connor, J.M. (1993). Dyskeratosis congenita. Three additional families show linkage to a locus in Xq28. *J. Med. Genet.*, **30**, 618–19.

Arnio, M., Salovaara, R., Aaltonen, L.A. et al. (1997). Features of gastric cancer in hereditary non-polyposis colorectal cancer syndromes. *Int. J. Cancer*, **74**, 551–5.

Arnold, A.C., Hepler, R.S., Yee, R.W., Maggiano, J., Eng, L.F. & Foos, R.Y. (1985). Solitary retinal astrocytoma. *Surv. Ophthalmol.*, **30**, 173–81.

Arunkumar, M.J., Ranjan, A., Jacob, M. & Rajshekhar, V. (2001). Neurocutaneous melanosis: a case of primary intracranial melanoma with metastasis. *Clin. Oncol.*, **13**, 52–4.

Arvanitis, M.L., Jagleman, D.G., Fazio, V.W. et al. (1990). Mortality in patients with familial adenomatous polyposis. *Dis. Colon Rectum*, **33**, 639–42.

Arvelier, B.G., de St Basile, Fischer, A. et al. (1990). Germ-line mosaicism simulates genetic heterogeneity in Wiskott–Aldrich syndrome. *Am. J. Hum. Genet.*, **46**, 906–11.

Ashcraft, K.W., Holder, T.M. & Harris, D.J. (1975). Familial presacral teratomas. *Birth Defect.*, **11**, 143–6.

Ashton, G.H., McLean, W.H., South, A.P. et al. (2004). Recurrent mutations in kindlin-1, a novel keratinocyte focal contact protein, in the autosomal recessive skin fragility and photosensitivity disorder, Kindler syndrome. *J. Invest. Dermatol.*, **122**, 78–83.

Astuti, D., Douglas, F., Lennard, T.W.J. et al. (2001a). Germline *SDHD* mutation in familial phaeochromocytoma. *Lancet*, **357**, 1181–2.

Astuti, D., Latif, F., Dallol, A. et al. (2001b). Mutations in the mitochondrial complex II subunit SDHB cause susceptibility to familial paraganglioma and pheochromocytoma. *Am. J. Hum. Genet.*, **69**, 49–54.

Atherton, D.J., Botcherby, P.K., Francis, A.J. et al. (1989). Familial keratoses of actinic distribution associated with internal malignancy and cellular hypersensitivity to UVA. *Br. J. Dermatol.*, **120**, 671–81.

Athma, P., Rappaport, R. & Swift, M. (1996). Molecular genotyping shows that ataxia-telangiectasia heterozygotes are predisposed to breast cancer. *Cancer Genet. Cytogenet.*, **92**, 130–4.

Attard-Montalto, S.P., Schuller, I., Lastowska, M.A. et al. (1994). Non-Hodgkin's lymphoma and Klinefelter syndrome. *Pediatr. Haematol. Oncol.*, **11**, 197–200.

Auerbach, A.D. (1993). Fanconi anemia diagnosis and the diepoxybutane (DEB) test. *Exp. Hematol.*, **21**, 731–3.

Auerbach, A.D., Sagi, M. & Adler, B. (1985). Fanconi anemia: prenatal diagnosis in 30 fetuses at risk. *Pediatrics*, **76**, 794–800.

Augustsson, A., Stierner, U., Rosdahl, I. & Suurkula, M. (1990). Common and dysplastic naevi as risk factors for cutaneous malignant melanoma in a Swedish population. *Acta. Derm. Venereol.*, **71**, 518–24.

Auranen, A., Pukkala, E., Makinen, J., Sankila, R., Grenman, S. & Salmi, T. (1996). Cancer incidence in the first-degree relatives of ovarian cancer patients. *Br. J. Cancer*, **74**, 280–4.

Auroy, S., Avril, M.F., Chompret, A. et al. (2001). Sporadic multiple primary melanoma cases: CDKN2A germline mutations with a founder effect. *Gene. Chromosome. Cancer*, **32**(3), 195–202.

Azizi, E., Friedman, J., Pavlotsky, F., Iscovich, J., Bornstein, A., Shafir, R., Trau, H., Brenner, H. & Nass, D. (1995). Familial cutaneous malignant melanoma and tumors of the nervous system. A hereditary cancer syndrome. *Cancer*, **76**, 1571–8.

Bader, J.L. & Miller, R.W. (1978). Neurofibromatosis and childhood leukaemia. *J. Pediatr.*, **92**, 925–9.

Bahmer, F.A., Fritsch, P., Kreusch, J. et al. (1990). Terminology in surface microscopy. *J. Am. Acad. Dermatol.*, **23**(6), 1159–62.

Bahuau, M., Vidaud, D., Kujas, M., Palangie, A., Assouline, B., Chaignaud-Lebreton, M., Prieur, M., Vidaud, M., Harpey, J.P., Lafourcade, J. & Caille, B. (1997). Familial aggregation of malignant melanoma/dysplastic naevi and tumours of the nervous system: an original syndrome of tumour proneness. *Ann. Genet.*, **40**, 78–91.

Bahuau, M., Vidaud, D., Jenkins, R.B., Bieche, I., Kimmel, D.W., Assouline, B., Smith, J.S., Alderete, B., Cayuela, J.M., Harpey, J.P., Caille, B. & Vidaud, M. (1998). Germ-line deletion involving the INK4 locus in familial proneness to melanoma and nervous system tumors. *Cancer Res.*, **58**, 2298–303.

Balch, C.M., Soong, S.J., Gershenwald, J.E. et al. (2001). Prognostic factors analysis of 17,600 melanoma patients: validation of the American joint committee on cancer melanoma staging system. *J. Clin. Oncol.*, **19**(16), 3622–34.

Baldinu, P., Cossu, A., Manca, A. et al. (2002). Microsatellite instability and mutation analysis of candidate genes in unselected Sardinian patients with endometrial carcinoma. *Cancer*, **94**, 3157–68.

Bale, S.J. (1999). The sins of the fathers: self-healing squamous epithelioma in Scotland. *J. Cutan. Med. Surg.*, **3**, 207–10.

Bale, S.J. & DiGiovanna, J.J. (1997). Genetic approaches to understanding the keratinopathies. *Adv. Dermatol.*, **12**, 99–113.

Bale, S.J., Dracopoli, N.C., Tucker, M.A. et al. (1989). Mapping the gene for hereditary cutaneous malignant melanoma dysplastic nevus syndrome to chromosome 1p. *New Engl. J. Med.*, **320**, 1367–72.

Bandera, C.A., Muto, M.G., Schorge, J.O., Berkowitz, R.S., Rubin, S.C. & Mok, S.C. (1998). BRCA1 gene mutations in women with papillary serous carcinoma of the peritoneum. *Obstet. Gynecol.*, **92**, 596–600.

Bandipalliam, P. (2005). Syndrome of early onset color cancer, hematologic malignancies and features of neurofibromatosis in HNPCC families with homozygous mismatch repair gene mutations. *Fam. Cancer.*, **4**(4), 323–33.

Barana, D., van der, K.H., Wijnen, J., Longa, E.D., Radice, P., Cetto, G.L., Fodde, R. & Oliani, C. (2004). Spectrum of genetic alterations in Muir–Torre syndrome is the same as in HNPCC. *Am. J. Med. Genet. A.*, **125**(3), 318–19.

Bardram, L. & Stage, J.G. (1985). Frequency of endocrine disorders in patients with the Zollinger–Ellison syndrome. *Scand. J. Gasteroenterol.*, **20**, 233–8.

Barker, D., Wright, E., Nguyen, K. et al. (1987). Gene for von Recklinghausen neurofibromatosis is in the pericentric region of chromosome 17. *Science*, **236**, 1100–2.

Barker, K., Zhou, X.-P., Araki, T. et al. (2001). PTEN mutations are uncommon in Proteus syndrome. *J. Med. Genet.*, **38**, 480–1.

Barker, K.T., Foulkes, W.D., Schwartz, C.E. et al. (2006). Is the EI11K allele of VG5Q associated with Klippel—Trenaunay and other overgrowth syndromes? *J. Med. Genet.*, **27**, epub. PMID 16443853.

Barsh, G.S. (1996). The genetics of pigmentation: from fancy genes to complex traits. *Trend. Genet.*, **12**, 299–305.

Barton, L.M., Roberts, P., Tranton, V. et al. (2004). Chediak–Higashi syndrome. *Br. J. Haematl.*, **125**, 2.

Bartsch, D.K., Langer, P., Wild, A. et al. (2000). Pancreatoduodenal endocrine tumours in multiple endocrine neoplasia type 1: surgery or surveillance? *Surgery*, **128**, 958–60.

Bartsch, D.K., Sina-Frey, M., Lang, S., Wild, A., Gerdes, B., Barth, P., Kress, R., Grutzmann, R., Colombo-Benkmann, M., Ziegler, A., Hahn, S.A., Rothmund, M. & Rieder, H. et al. (2002). CDKN2A germline mutations in familial pancreatic cancer. *Ann. Surg.*, **236**(6), 730–7.

Baser, M.E., Friedman, J.M., Aeschliman, D., Joe, H., Wallace, A.J., Ramsden, R.T. & Evans, D.G. (2002a). Predictors of the risk of mortality in neurofibromatosis 2. *Am. J. Hum. Genet.*, **71**, 715–23.

Baser, M.E., Friedman, J.M., Wallace, A.J., Ramsden, R.T., Joe, H. & Evans, D.G.R. (2002b). Evaluation of clinical diagnostic criteria for neurofibromatosis 2. *Neurology*, **59**, 1759–65.

Baser, M.E., Kuramoto, L., Joe, H., Friedman, J.M., Wallace, A.J., Gillespie, J.E., Ramsden, R.T. & Evans, D.G. (2004). Genotype–phenotype correlations for nervous system tumors in neurofibromatosis 2: a population-based study. *Am. J. Hum. Genet.*, **75**, 231–9.

Bassett, G.S. & Cowell, H.R. (1985). Metachondromatosis: report of four cases. *J. Bone Joint Surg. Am.*, **67A**, 811–14.

Bastiaens, M., ter Huurne, J., Gruis, N., Bergman, W., Westendorp, R., Vermeer, B.J. & Bouwes Bavinck, J.N. (2001). The melanocortin-1-receptor gene is the major freckle gene. *Hum. Mol. Genet.*, **10**(16), 1701–8.

Bataille, V., Newton Bishop, J.A., Sasieni, P., Swerdlow, A.J., Pinney, E., Griffiths, K. & Cuzick, J. (1996). Risk of cutaneous melanoma in relation to the numbers, types and sites of naevi: a case–control study. *Br. J. Cancer*, **73**(12), 1605–11.

Baumler, C., Duan, F., Onel, K. et al. (2003). Differential recruitment of caspase 8 to cFlip confers sensitivity or resistance to Fas-mediated apoptosis in a subset of familial lymphoma patients. *Leuk. Res.*, **27**, 841–51.

Baysal, B.E., Ferrell, R.E., Willett-Brozick, J.E. et al. (2000). Mutations in SDHD, a mitochondrial complex II gene, in hereditary paraganglioma. *Science*, **287**, 848–51.

Beckwith, J.B., Kiviat, N.B. & Bonadio, J.F. (1990). Nephrogenic rests, nephroblastomatosis and the pathogenesis of Wilms tumor. *Pediatr. Pathol.*, **10**, 1–36.

Beller, U., Halle, D., Catane, R., Kaufman, B., Hornreich, G. & Levy-Lahad, E. (1997). High frequency of BRCA1 and BRCA2 germline mutations in Ashkenazi Jewish ovarian cancer patients, regardless of family history [see comments]. *Gynecol. Oncol.*, **67**, 123–6.

Bender, B.U., Gutsche, M., Gläsker, S. et al. (2000). Differential genetic alterations in sporadic and von Hippel–Lindau syndrome-associated pheochromocytomas. *J. Clin. Endocrinol. Metab.*, **85**, 4568–74.

Benhamou, S. & Sarasin, A. (2005). ERCC2 /XPD gene polymorphisms and lung cancer: a HuGE review. *Am. J. Epidemiol.*, **161**, 1–14.

Ben-Izhak, O., Munichor, M., Malkin, L. & Kerner, H. (1998). Brenner tumour of the vagina. *Int. J. Gynae. Pathol.*, **17**, 79–82.

Berchuck, A., Heron, K.A., Carney, M.E., Lancaster, J.M., Fraser, E.G., Vinson, V.L, Deffenbaugh, A.M., Miron, A., Marks, J.R., Futreal, P.A. & Frank, T.S. (1998). Frequency of germline and somatic BRCA1 mutations in ovarian cancer. *Clin. Cancer Res.*, **4**, 2433–7.

Berchuck, A., Schildkraut, J.M., Marks, J.R. & Futreal, P.A. (1999). Managing hereditary ovarian cancer risk [Review] [62 refs]. *Cancer*, **86**, 1697–704.

Berendes, U., Kuhner, A. & Schnyder, U.W. (1971). Segmentary and disseminated lesions in multiple hereditary cutaneous leiomyoma. *Humangenetik*, **13**, 81–2.

Berends, M.J., Wu, Y., Sijmons, R.H., Mensink, R.G., van Der, S.T., Hordijk-Hos, J.M., de Vries, E.G., Hollema, H., Karrenbeld, A., Buys, C.H., van der Zee, A.G., Hofstra, R.M. & Kleibeuker, J.H. (2002). Molecular and clinical characteristics of MSH6 variants: an analysis of 25 index carriers of a germline variant. *Am. J. Hum. Genet.*, **70**(1), 26–37.

Berezin, M. & Karazik, A. (1995). Familial prolactinoma. *Clin. Endocrinol.* **42**, 483–6.

Bergman, L., Teh, B., Cardinal, J. et al. (2000). Identification of MEN1 gene mutations in families with MEN 1 and related disorders. *Br. J. Cancer*, **83**, 1009–14.

Bergman, W., Palan, A. & Went, L.N. (1986). Clinical and genetic studies in six Dutch kindreds with the Dysplastic Naevus syndrome. *Ann. Hum. Genet.*, **50**, 249–58.

Bergman, W., Watson, P., de Jong, J., Lynch, H.T. & Fusaro, R.M. (1990). Systemic cancer and the FAMMM syndrome. *Br. J. Cancer*, **61**, 932–6.

Bergman, W., Gruis, N.A. & Frants, R.R. (1992). The Dutch FAMMM family material: clinical and genetic data. *Cytogenet. Cell Genet.*, **59**, 161–4.

Berlin, N.I., Van Scott, E.J., Glendenning, W.E. et al. (1966). Basal cell nevus syndrome. *Ann. Int. Med.*, **64**, 403.

Berman, D.B., Costalas, J., Schultz, D.C., Grana, G., Daly, M. & Godwin, A.K. (1996). A common mutation in BRCA2 that predisposes to a variety of cancers is found in both Jewish Ashkenazi and non-Jewish individuals. *Cancer Res.*, **56**, 3409–14.

Bernends, R. (2003). Cancer: cues for migration. *Nature*, **425**, 247–8.

Berry, D.A., Iverson, E.S., Gudbjartsson, D.F. et al. (2002). BRCAPRO validation, sensitivity of genetic testing of BRCA1/BRCA2, and prevalence of other breast cancer susceptibility genes. *J. Clin. Oncol.*, **20**, 2701–12.

Bevan, S., Woodford-Richens, K., Rozen, P. et al. (1999). Screening SMAD1, SMAD2, SMAD3 and SMAD5 for germline mutations in juvenile polyposis syndrome. *Gut*, **45**, 406–8.

Beveridge, G.W. & Langlands, A.O. (1973). Familial hyperkeratosis lenticularis perstans associated with tumours of the skin. *Br. J. Dermatol.*, **88**, 453–8.

Bewtra, C., Watson, P. & Conway, T. (1992). Hereditary ovarian cancer: a clinicopathological study. *Int. J. Gynecol. Pathol.*, **11**, 180–7.

Bignami, M., Casorrlli, I., Karran, P. et al. (2003). Mismatch repair and response to DNA-damaging antitumour therapies. *Eur. J. Cancer*, **39**, 2142–9.

Biggs, P.J., Wooster, R., Ford, D. et al. (1995). Familial cylindromatosis (turban tumour syndrome) gene localised to chromosome 16q12–13: evidence for its role as a tumour suppressor gene. *Nat. Genet.*, **11**, 441–3.

Birch, J.M., Hartley, A.L., Marsden, H.B. et al. (1984). Excess risk of breast cancer in the mothers of children with soft tissue sarcomas. *Br. J. Cancer*, **49**, 324–31.

Birch, J.M., Hartley, A.L., Blair, V. et al. (1990). The Li–Fraumeni cancer family syndrome. *J. Pathol.*, **161**, 1–2.

Birch, J.M., Hartley, A.L., Tricker, K.J. et al. (1994). Prevalence and diversity of constitutional mutations in the p53 gene among 21 Li–Fraumeni families. *Cancer Res.*, **54**, 1298–304.

Birch, J.M., Blair, V., Kelsey, A.M., Evans, D.G., Harris, M., Tricker, K.J. & Varley, J.M. (1998). Cancer phenotype correlates with constitutional TP53 genotype in families with the Li–Fraumeni syndrome. *Oncogene*, **17**, 1061–8.

Birch, J.M., Alston, R.D., McNally, R.J.Q. et al. (2001). Relative frequency and morphology of cancers in carriers of germline *TP53* mutations. *Oncogene*, **20**, 4621–8.

Birt, A.R., Hogg, G.R. & Dube, W.J. (1977). Hereditary multiple fibrofolliculomas with trichodiscomas and acrochordons. *Arch. Dermatol.*, **113**(12), 1674–7.

Bishop, D.T. & Gardner, E.J. (1980). Analysis of the genetic predisposition of cancer in individual pedigrees. In *Cancer Incidence in Defined Populations*, eds. Cairns, J., Lyon, J.L. & Skolnick, M. Banbury Report 4. Cold Spring Harbor Laboratory Press, Cold Spring Harbor, NY, pp. 389–406.

Bishop, D.T., Demenais, F., Goldstein, A.M. et al. (2002). Geographical variation in the penetrance of CDKN2A mutations for melanoma. *J. Natl. Cancer. Inst.* **94**(12), 894–903.

Bjorge, T., Lie, A.K., Hovig, E., Gislefoss, R.E., Hansen, S., Jellum, E., Langseth, H., Nustad, K., Trope, C.G. & Dorum, A. (2004). BRCA1 mutations in ovarian cancer and borderline tumours in Norway: a nested case–control study. *Br. J. Cancer*, **91**, 1829–34.

Blattner, W.A., Garber, J.E., Mann, D.L. et al. (1980). Waldenstrom's macroglobulinaemia and autoimmune disease in a family. *Ann. Int. Med.*, **93**, 830–2.

Blaugrund, J.E., Johns, M.M., Eby, Y.J. et al. (1994). *RET* proto-oncogene mutations in inherited and sporadic medullary thyroid cancer. *Hum. Mol. Genet.*, **3**, 1895–7.

Bloom, D. (1966). The syndrome of congenital telangiectatic erythema and stunted growth. *J. Pediatr.*, **68**, 103–13.

Bluteau, O., Jeannot, E., Bioulac-Sage, P. et al. (2002). Bi-allelic inactivation of TCFI in hepatic adenomas. *Nat. Genet.*, **32**, 312–5.

Boardman, L.A., Thibodeau, S.N., Schaid, D.J. et al. (1998). Increased risk for cancer in patients with the Peutz–Jeghers syndrome. *Ann. Int. Med.*, **128**, 896–9.

Bocker, W., Bier, B., Freytag, G., Brommelkamp, B., Jarasch, E.D., Edel, G., Dockhorndworniczak, B. & Schmid, K.W. (1992). An immunohistochemical study of the breast using antibodies to basal and luminal keratins, alpha-smooth muscle actin, vimentin, collagen-Iv and laminin. 2. Epitheliosis and ductal carcinoma in situ. *Virchows Arch. A.-Pathol. Anat. Histopathol.*, **421**, 323–30.

Boland, et al. (1998). A National Cancer Institute Workshop on Microsatellite for cancer detection and familial predisposition: development of international criteria for determination of microsatellite instability in colorectal cancer. *Cancer Res.*, **58**, 5248–57.

Bolger, G.B., Stamberg, J., Kirsch, I.L. et al. (1985). Chromosome translocation t(14;22) and oncogene (c-sis) variant in a pedigree with familial meningioma. *New Engl. J. Med.*, **312**, 564–7.

Bolino, A., Schuffenecker, I., Luo, Y., et al. (1995). *RET* mutations in exons 13 and 14 of FMTC patients. *Oncogene*, **10**, 2415–9.

Bongarzone, I., Monzini, N., Borrello, M.G., et al. (1993). Molecular characterisation of a thyroid tumor-specific transforming sequence formed by the fusion of *ret* tyrosine kinase and the regulatory subunit RI of cyclic AMP-dependent protein kinase A. *Mol. Cell Biol.*, **13**, 358–66.

Bongarzone, I., Butti, M.G., Coronelli, S. et al. (1994). Frequent activation of the *ret* protooncogene by fusion with a new activating gene in papillary thyroid carcinomas. *Cancer Res.*, **54**, 2979–85.

Bonifas, J.M., Rothman, A.L., Epstein, E.H. et al. (1991). Epidermolysis bullosa simplex: evidence in two families for keratin gene abnormalities. *Science*, **254**, 1202–5.

Boocock, G.R.B., Morrison, J.A., Popovic, M., Richards, N., Ellis, L., Durie, P.R. & Rommens, J.M. (2003). Mutations in SBDS are associated with Shwachman–Diamond syndrome. *Nat. Genet.*, **33**, 97–101.

Borg, A., Sandberg, T., Nilsson, K. et al. (2000). High frequency of multiple melanomas and breast and pancreas carcinomas in CDKN2A mutation-positive melanoma families. *J. Natl. Cancer Inst.*, **92**(15), 1260–6.

Borresen, A.L. (1992). Oncogenesis in ovarian cancer. [Review]. *Acta Obstetricia et Gynecologica Scandinavica*, Supplement **155**, 25–30.

Borresen, A.L., Andersen, T.I., Garber, J. et al. (1992). Screening for germline TP53 mutations in breast cancer patients. *Cancer Res.*, **52**, 3234–6.

Bougeard, G., Charbonnier, F., Moerman, A. et al. (2003). Early onset brain tumour and lymphoma in MSH2 deficient children. *Am. J. Hum. Genet.*, **72**, 213–6.

Boulikas, T. (1996). Xeroderma pigmentosum and molecular cloning of DNA repair genes. *Anticancer Res.*, **16**, 693–708.

Bourgeois, J.M. et al. (2001). Plexiform neurofibroma of the submandibular salivary gland in a child. *Can. J. Gastroenterol.*, **15**(12), 835–7.

Bourne, H.R. (1991). Consider the coiled coil. *Nature*, **351**, 188–90.

Box, N.F., Duffy, D.L., Chen, W., Stark, M., Martin, N.G., Sturm, R.A. & Hayward, N.K. (2001). MC1R genotype modifies risk of melanoma in families segregating CDKN2A mutations. *Am. J. Hum .Genet.*, **69**(4), 765–73.

Boyd, J., Sonoda, Y., Federici, M.G., Bogomolniy, F., Rhei, E., Maresco, D.L., Saigo, P.E., Almadrones, L.A., Barakat, R.R., Brown, C.L., Chi, D.S., Curtin, J.P., Poynor, E.A. & Hoskins, W.J. (2000). Clinicopathologic features of BRCA-linked and sporadic ovarian cancer. *J. Am. Med. Assoc.*, **283**, 2260–5.

Brandi, M., Gagel, R., Angeli, A. et al. (2001). Guidelines for diagnosis and therapy of MEN type 1 and type 2. *J. Clin. Endocrinol. Metab.*, **86**, 5658–71.

Brandi, M.L., Marx, S.J., Aurbach, G.D. & Fitzpatrick, L.A. (1987). Familial multiple endocrine neoplasia type 1. A new look at pathophysiology. *Endocrinol. Rev.*, **8**, 391–405.

Brassett, C., Joyce, J.A., Froggatt, N.J. et al. (1996). Microsatellite instability in early onset and familial colorectal cancer. *J. Med. Genet.*, **33**, 981–5.

Breast Cancer Linkage Consortium (1997). Pathology of familial breast cancer: differences between breast cancers in carriers of BRCA1 or BRCA2 mutations and sporadic cases. *Lancet*, **349**, 1505–10.

Breast Cancer Linkage Consortium (1999). Cancer risks in BRCA2 mutation carriers. *J. Natl. Cancer Inst.*, **91**(15), 1310–6.

Brekelmans, C.T., Seynaeve, C., Bartels, C.C., Tilanus-Linthorst, M.M., Meijers-Heijboer, E.J., Crepin, C.M., van Geel, A.A., Menke, M., Verhoog, L.C., van den, O.A., Obdeijn, I.M., & Klijn, J.G. (2001). Effectiveness of breast cancer surveillance in BRCA1/2 gene mutation carriers and women with high familial risk. *J. Clin. Oncol.* **19**, 924–30.

Brenner, S.H. & Wallach, R.C. (1983). Familial benign cystic teratoma. *Int. J. Gynaecol. Obstet.*, **21**, 167–9.

Brentnall, T.A., Bronner, M.P., Byrd, D.R., Haggitt, R.C. & Kimmey, M.B. (1999). Early diagnosis and treatment of pancreatic dysplasia in patients with a family history of pancreatic cancer. *Ann. Int. Med.*, **131**, 247–55.

Breslow, N.E. & Beckwith, J.B. (1982). Epidemiological features of Wilms' tumor: results of the national Wilms' tumor study. *J. Natl. Cancer Inst.*, **68**, 429–36.

Breslow, N.E., Olson, J., Moksness, J., Beckwith, J.B. & Grundy, P. (1996). Familial Wilms' tumor: a descriptive study. *Med. Pediatr. Oncol.*, **27**, 398–403.

Breslow, N.E. et al. (2000). Renal failure in the Denys-Drash and Wilms' tumor-aniridia syndromes. *Cancer Res.*, **60**(15), 4030–2.

Brind, A.M. & Bassendine, M.F. (1990). Molecular genetics of chronic liver disease. *Baillières Clin. Gastroenterol.*, **4**, 233–53.

Broca, P.P. (1866). *Traité des Tumeurs* 1. Paris: P. Asselin, p. 80.

Brodeur, G.M. (1990). Neuroblastoma: clinical significance of genetic abnormalities. *Cancer Surv.*, **9**, 673–88.

Brodeur, G.M. & Fong, C.T. (1989). Molecular biology and genetics of human neuroblastoma. *Cancer Genet. Cytogenet.*, **41**, 153–74.

Brody, L.C. (2005). Treating cancer by targeting a weakness. *New Engl. J. Med.*, **353**(9), 949–50.

Brook-Carter, P.T., Peral, B., Ward, C.J., Thompson, P., Hughes, J., Maheshwar, M.M., Nellist, M., Gamble, V., Harris, P.C. & Sampson, J.R. (1994). Deletion of the TSC2 and PKD1 genes associated with severe infantile polycystic kidney disease – a contiguous gene syndrome. *Nat. Genet.*, **8**, 328–32.

Brooks-Wilson, A.R., Kaurah, P., Suriano, G. et al. (2004). Germline E-cadherin mutations in hereditary diffuse gastric cancer: assessment of 42 new families and review of genetic screening criteria. *J. Med. Genet.*, **41**(7), 508–17.

Brown, G.C. & Shields, J.A. (1985). Tumors of the optic nerve head. *Surv. Ophthalmol.*, **29**, 239–64.

Brummelkamp, T.R., Nijman, S.M.B., Dirac, A.M.G. & Bernards, R. (2003). Loss of the cylindromatosis tumour suppressor inhibits apoptosis by activating NF-kB. *Nat.*, **424**, 797–801.

Brzustowicz, L.M., Farrell, S., Khan, M.B. & Weksberg, R. (1999). Mapping of a new SGBS locus to chromosome Xp22 in a family with a severe form of Simpson-Golabi-Behmel syndrome. *Am. J. Hum. Genet.* **65**, 779–83.

Bubb, V.J., Curtis, L.J., Cunningham, C., Dunlop, M.G., Carothers, A.D., Morris, R.G., White, S., Bird, C.C. & Wyllie, A.H. (1996). Microsatellite instability and the role of hMSH2 in sporadic colorectalcancer. *Oncogene*, **12**(12), 2641–9.

Buckley, R.H. (2004a). The multiple causes of human SCID. *J. Clin. Invest.* **114**, 1409–11.

Buckley, R.H. (2004b). Molecular defects in human severe combined immunodeficiency and approaches to immune reconstitution. *Annu. Rev. Immunol.*, **22**, 625–55.

Buhler, E.M. & Malik, N.J. (1984). The tricho-rhino-phalangeal syndrome(s); chromosome 8 long arm deletion; is there a shortest region of overlap between reported cases? TRPI and TRPII syndromes; are they separate entities? [Editorial]. *Am. J. Med Genet.*, **19**, 113–19.

Buhler, E.M., Buhler, U.K., Beutler, C. et al. (1987). A final word on the tricho-rhino-phalangeal syndrome. *Clin. Genet.*, **31**, 273–5.

Buller, R.E., Skilling, J.S., Kaliszewski, S., Niemann, T. & Anderson, B. (1995). Absence of significant germ line p53 mutations in ovarian cancer patients. *Gynecol. Oncol.* **58**, 368–74.

Bulow, S. (1984). The risk of developing cancer after colectomy and ileorectal anastomosis in Danish patients with polyposis coli. *Dis. Colon Rectum*, **27**, 726–9.

Bunyan, D.J., Shea-Simmonds, J., Reck, A.C. et al. (1995). Genotype/phenotype correlations of new causative APC gene mutations in patients with familial adenomatous polyposis. *J. Med. Genet.*, **32**, 728–31.

Burch, J.D, Craib, K.J.P, Choi, B.C.K, Miller, A.B., Risch, H.A. & Howe, G.R. (1987). An exploratory case–control study of brain tumors in adults. *J. Natl. Cancer Inst.*, **78**, 601–9.

Burgess, J.R., Harle, R.A., Tucker, P. et al. (1996a). Adrenal lesions in a large kindred with multiple endocrine neoplasia type 1. *Arch. Surg.*, **131**, 699–702.

Burgess, J.R., Shepherd, J.J., Parameswaran, V., Hoffman, L. & Greenaway, T.M. (1996b). Spectrum of pituitary disease in multiple endocrine neoplasia type 1 (MEN 1): clinical, biochemical, and radiological features of pituitary disease in a large MEN 1 kindred. *J. Clin. Endocrinol. Metab.*, **81**, 2642–6.

Burke, E., Li, F., Janov, A.J. et al. (1991). Cancer in relatives of survivors of childhood sarcoma. *Cancer*, **67**, 1467–9.

Burke, W., Daly, M., Garber, J., Botkin, J., Kahn, M.J., Lynch, P., McTiernan, A., Offit, K., Perlman, J., Petersen, G., Thomson, E. & Varricchio, C. (1997). Recommendations for follow-up care of individuals with an inherited predisposition to cancer. II. BRCA1 and BRCA2. Cancer Genetics Studies Consortium. *J. Am. Med. Assoc.*, **277**, 997–1003.

Burki, N., Gencik, A., Torhost, J.K.H. et al. (1987). Familial and histological analyses of 138 breast cancer patients. *Breast Cancer Res. Treat.*, **10**, 159–67.

Burkland, C.E. & Juzek, R.H. (1966). Familial occurrence of carcinoma of the ureter. *J. Urol.*, **96**, 697–701.

Burn, J., Chapman, P., Delhanty, J. et al. (1991). The UK northern region genetic register for familial adenomatous polyposis coli: use of age of onset, CHRPE and DNA markers in risk calculations. *J. Med. Genet.*, **28**, 289–96.

Burt, R.D., Vaughan, T.L., McKnight, B. et al. (1996). Associations between human leukocyte antigen type and nasopharyngeal carcinoma in Caucasians in the United States. *Cancer Epidemiol. Biomark. Prev.*, **5**, 879–87.

Burt, R.W., Berenson, M.M., Lee, R.G. et al. (1994). Upper gastrointestinal polyps in Gardner's syndrome. *Gastroenterology*, **86**, 295–301.

Bussey, H.J.R., Veale, A.M.O. & Morson, B.C. (1978). Genetics of gastrointestional polyposis. *Gastroenterology*, **74**, 1325–30.

Bussey, H.U.F. (1975). *Familial Polyposis Coli: Family Studies, Histopathology, Differential Diagnosis and Results of Treatment*. Johns Hopkins University Press, Baltimore.

Buzzi, F., Badolato, R., Mazza, C., et al. (2003). Autoimmune polyendocrinopathy C-ED syndrome; time to review diagnostic criteria. *J. Clin. Endo. Metab.*, **88**, 3146–8.

Cahill, D.P., Lengauer, C., Yu, J., Riggins, G.J., Willson, J.K., Markowitz, S.D., Kinzler, K.W. & Vogelstein, B. (1998). Mutations of mitotic checkpoint genes in human cancers. *Nature*, **392**(6673), 300–3.

Cairney, A.E.L., Andrews, M., Greenberg, M., Smith, D. & Weksberg, R. (1987). Wilms' tumour in three patients with Bloom syndrome. *J. Pediatr.*, **111**, 414–16.

Caldas, C., Carneiro, F., Lynch, H.T. et al. (1999). Familial gastric cancer: overview and guidelines for management. *J. Med. Genet.*, **36**, 873–80.

Calin, G., Herlea, V., Barbanti-Brodano, G. & Negrini, M. (1998). The coding region of the Bloom syndrome BLM gene and of the CBL proto-oncogene is mutated in genetically unstable sporadic gastrointestinal tumors. *Cancer Res.*, **58**(17), 3777–81.

Calin, G.A., Gafa, R., Tibiletti, M.G., Herlea, V., Becheanu, G., Cavazzini, L., Barbanti-Brodano, G., Nenci, I., Negrini, M. & Lanza, G. (2000). Genetic progression in microsatellite instability high (MSI-H) colon cancers correlates with clinico-pathological parameters: a study of the TGRbetaRII, BAX, hMSH3, hMSH6, IGFIIR and BLM genes. *Int. J. Cancer*, **89**(3), 230–5.

Callebaut, I. & Mornon, J.P. (1997). From BRCA1 to RAP1: a widespread BRCT module closely associated with DNA repair. *FEBS Lett.*, **400**, 25–30.

Campbell, S., Bhan, V., Royston, P., Whitehead, M.I. & Collins, W.P. (1989). Transabdominal ultrasound screening for early ovarian cancer. *Br. Med. J.*, **299**, 1363–7.

Canning, C.R. & Hungerford, J. (1988). Familial uveal melanoma. *Br. J. Ophthalmol.*, **72**, 241–3.

Cannon, L., Bishop, D.T., Skolnick, M., Hunt, S., Lyon, J.L. & Smart, C.R. (1982). Genetic epidemiology of prostate cancer in the Utah Mormon genealogy. *Cancer Surv.*, **1**, 47–69.

Cannon-Albright, L., Goldgar, D., Meyer, L. et al. (1992). Assignment of a locus for familial melanoma MLM, to chromosome 9P13–22. *Science*, **258**, 1148–52.

Cannon-Albright, L.A., Goldgar, D.E., Wright, E.C. et al. (1990). Evidence against the reported linkage of the cutaneous melanoma-dysplastic nevus syndrome locus to chromosome 1p36. *Am. J. Hum. Genet.*, **46**, 912–18.

Cantor, S.B., Bell, D.W., Ganesan, S., Kass, E.M., Drapkin, R., Grossman, S., Wahrer, D.C., Sgroi, D.C., Lane, W.S., Haber, D.A. & Livingston, D.M. (2001). BACH1, a novel helicase-like protein, interacts directly with BRCA1 and contributes to its DNA repair function. *Cell*, **105**, 149–60.

Carbano, M., Rizzo, P., Powers, A. et al. (2002). Molecular analyses, morphology and immuno-histochemistry together differentiate pleural synovial sarcomas from mesotheliomas: clinical implications. *Anticancer Res.*, **22**(6B), 3443–8.

Carcangiu, M.L., Radice, P., Manoukian, S., Spatti, G., Gobbo, M., Pensotti, V., Crucianelli, R. & Pasini, B. (2004). Atypical epithelial proliferation in fallopian tubes in prophylactic salpingo-oophorectomy specimens from BRCA1 and BRCA2 germline mutation carriers. *Int. J. Gynecol. Pathol.*, **23**, 35–40.

Carlson, J.A., Ambros, R., Malfetano. J. et al. (1998). Vulvar lichen sclerosis and squamous cell carcinoma: a cohort , case control, and investigational study with historical perpective; implications for chronic inflammation and sclerosis in the development of neoplasia. *Hum. Pathol.*, **29**, 932–48.

Carney, J.A. (1995). Carney complex; the complex of myxomas, spotty pigmentation. Endocrine overactivity and schwannomas. *Semin. Dermatol.*, **14**, 90–8.

Carney, J.A. (1999). Gastric stromal sarcoma, pulmonary chondroma and extra-adrenal para-ganglioma (Carney Triad): natural history, adrenocortoical component and possible familial occurrence. *Mayo Clin. Proc.*, **74**, 543–52.

Carney, J.A., Go, V.L., Sizemore, G.W. & Hayles, A.B. (1976). Alimentary-tract gan-glioneuromatosis. A major component of the syndrome of multiple endocrine neoplasia, type 2b. *New Engl. J. Med.*, **295**, 1287–91.

Carney, J.A., Gordon, H., Carpenter, P.C., Shenoy, B.V. & Go, V.L. (1985). The complex of myxomas, spotty pigmentation and endocrine overactivity. *Medicine*, **64**, 270–83.

Carney, J.A., Hruska, L.S., Beauchamp, G.D. & Gordon, H. (1986). Dominant inheritance of the complex of myxomas, spotty pigmentation and endocrine overactivity. *Mayo Clin. Proc.*, **61**, 165–72.

Carpten, J.D., Robbins, C.M., Villablanca, A. *et al.* (2002). HRPT 2, encoding parafibromin is mutated in hyperparathyroidism – Jaw tumor syndrome. *Nat. Genetics*, **32**, 676–80.

Carrucci, J.A. (2004). Squamous cell carcinoma in organ transplant recipients; approach to management. *Skin Therapy*, Lett **9**, 5–7.

Carter, C.L., Corle, D.K. & Micozzi, M.S. (1988). A prospective study of the development of breast cancer in 16,692 women with benign breast disease. *Am. J. Epidemiol.*, **128**, 467–77.

Carter, C.L., Hu, N., Wu, M., Lin, P.Z., Murigande, C. & Bonney, G.E. (1992). Segregation analysis of esophageal cancer in 221 high-risk Chinese families. *J. Natl. Cancer Inst*, **84**, 771–6.

Cartpten, J.D. et al. (2002). HRPT2, encoding parafibromin, is mutated in hyperparathyroidism-jaw tumor syndrome. *Nat. Genet.*, **32**(4), 676–80.

Cartwright, R.A., Bernard, S.M., Bird, C.C. et al. (1987). Chronic lymphocytic leukaemia: case–control epidemiological study in Yorkshire. *Br. J. Cancer*, **56**, 79–82.

Cartwright, R.A., McKinney, P.A., O'Brien, C. et al. (1988). Non-Hodgkin's lymphoma: case–control epidemiological study in Yorkshire. *Leuk. Res.*, **12**, 81–8.

Casagrande, J.T., Louie, E.W., Pike, M.C., Roy, S., Ross, R.K. & Henderson, B.E. (1979). "Incessant ovulation" and ovarian cancer. *Lancet*, **2**, 170–3.

Cavanee, W.K. (1991). The Beckwith-Wiedemann syndrome: lessons for developmental oncology. In *Hereditary Tumors*, eds. Brandi, M.L. & White, R. Raven Press, New York.

Cave-Riant, F. Benier, C., Labange, P. et al. (2002). Spectrum and expression analysis of KRIT1 mutations in 121 consecutive and unrelated patients with cerebral cavernous malformations. *Eur. J. Hum. Genet.*, **10**, 733–40.

Cawthon, R.M., Weiss, R., Xu, G. et al. (1990). A major segment of the neurofibromatosis type 1 gene: cDNA sequence, genomic structure and point mutations. *Cell*, **62**, 193–201.

Cetiner, M., Adiguzel, C., Argon, D., Ratip, S., Eksioglu-Demiralp, E., Tecimer, T. & Bayik, M. (2003). Hairy cell leukemia in father and son. *Med. Oncol.*, **20**(4), 375–8.

Chak, A., Lee, T., Kinnard, M.F., Brock, W., Faulx, A., Willis, J., Cooper, G.S., Sivak Jr, M.V. & Goddard, K.A. (2002). Familial aggregation of Barrett's oesophagus, oesophageal adenocarcinoma, and oesophagogastric junctional adenocarcinoma in Caucasian adults. *Gut*, **51**, 323–8.

Chakravarti, A., Halloran, S.L., Bale, S.J. & Tucker, M.A. (1986). Etiological heterogeneity in Hodgkin's disease: HLA linked and unlinked determinants of susceptibility independent of histological concordance. *Genet. Epidemiol.*, **3**, 407–15.

Chan, E.F., Gat, U., McNoff, J.M. & Fuchs, E. (1999). A common human skin tumour is caused by activating mutation in beta catenin. *Nat. Genet.*, **21**, 410–13.

Chandrasekharappa, S.C., Guru, S.C., Manickam, P. et al. (1997). Positional cloning of the gene for multiple endocrine neoplasia type 1 (MEN 1) gene. *Science*, **276**, 404–7.

Chang, H., Tunq, R.C., Schlesinger, T., et al. (2001). Familial cutaneous mastocytosis. *Paed. Dermatol.*, **18**(4), 271–6.

Chang, S. & Prados, M.G. (1994). Identical twins with Ollier's disease and intracranial gliomas: case report. *Neurosurgery*, **34**, 903–6.

Chappuis, P.O., Rosenblatt, J. & Foulkes, W.D. (1999). The influence of familial and hereditary factors on the prognosis of breast cancer. *Ann. Oncol.*, **10**, 1163–70.

Chappuis, P.O., Nethercot, V. & Foulkes. W.D. (2000). Clinico-pathological characteristics of *BRCA1*- and *BRCA2*-related breast cancer. *Semin. Surg. Oncol.*, **18**, 287–95.

Charbonnier, F., Olschwang, S., Wang, Q., Boisson, C., Martin, C., Buisine, M.P., Puisieux, A. & Frebourg, T. (2002). MSH2 in contrast to MLH1 and MSH6 is frequently inactivated by exonic and promoter rearrangements in hereditary nonpolyposis colorectal cancer. *Cancer Res.*, **62**, 848–53.

Chen, C., Cook, L.S., Li, X.Y. et al. (1999). CYP2D6 genotype and the incidence of anal and vulvar cancer. *Cancer Epidemiol. Biomark. Prev.*, **8**, 839–40.

Chen, J.D., Morrison, C.D., Zhang, C., Kahnoski, K., Carpten, J.D. & Teh, B.T. (2003). Hyperparathyroidism-jaw tumour syndrome. *J. Int. Med.*, **253**, 634–42.

Chen, L., Lee, L., Kudlow, B.A., et al. (2003). LMNA mutations in atypical Werner's syndrome. *Lancet*, **362** (9382), 440–5.

Chenevix-Trench, G., Spurdle, A.B., Gatei, M., Kelly, H., Marsh, A., Chen, X., Donn, K., Cummings, M., Nyholt, D., Jenkins, M.A., Scott, C., Pupo, G.M., Dork, T., Bendix, R., Kirk, J., Tucker, K., McCredie, M.R., Hopper, J.L., Sambrook, J., Mann, G.J. & Khanna, K.K. (2002). Dominant negative ATM mutations in breast cancer families. *J. Natl. Cancer Inst.*, **94**, 205–15.

Chitayat, D., Friedman, J.M. & Dimmick, J.E. (1990). Neuroblastoma in a child with Wiedemann–Beckwith syndrome. *Am. J. Med. Genet.*, **35**, 433–6.

Choi, N.W., Schuman, I.M. & Gullen, W.H. (1970). Epidemiology of primary central nervous system neoplasmas. II. Case–control study. *Am. J. Epidemiol.*, **91**, 467–85.

Christian, J.E. & Ballon, S.C. (1990). Ovarian fibrosarcoma associated with Maffucci's syndrome. *Gynaecol. Oncol.*, **37**, 290–1.

Chu, G. & Mayne, L. (1996). Xeroderma pigmentosum, Cockayne syndrome and trichothiodystrophy: do the genes explain the disease? *Trend. Genet.*, **12**, 187–92.

Cirillo Silengo, M., Dan, G.F., Bianco, M.C. et al. (1982). Distinctive hair changes (pili torti) in Rapp Hodgkin ectodermal dyslasia syndrome. *Clin. Genet.*, **21**, 297–300.

Clark, A.J., Barnetson, S.M., Farrington, S.M. & Dunlop, M.G. (2004) Prognosis I DNA mismatch repair defiecient colorectal cancer: are all MSI tumours equivalent? *Fam. Cancer*, **3**, 85–91.

Clark, R.D. & Hutter, J.J. (1982). Familial neurofibromatosis and juvenile chronic myelogenous leukemia. *Hum. Genet.*, **60**, 230–2.

Clarke, J., Loffreda, M. & Helm, K.F. (2002). Multiple familial trichoepitheliomas: a folliculosebaceous-apocrine genodermatosis. *Am. J. Dermopath.*, **24**, 402–5.

Claus, E., Risch, N. & Thompson, W.D. (1994). Autosomal dominant inheritance of early-onset breast cancer. Implications for risk prediction. *Cancer*, **73**, 643–51.

Claus, E.B., Risch, N.J. & Thompson, W.D. (1991). Genetic analysis of breast cancer in the Cancer and Steroid Hormone Study. *Am. J. Hum. Genet.*, **48**, 232–42.

Cloos, J., Leemans, C.R., van der Sterre, M.L., Kuik, D.J., Snow, G.B. & Braakhuis, B.J. (2000). Mutagen sensitivity as a biomarker for second primary tumors after head and neck squamous cell carcinoma. *Cancer Epidemiol. Biomark. Prev.*, **9**, 713–17.

Coburn, M.C., Pricolo, V.E., DeLuca, F.G. & Bland, K.I. (1995). Malignant potential in intestinal juvenile polyposis syndromes. *Ann. Surg. Oncol.*, **2**, 386–91.

Coene, E., Van Oostveldt, P., Williams, K. et al. (1997). BRCA1 is localised in cytoplasmic tube-like invaginations in the nucleus. *Nat. Genet.*, **16**, 122–4.

Cohen, A.J., Li, F.P., Berg, S. et al. (1979). Hereditary renal cell carcinoma associated with a chromosomal translocation. *New Engl. J. Med.*, **301**, 592–5.

Cohen, M.M. (1989). A comprehensive and critical assessment of overgrowth and overgrowth syndromes. *Adv. Hum. Genet.*, **18**(4), 181–304.

Cohen, M.M. & Levy, H.P. (1989). Chromosome instability syndromes. *Adv. Hum. Genet.*, **18**, 43–150.

Cohen, P.R., Kohn, S.R. & Kurzrock, R. (1991). Association of sebaceous gland tumours and internal malignancy: the Muir–Torre syndrome. *Am. J. Med.*, **90**, 606–13.

Colditz, G.A., Hankinson, S.E., Hunter, D.J. et al. (1995). The use of oestrogens and protestins and the risk of breast cancer in postmenopausal women. *New Engl. J. Med.*, **332**, 1589–93.

Colditz, G.A., Rosner, B.A. & Speizer, F.E. (1996). Risk factors for breast cancer according to family history of breast cancer. *J. Natl. Cancer Inst.*, **88**, 365–71.

Coleman, R. & Hay, R.J. (1997). Chronic mucocutaneous candidiasis associated with hypothyroidism: a distinct syndrome? *Br. J. Dermatol.*, **136**, 24–9.

Colgan, T.J., Murphy, J., Cole, D.E., Narod, S. & Rosen, B. (2001). Occult carcinoma in prophylactic oophorectomy specimens: prevalence and association with BRCA germline mutation status. *Am. J. Surg. Pathol.*, **25**, 1283–9.

Collaborative Group on Hormonal factors in breast cancer (Beral, V., Bull, D., Doll, R. et al.) (2001). Familial breast cancer. Lancet, **358**(9291), 1389–99.

Collins, F.S. (1996). BRCA1 – lots of mutations, lots of dilemmas. *New Engl. J. Med.*, **334**, 186–8.

Collins, N., McManus, R., Wooster, R. et al. (1995). Consistent loss of the wild type allele in breast cancers from a family linked to BRCA2 gene on chromosome 13q12–13. *Oncogene*, **10**, 1673–5.

Colovic, M.D., Jankovic, G.M. & Wiernik, P.H. (2001). Hairy cell leukemia in first cousins and review of the literature. *Eur. J. Haematol.*, **67**(3), 185–8.

Comotti, B., Bassan, R., Buzzeti, M., Finazzi, G. & Barbui, T. (1987). Multiple myeloma in a pair of twins. *Br. J. Haematol.*, **65**, 123–4.

Conley, C.L., Misiti, J. & Laster, A.J. (1980). Genetic factors predisposing to chronic lymphocytic leukemia and to autoimmune disease. *Medicine*, **59**, 323–34.

Connor, J.M., Gatherer, D., Gray, F.C. et al. (1986). Assignment of the gene for dyskeratosis congenita to Xq28. *Hum. Genet.*, **72**, 348–51.

Conte, R., Lauria, F. & Zucchelli, P. (1983). HLA in familial Hodgkin's disease. *J. Immunogenet.*, **10**, 251–5.

Cook, J.A., Oliver, K., Mueller, R.F. et al. (1996). A cross-sectional study of renal involvement in tuberous sclerosis. *J. Med. Genet.*, **33**, 480–4.

Cooper, W.N., Luharia, A., Evans, G.A. et al. (2005). Molecular subtypes and phenotypic expression of Beckwith–Wiedemann syndrome. *Eur. J. Hum. Genet.*, **13**, 1025–32.

Coppes, M.J., Huff, V. & Pelletier, J. (1993). Denys–Drash syndrome: relating a clinical disorder to genetic alterations in the tumour suppressor gene WT1. *J. Pediatr.*, **123**, 673–8.

Corbetta, S., Pizzocaro, A., Peracchi, M. et al. (1997). Multiple endocrine neoplasia type 1 in patients with recognized pituitary tumours of different types. *Clin. Endocrinol.*, **47**, 507–12.

Corden, L.D. & McLean, W.H. (1996). Human keratin diseases: hereditary fragility of specific epithelial tissues. *Exp. Dermatol.*, **5**, 297–307.

Corello, S.P., Smith, F.J., Sittevis-Smith, J.H. et al. (1998). Keratin muations cause either steatocystoma multiplex or pachonychia congenital type 2. *Br. J. Dermatol.*, **39**, 475–80.

Corrao, G., Corazza, G.R., Bagnardi, V., Brusco, G., Ciacci, C., Cottone, M., Sategna Guidetti, C., Usai, P., Cesari, P., Pelli, M.A., Loperfido, S., Volta, U., Calabro, A. & Certo, M. Club del Tenue Study Group (2001). Mortality in patients with coeliac disease and their relatives: a cohort study. *Lancet*, **358**(9279), 356–61.

Correa, P. & Shiao, Y.H. (1994). Phenotypic and genotypic events in gastric carcinogenesis. *Cancer Res.*, **54**, 1941s–3s.

Costa, O.L., Silva, D.M., Colnago, F.A., Vieira, M.S. & Musso, C.M. (1987). Turcot syndrome. Autosomal dominant or recessive transmission? *Dis. Colon Rectum.*, **30**, 391–4.

Cotton, J.L., Kavey, R.W., Palmier, C.E. et al. (1991). Cardiac tumours and the nevoid basal cell carcinoma syndrome. *Pediatrics*, **87**, 725–8.

Couch, F.J., Farid, L.M., DeShano, M.L. et al. (1996). BRCA2 germline mutations in male breast cancer cases and breast cancer families. *Nat. Genet.*, **13**, 123–5.

Couch, F.J., DeShano, M.L., Blackwood, M.A. et al. (1997). BRCA1 mutations in women attending clinics that evaluate the risk of breast cancer. *New Engl. J. Med.*, **336**, 1409–15.

Coulombe, P.A., Hutton, M.E., Letai, A. et al. (1991). Point mutations in human keratin 14 genes of epidermolysis bullosa simplex patients: genetic and functional analyses. *Cell*, **66**, 1301–11.

Courtois, G., Smahi, A., Reichenbach, J. et al. (2003). A hypermorphic 1 kappa B alpha mutation is associated with autosomal dominant anhydrotic ectodermal dysplasia and T cell immunodeficiency. *J. Clin. Invest.*, **112**, 1108–15.

Cowell, J.K., Bia, B. & Akoulitchev, A. (1996). A novel mutation in the promoter region in a family with a mild form of retinoblastoma indicates the location of a new regulatory domain for the RB1 gene. *Oncology*, **12**, 431–6.

Crabtree, M.D., Tomlinson, I.P., Hodgson, S.V. et al. (2002). Explaining variation in familial adenomatous polyposis: relationship between genotype and phenotype and evidence for modifier genes. *Gut*, **51**, 420–3.

Crabtree, M., Sieber, O.M., Lipton, L. et al. (2003). Refining the relation between "first hits" and "second hits" at the APC locus: the "loose fit" model and evidence for differences in somatic mutation spectra among patients. *Oncogene*, **22**, 4257–65.

Crabtree, M.D., Fletcher, C., Churchman, M. et al. (2004). Analysis of candidate modifier loci for the severity of colonic familial adenomatous polyposis, with evidence for the importance of the N-acetyltransferases. *Gut*, **53**, 271–6.

Craig, H.D., Gunel, M., Cepeda, O. et al. (1998). Multilocus linkage identifies two new loci for a mendelian form of stroke, cerebral cavernous malformation, at 7p15–13 and 3q25.2–27. *Hum. Mol. Genet.*, **7**(12), 1851–8.

Cramer, D.W., Hutchison, G.B., Welch, W.R., Scully, R.E. & Ryan, K.J. (1983). Determinants of ovarian cancer risk. I. Reproductive experiences and family history. *J. Natl. Cancer Inst.*, **71**, 711–16.

Creagen, E.T. & Fraumeni, J.F.J. (1973). Familial gastric cancer and immunologic abnormalities. *Cancer*, **32**, 1325–31.

Crist, W.M. & Kun, L.E. (1991). Common solid tumours of childhood. *New Engl. J. Med.*, **324**, 461–71.

Cristofaro, G., Lynch, H.T., Caruso, M.L. et al. (1987). New phenotypic aspects in a family with Lynch syndrome II. *Cancer*, **60**, 51–8.

Crockford, G.P., Linger, R., Hockley, S. et al. (2006). Genome-wide linkage screen for testicular germ cell tumour susceptibility loci. *Hum. Mol. Genet.*, **15**(3), 443–51.

Cuckle, H.S. & Wald, N.J. (1990). The evaluation of screening tests for ovarian cancer. In Ovarian Cancer: Biological and Therapeutic Challenges, eds. Sharp, F., Mason, P. & Leake, R.E. Chapman and Hall, London.

Cumin, I., Cohen, J.Y., David, A. et al. (1996). Rothmund–Thomson syndrome and osteosarcoma. *Med. Pediatr. Oncol.*, **26**, 414–16.

Cunliffe, I.A., Moffat, D., Hardy, D. & Moore, A.T. (1991). Bilateral optic sheath meningiomas in a patient with neurofibromatosis type 2. *Br. J. Ophthalmol.*, **76**, 310–12.

Cuzick, J., Harris, R. & Mortimer, P.S. (1984). Palmar keratoses and cancers of the bladder and lung. *Lancet*, **i**, 530–3.

Cybulski, C., Gorski, B., Debniak, T., Gliniewicz, B., Mierzejewski, M., Masojc, B., Jakubowska, A., Matyjasik, J., Zlowocka, E., Sikorski, A., Narod, S.A. & Lubinski, J. (2004). NBS1 is a prostate cancer susceptibility gene. *Cancer Res.*, **64**, 1215–19.

Daghistani, D., Toledano, S.R. & Curless, R. (1990). Monosomy 7 syndrome. *Cancer Genet. Cytogenet.*, **44**, 263–9.

Dahele, M.R. et al. (2004). A patient with Rothmund–Thomson syndrome and tongue cancer – experience of radiation toxicity. *Clin. Oncol. (R. Coll. Radiol.)*, **16**(5), 371–2.

Daling, J.R., Madeleine, M.M., Schwartz, S.M. et al. (2002). A population based study of squamous cell vaginal cancer: HPV and cofactors. *Gynaecol. Oncol.*, **84**, 263–70.

Daniel, E.S., Ludvig, S.L., Levin, K.J., Ruprecht, R.M., Rajachich, G.M. & Schwabwe, A.D. (1982). The Cronkhite Canada syndrome. An analysis of clinical and pathologic features and therapy in 55 cases. *Medicine*, **61**, 293–309.

Dasouki, M.J., Ishmael, H. & Eng, C. (2001). Macrocephaly, macrosomia and autistic behavior due to a *de novo PTEN* germline mutation. *Am. J. Hum. Genet.*, **69S**, 280 [Abstract 564].

Davidson, H.R. & Connor, J.M. (1988). Dyskeratosis congenita. *J. Med. Genet.*, **25**, 843–6.

Davies, H., Bignell, G.R., Cox, C., Stephens, P., Edkins, S., Clegg, S., Teague, J., Woffendin, H., Garnett, M.J., Bottomley, W., Davis, N., Dicks, E., Ewing, R., Floyd, Y., Gray, K., Hall, S., Hawes, R., Hughes, J., Kosmidou, V., Menzies, A., Mould, C., Parker, A., Stevens, C., Watt, S., Hooper, S., Wilson, R., Jayatilake, H., Gusterson, B.A., Cooper, C., Shipley, J., Hargrave, D., Pritchard-Jones, K., Maitland, N., Chenevix-Trench, G., Riggins, G.J., Bigner, D.D., Palmieri, G., Cossu, A., Flanagan, A., Nicholson, A., Ho, J.W., Leung, S.Y., Yuen, S.T., Weber, B.L., Seigler, H.F., Darrow, T.L., Paterson, H., Marais, R., Marshall, C.J., Wooster, R., Stratton, M.R. & Futreal, P.A. (2002). Mutations of the BRAF gene in human cancer. *Nature*, **417**, 949–54.

Davies, H.D., Leusink, G.L., McConnell, A., Deyell, M., Cassidy, S.B., Fick, G.H. & Coppes, M.J. (2003). Myeloid leukemia in Prader–Willi syndrome. *J. Pediatr.*, **142**, 174–8.

De Andrade, D.O., Dravet, C., Rayboud, C. et al. (2004). An unusual case of neurocutaneous melanosis. *Epileptic Dis.*, **6**, 145–52.

De la Chapelle, A. (2004). Genetic predisposition to colorectal cancer. *Nat. Rev. Cancer*, **4**, 769–80.

De la Torre, C., Pincheria, J., Lopez-Saez, J.F. et al. (2003). Human syndromes with genomic instability and multiprotein machines that repair DNA double-strand breaks. *Histol. histopathol.*, **18**, 225–43.

De Moor, P., Boogaerts, M. & Louwagie, A. (1988). More familial leukaemia in patients with both unexplained high transcortin levels and an HLA antigen Cw3. *Br. J. Haematol.*, **69**, 225–7.

De Pietri, S., Sassatelli, R., Roncucci, L. et al. (1995). Clinical and biological features of adenomatosis coli in northern Italy. *Scand. J. Gastroenterol.*, **30**, 771–9.

De Pina Neto, J.M., de Souza, N.V., Velludo, M.A. et al. (1998). Retinal changes and tumourigenesis in ramon syndrome: follow-up of a Brazilian family. *Am. J. Med. Genet.*, **77**, 43–6.

De Raedt, T., Brems, H., Wolkenstein, P., Vidaud, D., Pilotti, S., Perrone, F., Mautner, V., Frahm, S., Sciot, R. & Legius, E. (2003). Elevated risk for MPNST in NF1 microdeletion patients. *Am. J. Hum. Genet.*, **72**, 1288–92.

De Rosa, M., Fasano, C., Panariello, L. et al. (2000). Evidence for a recessive inheritance of Turcot's syndrome caused by compound heterozygous mutations within the PMS2 gene. *Oncogene*, **19**, 1719–23.

de Snoo, F.A., Bergman, W. & Gruis, N.A. (2003). Familial melanoma: a complex disorder leading to controversy on DNA testing. *Fam. Cancer*, **2**(2), 109–16.

De Vos, M., Hayward, B.E., Picton, S., Sheridan, E. & Bonthron, D.T. (2004). Novel PMS2 pseudogenes can conceal recessive mutations causing a distinctive childhood cancer syndrome. *Am. J. Hum. Genet.*, **74**(5), 954–64.

de Vos tot Nederveen Cappel, W.H., Offerhaus, G.J., van Puijenbroek, M., Caspers, E., Gruis, N.A., De Snoo, F.A., Lamers, C.B., Griffioen, G., Bergman, W., Vasen, H.F. & Morreau, H. (2003). Pancreatic carcinoma in carriers of a specific 19 base pair deletion of CDKN2A/p16 (p16-leiden). *Clin. Cancer Res.*, **9**(10 Pt 1), 3598–605.

DeBauche, D.M., Pai, G.S. & Stanley, W.S. (1988). Hypersensitivity to X-irradiation-induced G2 chromatid damage in dyskeratosis congenita. *Am. J. Hum. Genet.*, Suppl 43, A22.

DeBaun, M.R. (2002). Screening for cancer in children with Costello syndrome. *Am. J. Med. Genet.*, **108**, 88–90.

DeBaun, M.R., Niemitz, E.L., McNeil, D.E., Brandenburg, S.A., Lee, M.P. & Feinberg, A.P. (2002). Epigenetic alterations of H19 and LIT1 distinguish patients with Beckwith–Wiedemann syndrome with cancer and birth defects. *Am. J. Hum. Genet.*, **70**, 604–11.

DeBaun, M.R., Niemitz, E.L. & Feinberg, A.P. (2003). Association of in vitro fertilization with Beckwith–Wiedemann syndrome and epigenetic alterations of LIT1 and H19. *Am. J. Hum. Genet.*, **72**, 156–60.

Debinski, H.S., Spigelman, A.D., Hatfield, A. et al. (1995) Upper Intestinal surveillance in FAP, *Eur. J. Cancer*, **31A**(7–8), 1149–53.

Decker, R.A., Peacock, M.L., Borst, M.J., Sweet, J.D. & Thompson, N.W. (1995). Progress in genetic screening of multiple endocrine neoplasia type 2A: is calcitonin testing obsolete? *Surgery*, **118**, 257–64.

Delahunt, B. & Eble, J.N. (1997). Papillary renal cell carcinoma: a clinicopathologic and immunohistochemical study of 105 tumors. *Mod. Pathol.*, **10**(6), 537–44.

Delaporte, E., N'guyen-Mailfer, C., Janin, A. et al. (1995). Keratoderma with scleroatrophy of the extremities or sclerotylosis (Huriez syndrome): a reappraisal. *Br. J. Dermatol.*, **133**, 409–16.

deLeeuw, B., Balemans, M., Weghuis, D.O.O. et al. (1994). Molecular cloning of the synovial sarcoma-specific molecular translocation (X:18)(p.11.2:q11.2) breakpoint. *Hum. Mol. Genet.*, **3**, 745–9.

Deligdisch, L., Gil, J., Kerner, H., Wu, H.S., Beck, D. & Gershoni-Baruch, R. (1999). Ovarian dysplasia in prophylactic oophorectomy specimens: cytogenetic and morphometric correlations. *Cancer*, **86**, 1544–50.

Della Torre, G., Pasini, B., Frigerio, S. et al. (2001). CDKN2A and CDK4 mutation analysis in Italian melanoma-prone families: functional characterization of a novel CDKN2A germ line mutation. *Br. J. Cancer*, **85**(6), 836–44.

Delleman, J., De Jong, J.G.Y. & Bleeker, G.M. (1978). Meningiomas in five members of a family over two generations, in one member simultaneously with acoustic neurinomas. *Neurology*, **28**, 567–70.

Department of Health (1995). *Calman the Hine Report: A Policy for Commissioning Cancer Services.* Report of the Expert Advisory Group on Cancer. London, UK.

Department of Health (1999). *A Policy Framework for Commissioning Cancer Services.* Report of the Expert Advisory Group on Cancer. England and Wales, UK.

Der Kaloustian, V.M., McGill, J.J., Vekemans, M. & Kopelman, H.R. (1990). Clonal lines of aneuploid cells in Rothmund–Thomson syndrome. *Am. J. Med. Genet.*, **37**, 336–9.

Derenoncourt, A.N., Castro Magana, M. & Jones, K.L. (1995). Mediastinal teratoma and precocious puberty in a boy with mosaic Klinefelter syndrome. *Am. J. Med. Genet.*, **55**, 38–42.

Derry, J.M., Ochs, H.D. & Francke, U. (1994). Isolation of a novel gene mutated in Wiskott–Aldrich syndrome. *Cell*, **75**, 635–4.

DeVivo, I., Gertig, D., Nagase, S. et al. (2000). Novel germline mutations in the *PTEN* tumour suppressor gene found in women with multiple cancers. *J. Med. Genet.*, **37**, 336–41.

Devor, E.J. & Buechley, P.W. (1979). Gallbladder cancer in Hispanic New Mexicans. II. Familial occurrence in two northern New Mexico kindreds. *Cancer Cell Cytogenet.*, **1**, 139–45.

Dhillon, P.K., Farrow, D.C., Vaughan, T.L., Chow, W.H., Risch, H.A., Gammon, M.D., Mayne, S.T., Stanford, J.L., Schoenberg, J.B., Ahsan. H., Dubrow, R., West, A.B., Rotterdam, H., Blot, W.J. & Fraumeni Jr, J.F. (2001). Family history of cancer and risk of esophageal and gastric cancers in the United States. *Int. J. Cancer*, **93**, 148–52.

DiFiore, F., Charbonnier, F., Martin, C. et al. (2004). Screening for genomic rearrangements of the MMR genes must be included in the routine diagnosis of HNPCC. *J. Med. Genet.*, **41**, 18–20.

DiGiovanna, J.J. & Safai, S. (1981). Kaposi's sarcoma. *Am. J. Med.*, **71**, 779–83.

Diller, L., Sexsmith, E., Gottlieb, A. et al. (1995). Germline p53 mutations are frequently detected in young children with rhabdomyosarcoma. *J. Clin. Invest.*, **95**, 1606–11.

Distante, S., Nasoulias, S., Somers, G.R. et al. (1996). Familial adenomatous polyposis in a 5 year old child: a clinical pathological and molecular genetic study. *J. Med. Genet.*, **33**, 157–60.

Dobru, D., Seuchea, N., Dorin, M. & Careinau, V. (2004). Blue Rubber Bleb syndrome: a case report and literature review. *Rom. J. Gastro.*, **13**, 237–40.

Domingo, E., Laiho, P., Ollikainen, M., Pinto, M., Wang, L., French, A.J., Westra, J., Frebourg, T., Espin, E., Armengol, M., Hamelin, R., Yamamoto, H., Hofstra, R.M., Seruca, R., Lindblom, A., Peltomaki, P., Thibodeau, S.N., Aaltonen, L.A. & Schwartz Jr, S. (2004). BRAF screening as a low-cost effective strategy for simplifying HNPCC genetic testing. *J. Med. Genet.*, **41**, 664–8.

Domizio, P., Talbot, I.C., Spigelman, A.D. et al. (1990). Upper gastrointestinal pathology in familial adenomatous polyposis: results from a prospective study of 102 patients. *J. Clin. Pathol.*, **43**, 738–43.

Dong, C., Lonnstedt, I. & Hemminki, K. (2001). Familial testicular cancer and second primary cancers in testicular cancer patients by histological type. *Eur. J. Cancer*, **37**, 1878–85.

Dong, S.M., Traverso, G., Johnson, C., Geng, L., Favis, R., Boynton, K., Hibi, K., Goodman, S.N., D'Allessio, M., Paty, P., Hamilton, S.R., Sidransky, D., Barany. F., Levin, B., Shuber, A., Kinzler, K.W., Vogelstein, B. & Jen, J. (2001). Detecting colorectal cancer in stool with the use of multiple genetic targets. *J. Natl. Cancer Inst.*, **93**, 858–65.

Dorum, A., Moller, P., Kamsteeg, E.J., Scheffer, H., Burton, M., Heimdal, K.R., Maehle, L.O., Hovig, E., Trope, C.G., van der Hout, A.H., van der Meulen, M.A., Buys, C.H. & te, M.G. (1997). A BRCA1 founder mutation, identified with haplotype analysis, allowing genotype/phenotype determination and predictive testing. *Eur. J. Cancer*, **33**, 2390–2.

Dorum, A., Hovig, E., Trope, C., Inganas, M. & Moller, P.(1999). Three per cent of Norwegian ovarian cancers are caused by BRCA1 1675delA or 1135insA. *Eur. J. Cancer*, **35**, 779–81.

dos Santos, J.G. & de Magalhes, J. (1980). Familial gastric polyposis: a new entity. *J. Genet. Hum.*, **28**, 293–7.

Douglass, E.G., Valentine, M., Etcubanas, E. et al. (1987). A specific chromosomal abnormality in rhabdomyosarcoma. *Cytogenet. Cell Genet.*, **45**, 148–55.

Downs, A.M. & Kennedy, C.T. (1998). Scleroatrophic syndrome of Huriez in an infant. *Paed. Dematol.*, **15**, 207–9.

Dowton, S.B., Beardsley, D., Jamison, D., Blattner, S. & Lie, F.P. (1985). Studies of a familial platelet disorder. *Blood*, **65**, 557–65.

Dozois, R.R., Kempers, R.D., Dahlin, D.C. et al. (1970). Ovarian tumours associated with Peutz–Jeghers syndrome. *Ann. Surg.*, **172**, 233–8.

Dracopoli, N. & Fountain, J. (1996). CDKN2 mutations in melanoma. *Cancer Surv.*, **26**, 115–32.

Draper, G.J., Sanders, B.M. & Kingston, J.E. (1986). Second primary neoplasms in patients with retinoblastoma. *Br. J. Cancer*, **53**, 661–71.

Draper, G.J., Sanders, B.M., Brownbill, P.A. & Hawkins, M.M. (1992). Patterns of risk of hereditary retinoblastoma and applications to genetic counselling. *Br. J. Cancer*, **66**, 211–19.

Draptchinskaia, N., Gustavsson, P., Andersson, B., Pettersson, M., Willig, T.N., Dianzani, I., Ball, S., Tchernia, G., Klar, J., Matsson, H., Tentler, D., Mohandas, N., Carlsson, B. & Dahl, N. (1999). The gene encoding ribosomal protein S19 is mutated in Diamond-Blackfan anaemia. *Nat. Genet.*, **21(2)**, 169–75.

Dreijerink, K.M. & Lips, C.J. (2005). Diagnosis and management of multiple endocrine neoplasia type 1 (MEN1). *Heredit. Cancer Clin. Pract.*, **3**, 1–6.

Drinkwater, N.R. & Lee, G.-H. (1995). Genetic susceptibility to liver cancer. In *Liver Regeneration and Carcinogenesis*. Academic Press, San Diego, pp. 301–21.

Dror, Y. & Freedman, M.H. (1999). Swachman—Diamond syndrome: an inherited preleukaemic bone-marrow failure disorder with aberrant hematopoietic progenitors and faulty marrow microenvironment. *Blood*, **94**, 3048–54.

Drovdlic, C.M., Goddard, K.A., Chak, A., Brock, W., Chessler, L., King, J.F., Richter, J., Falk, G.W., Johnston, D.K., Fisher, J.L., Grady, W.M., Lemeshow, S. & Eng, C. (2003). Demographic and phenotypic features of 70 families segregating Barrett's oesophagus and oesophageal adenocarcinoma. *J. Med. Genet.*, **40**, 651–6.

Dudok-deWit, A.C., Tibben, A. & Duivenvoorden, H.J. (1997a). Distress in individuals facing predictive DNA testing for autosomal dominant late-onset disorders: comparing questionnaire results with in-depth interviews. Rotterdam/Leiden Genetics Workshop. *Am. J. Med. Genet*, **75**, 62–74.

Dudok-deWit, A.C., Tibben, A. & Duivenvoorden, H.J. (1997b). Psychological distress in applicants for predictive DNA testing for autosomal dominant, heritable, late-onset disorders. II. The Rotterdam/Leiden Genetics Workshop. *J. Med. Genet.*, **34**, 382–90.

Duggan, B.D. & Dubeau, L. (1998). Genetics and biology of gynaecologic cancer. *Curr. Opin. Oncol.*, **10**, 439–46.

Duhaime, A.C., Bunin, G., Sutton, L., Rorke, L.B. & Packer, R. (1989). Simultaneous presentation of glioblastoma multiforme in siblings two and five years old: case report. *Neurosurgery*, **24**, 434–9.

Duker, N.J. (2002). Chromosome breakage syndromes and cancer. *Am. J. Med. Genet.*, **115**, 125–9.

Dumont-Herskowitz, R.A., Safaii, H.S. & Senior, B. (1978). Ovarian fibromata in four successive generations. *J. Pediatr.*, **93**, 621–4.

Dunlop, M.G. (2002). Guidance on gastroenterological surveillance for hereditary non-polyposis colorectal cancer, familial adenomatous polyposis, juvenile polyposis and Peutz–Jegher syndrome. *Gut*, **51**(Suppl. V), v21–7.

Dunlop, M.G., Farrington, S.M., Carothers, A.D., Wyllie, A.H., Sharp, L., Burn, J., Liu, B., Kinzler, K.W. & Vogelstein, B. (1997). Cancer risk associated with germline DNA mismatch repair gene mutations. *Hum. Mol. Genet.*, **6**(1), 105–10.

Duperrat, B. & Albert, N.I. (1948). Forme familiale d'epithelioma de Malherbe. *Bull. Soc. Franc. Derm. Syph.*, **5**, 196–7.

Dupont, W.D. & Page, D.L. (1985). Risk factors for breast cancer in women with proliferative breast disease. *New Engl. J. Med.*, **312**, 146–51.

Dupont, W.D. & Page, D.L. (1987). Breast cancer risk associated with proliferative disease, age at first birth, and a family history of breast cancer. *Am. J. Epidemiol.*, **125**, 769–79.

Durocher, F., Tonin, P., Shattuck-Eidens, D. et al. (1996). Mutation analysis of the BRCA1 gene in 23 families with cancer of the breast, ovary and multiple other sites. *J. Med. Genet.*, **33**, 814–19.

Dutz, J.P., Benoit, L., Wang, X., Demetrick, D.J., Junker, A., de Sa, D. & Tan, R. (2001). Lymphocytic vasculitis in X-linked lymphoproliferative disease. *Blood*, **97**, 95–100.

Eady, R.A. & Dunnill, M.G. (1994). Epidermolysis bullosa: hereditary skin fragility diseases as paradigms in cell biology. *Arch. Derm. Res.*, **287**, 2–9.

Eady, R.A.J., Gunner, D.B., Tidman, M.J. et al. (1985). Prenatal diagnosis of genetic skin disease by fetoscopy and electron microscopy: report on five years experience. *Br. J. Dermatol.*, **113**(Suppl 29), 45.

Easton, D. & Peto, J. (1990). The contribution of inherited predisposition to cancer incidence. *Cancer Surv.*, **9**, 395–416.

Easton, D., Ford, D. & Peto, J. (1993a). Inherited susceptibility to breast cancer. *Cancer Surv.*, **18**, 95–113.

Easton, D.E., Ponder, M.A., Huson, S.M. & Ponder, B.A.J. (1993b). An analysis of variation in expression of neurofibromatosis (NF) type 1 (NF1): evidence for modifying genes. *Am. J. Hum. Genet.*, **53**, 303–13.

Easton, D.E., Ford, D., Bishop, D.T. & The Breast Cancer Linkage Consortium (1995). Breast and ovarian cancer incidence in BRCA1 mutation carriers. *Am. J. Hum. Genet.*, **56**, 265–71.

Easton, D.F., Ponder, M.A., Cummings, T. et al. (1989). The clinical and age-at-onset distribution for the MEN-2 syndrome. *Am. J. Hum. Genet.*, **44**, 208–15.

Easton, D.F., Matthews, F.E., Ford, D., Swerdlow, A.J. & Peto, J. (1996). Cancer mortality in relatives of women with ovarian cancer – the OPCS study. *Int. J. Cancer*, **65**, 284–94.

Easton, D.F., Steele, L., Fields, P., Ormiston, W., Averill, D., Daly, P.A., McManus, R., Neuhausen, S.L., Ford, D., Wooster, R., Cannon-Albright, L.A., Stratton, M.R. & Goldgar, D.E. (1997). Cancer risks in two large breast cancer families linked to BRCA2 on chromosome 13q12–13. *Am. J. Hum. Genet.*, **61**, 120–8.

Eberle, M.A., Pfutzer, R., Pogue-Geile, K.L., Bronner, M.P., Crispin, D., Kimmey, M.B., Duerr, R.H., Kruglyak, L., Whitcomb, D.C. & Brentnall, T.A. (2002). A new susceptibility locus for autosomal dominant pancreatic cancer maps to chromosome 4q32–34. *Am. J. Hum. Genet.*, **70**, 1044–8.

Edwards, C.L., Tortolero-Luna, G., Linares, A.C. et al. (1996). Vulvar intraneoplasia and vulvar cancer. *Obstet. Gynecol. Clin. North Am.*, **23**, 295–324.

Edwards, C.Q., Dalone, M.M., Skolnick, M.H. et al. (1982). Hereditary hemochromatosis. *Clin. Haematol.*, **11**, 411–36.

Edwards, S.M., Kote-Jarai, Z., Meitz, J. et al. (2002). Two percent of men with early-onset prostate cancer harbor germline mutations in the BRCA2 gene. *Am. J. Hum. Genet.*, **72**(1), 1–12.

Eeles, R.A. (1995). Germline mutations in the *TP53* gene. *Cancer Surv.*, **25**, 101–24.

Eerola, I., Boon, L.M., Mulliken, J.B. et al. (2003). Capillary malformation–arteriovenous malformation, a new clinical and genetic disorder caused by RASA1 mutations. *Am. J. Hum. Genet.*, **73**, 1240–9.

Ehrenthal, D., Haeger, L., Griffin, T. et al. (1987). Familial pancreatic carcinoma in three generations: a case report and a review of the literature. *Cancer*, **59**, 1661–4.

Eide, T.J. (1986). Risk of colorectal cancer in adenoma-bearing individuals within a defined population. *Int. J. Cancer*, **38**, 173–6.

Eisen, A. & Weber, B.L. (1998). Primary peritoneal carcinoma can have multifocal origins: implications for prophylactic oophorectomy [editorial; comment]. *J. Natl. Cancer Inst.*, **90**, 797–9.

Elliott, M.L. & Maher, E.R. (1994). Syndrome of the month: Beckwith–Wiedemann syndrome. *J. Med. Genet.*, **31**, 560–4.

Elliott, M., Bayly, R., Cole, T. et al. (1994). Clinical features and natural history of Beckwith—Wiedemann syndrome: presentation of 74 new cases. *Clin. Genet.*, **46**, 168–74.

Ellis, N.A. & German, J. (1996). Molecular genetics of Bloom's syndrome. *Hum. Mol. Genet.*, **5**, 1457–63.

Ellis, N.A., Groden, J., Ye, T.Z., Straughen, J., Kennon, D.J., Ciocci, S., Proytcheva, M. & German, J. (1995). The Bloom's syndrome gene product is homologous to RecQ helicases. *Cell*, **83**(4), 655–66.

Elsaleh, H.I.B. et al. (2001). Microsatellite instability is a predictive marker for survival benefit from adjuvant chemotherapy in a population-based series of stage III colorectal carcinoma. *Clin. Colorectal Cancer*, **1**, 103–9.

Elwood, J.M., Whitehead, S.M., Davison, J., Stewart, M. & Galt, M. (1990). Malignant melanoma in England: risks associated with naevi, freckles, social class, hair colour, and sunburn. *Int. J. Epidemiol.*, **19**(4), 801–10.

Eng, C. (1999). *RET* proto-oncogene in the development of human cancer. *J. Clin. Oncol.*, **17**, 380–93.

Eng, C. (2000a). Familial papillary thyroid cancer – many syndromes, too many genes? *J. Clin. Endocrinol. Metab.*, **85**, 1755–7.

Eng, C. (2000b). Multiple endocrine neoplasia type 2 and the practice of molecular medicine. *Rev. Endocrinol. Metab. Dis.*, **1**, 283–90.

Eng, C. (2000c). Will the real Cowden syndrome please stand up: revised diagnostic criteria. *J. Med. Genet.*, **37**, 828–30.

Eng, C. (2001). News and views: to be or not to BMP. *Nat. Genet.*, **28**, 105–7.

Eng, C. (2003). PTEN: one gene, many syndromes. *Hum. Mutat.*, **22**,183–98.

Eng, C. & Parsons, R. (1998). Cowden syndrome. In *The Genetic Basis of Human Cancer*, eds. Vogelstein, B. & Kinzler, K.W. McGraw-Hill, New York, 519–26.

Eng, C. & Peacocke, M. (1998). *PTEN* and inherited hamartoma-cancer syndromes. *Nat. Genet.*, **19**, 223.

Eng, C., Li, F.P., Abramson, D.H. et al. (1993). Mortality from second tumors among long-term survivors of retinoblastoma. *J. Natl. Cancer Inst.*, **85**, 1121–8.

Eng, C., Murday, V., Seal, S. et al. (1994a). Cowden syndrome and Lhermitte–Duclos disease in a family: a single genetic syndrome with pleiotropy? *J. Med. Genet.*, **31**, 458–61.

Eng, C., Smith, D.P., Mulligan, L.M. et al. (1994b). Point mutation within the tyrosine kinase domain of the *RET* proto-oncogene in multiple endocrine neoplasia type 2B and related sporadic tumours. *Hum. Mol. Genet.*, **3**, 237–41.

Eng, C., Crossey, P.A., Mulligan, L.M. et al. (1995a). Mutations of the *RET* proto-oncogene and the von Hippel–Lindau disease tumour suppressor gene in sporadic and syndromic phaeochromocytoma. *J. Med. Genet.*, **32**, 934–7.

Eng, C., Mulligan, L.M., Smith, D.P. et al. (1995b). Low frequency of germline mutations in the *RET* proto-oncogene in patients with apparently sporadic medullary thyroid carcinoma. *Clin. Endocrinol.*, **43**, 123–7.

Eng, C., Mulligan, L.M., Smith, D.P. et al. (1995c). Mutation in the *RET* proto-oncogene in sporadic medullary thyroid carcinoma. *Gene. Chrom. Cancer*, **12**, 209–12.

Eng, C., Smith, D.P., Mulligan, L.M. et al. (1995d). A novel point mutation in the tyrosine kinase domain of the *RET* proto-oncogene in sporadic medullary thyroid carcinoma and in a family with FMTC. *Oncogene*, **10**, 509–13.

Eng, C., Clayton, D., Schuffenecker, I. et al. (1996a). The relationship between specific *RET* proto-oncogene mutations and disease phenotype in multiple endocrine neoplasia type 2: International *RET* Mutation Consortium analysis. *J. Am. Med. Assoc.*, **276**, 1575–9.

Eng, C., Mulligan, L.M., Healey, C.S. et al. (1996b). Heterogeneous mutation of the *RET* proto-oncogene in subpopulations of medullary thyroid carcinoma. *Cancer Res.*, **56**, 2167–70.

Eng, C., Schneider, K., Fraumeni, J.F. & Li, F.P. (1997). Third International Workshop on collaborative interdisciplinary studies of *p53* and other predisposing genes in Li–Fraumeni syndrome. *Cancer Epidemiol. Biomark. Prev.*, **6**, 379–83.

Eng, C., Thomas, G.A., Neuberg, D.S. et al. (1998). Mutation of the *RET* proto-oncogene is correlated with RET immunostaining in subpopulations of cells in sporadic medullary thyroid carcinoma. *J. Clin. Endocrinol. Metab.*, **83**, 4310–3.

Eng, C., Hampel, H. & de la Chapelle, A. (2001). Genetic testing for cancer predisposition. *Annu. Rev. Med.*, **52**, 371–400.

Eng, C., Kiuru, M., Fernandez, M.J. & Aaltonen, L.A. (2003). A role for mitochondrial enzymes in inherited neoplasia and beyond. *Nat. Rev. Cancer*, **3**, 193–202.

Engel, J.R., Smallwood, A., Harper, A., Higgins, M.J., Oshimura, M., Reik, W., Schofield, P.N. & Maher, E.R. (2000). Epigenotype-phenotype correlations in Beckwith–Wiedemann syndrome. *J. Med. Genet.*, **37**, 921–6.

Engelman, D.E., Andrade, L.A. & Vassallo, J.(2003). Human papillomavirus infection and p53 protein expression vulvar intraepithelial neoplasia and invasive squamous cell carcinoma. *Braz. J. Med. Biol. Res.*, **36**, 1159–65.

Enzi, G. (1984). Multiple lipomatosis: an updated clinical report. *Medicine*, **63**, 56–64.

Epstein, C.J., Martin, G.M., Schultz, A.L. et al. (1966). Werner's syndrome. *Medicine*, **45**, 177–221.

Erdman, S.H. & Barnard, J.A. (2002). Gastrointestinal polyps and polyposis syndromes in children. *Curr. Opin. Paeds.*, **14**, 576–82.

Eriksson, S., Carlson, J. & Velez, R. (1986). Risk of cirrhosis and primary liver cancer in Alpha-1 antitrypsin deficiency. *New Engl. J. Med.*, **314**, 736–9.

Escobar, V., Goldblatt, L.I., Bixler, D. et al. (1983). Clouston syndrome: an ultrastructural study. *Clin. Genet.*, **24**, 140–6.

Esposito, F., el Quandi, F.Z., Ghi, M.E. & Cherchi, P.L. (1995). Association of Morris' syndrome with squamous cell carcinoma of the vulva. *J. Gynecol. Obstet. Biol. Reprod. (Paris)*, **24**, 816–18.

Evans, D.B. & Critchlow, R.W. (1987). Carcinoma of the male breast and Klinefelter syndrome: is there an association? *CA Cancer J. Clin.*, **37**, 246–51.

Evans, D.G. & Howell, A. (2004). Are BRCA1- and BRCA2-related breast cancers associated with increased mortality? *Breast Cancer Res.*, **6**, E7.

Evans, D.G., Mason, S., Huson, S.M., Ponder, M., Harding, A.E. & Strachan, T. (1997a). Spinal and cutaneous schwannomatosis is a variant form of type 2 neurofibromatosis: a clinical and molecular study. *J. Neurol. Neurosurg. Psychiat.*, **62**, 361–6.

Evans, D.G., Walsh, S., Jeacock, J., Robinson, C., Hadfield, L., Davies, D.R. & Kingston. R. (1997b). Incidence of hereditary non-polyposis colorectal cancer in a population-based study of 1137 consecutive cases of colorectal cancer. *Br. J. Surg.*, **84**, 1281–5.

Evans, D.G., Baser, M.E., McGaughran, J., Sharif, S., Howard, E. & Moran, A. (2002). Malignant peripheral nerve sheath tumours in neurofibromatosis 1. *J. Med. Genet.*, **39**, 311–4.

Evans, D.G., Eccles, D.M., Rahman, N., Young, K., Bulman, M., Amir, E., Shenton, A., Howell, A. & Lalloo, F. (2004). A new scoring system for the chances of identifying a BRCA1/2 mutation outperforms existing models including BRCAPRO. *J. Med. Genet.*, **41**, 474–80.

Evans, D.G., Moran, A., King, A., Saeed, S., Gurusinghe, N. & Ramsden, R. (2005). Incidence of vestibular schwannoma and neurofibromatosis 2 in the north west of England over a 10-year period: higher incidence than previously thought. *Otol Neurotol.* **26**, 93–7.

Evans, D.G.R., Huson, S., Donnai, D. et al. (1992a). A genetic study of type 2 neurofibromatosis in the north west of England and the UK: prevalence, mutation rate, fitness and confirmation of maternal gene effect. *J. Med. Genet.*, **29**, 847–52.

Evans, D.G.R., Huson, S., Donnai, D. et al. (1992b). A clinical study of type 2 neurofibromatosis. *Q. J. Med.*, **84**, 603–18.

Evans, D.G.R., Ladisans, E.J., Rimmer, S., Burnell, L.D., Thakker, N. & Farndon, P.A. (1993). Complications of the nevoid basal cell carcinoma syndrome: results of a population based study. *J. Med. Genet.* **30**, 460–4.

Evans, J.P., Burke, W., Chen, R. et al. (1995). Familial pancreatic adenocarcinoma: association with diabetes and early molecular diagnosis. *J. Med. Genet.*, **32**, 330–5.

Evans, S.C. & Lozano, C. (1997). The Li–Fraumeni syndrome: an inherited susceptibility to cancer. *Mol. Med. Today*, **September**, 390–5.

Eyster, M., Saletan, S.L., Rabellino, E.M. et al. (1986). Familial essential thrombocythemia. *Am. J. Med.*, **89**, 497–502.

Fackenthal, J., Marsh, D.J., Richardson, A.L., et al. (2001). Male breast cancer in Cowden syndrome patients with germline *PTEN* mutations. *J. Med. Genet.*, **38**: 159–64.

Farmer, K.C.R., Spigelman, A.D., Williams, C.B. et al. (1991). Prospective placebo controlled double blind trial of sulindac in the management of upper gastro-intestinal polyps in FAP. Abstract, Leeds Castle Polyposis Group Meeting, Fort Lauderdale.

Farndon, J.R., Leight, G.S., Dilley, W.G. et al. (1986). Familial medullary thyroid carcinoma without associated endocrinopathies: a distinct clinical entity. *Br. J. Surg.*, **73**, 278–81.

Farndon, P.A., Del Mastro, R.G., Evans, D.G.R. et al. (1992). Location of gene for Gorlin syndrome. *Lancet*, **339**, 581–2.

Farrington, S.M., McKinley, A.J., Carothers, A.D., Cunningham, C., Bubb, V.J., Sharp, L., Wyllie, A.H. & Dunlop, M.G. (2002). Evidence for an age-related influence of microsatellite instability on colorectal cancer survival. *Int. J. Cancer*, **98**(6), 844–50.

Fathalla, M.F. (1971). Incessant ovulation – a factor in ovarian neoplasia? *Lancet*, **2**, 163.

Fayad, M.N., Yacoub, A., Salman, S. et al. (1987). Juvenile hyaline fibromatosis: two new patients and review of the literature. *Am. J. Med. Genet.*, **26**, 123–31.

Fearnhead, N.S., Wilding, J.L., Winney, B. et al. (2004). Multiple rare variants in different geness account for multifactorial inherited susceptibility to colorectal adenomas. *Proc. Natl. Acad. Sci. USA*, **101**, 15992–7.

Fearon, E.R. (1997). Human cancer syndromes: clues on the origin and nature of cancer. *Science*, **278**, 1043–50.

Fearon, E.R. & Vogelstein, B. (1990). A genetic model for colorectal tumorigenesis. *Cell*, **61**, 759–67.

Feder, J.N., Gnirke, A., Thomas, W. et al. (1996). A novel MHC class I-like gene is mutated in patients with hereditary haemochromatosis. *Nat. Genet.*, **13**, 399–407.

Feinstein, A., Friedman, J. & Schewach-Millet, M. (1988). Pachonychia congenita. *J. Am. Acad. Dermatol.*, **19**, 705–11.

Feldmann, J., Callebaut, I., Raposo, G. et al. (2003). Munc13–4 is essential for cytolytic granules fusion and is mutated in a form of familial hemophagocytic lymphohistiocytosis (FHL3). *Cell*, **115**, 461–73.

Felix, C.A., Slavc, L., Dunn, M. et al. (1995). *p53* gene mutations in pediatric brain tumors. *Med. Pediatr. Oncol.*, **25**, 431–6.

Feng, B.J., Huang, W., Shugart, Y.Y.et al. (2002). Genome-wide scan for familial nasopharyngeal carcinoma reveals evidence of linkage to chromosome 4. *Nat. Genet.*, **31**, 395–9.

Fenske, C., Banergee, P., Holden, C. & Carter, N. (2000). Brook–Spiegler syndrome locus assigned to 16q 12–13. *J. Invest. Dermatol.*, **114**, 1057–8.

Fenton, P.A., Clarke, S.E.M., Owen, W. et al. (2001). Cribriform variant papillary thyroid cancer: a characteristic of familial adenomatous polyposis. *Thyroid*, **11**, 193–7.

Ferger, F., Ribadean, D.A., Leriche, L. et al. (2002). Kit and c-kit mutations in mastocytosis: a short overview with special reference to novel molecular and diagnostic concepts. *Int. Arch. Allergy Immunol.*, **127**, 110–14.

Ferguson, A. & Kingstone, K. (1996). Coeliac disease and malignancies. *Acta Paediatr.* Suppl **412**, 78–81.

Ferguson-Smith, M.A., Wallace, D.C., James, Z.H. et al. (1971). Multiple self-healing squamous epithelioma. *Birth Defect.*, **7**(8), 157–63.

Fernandez, E., La Vecchia, C., D'Avanzo, B. et al. (1994). Family history and the risk of liver, gall bladder and pancreatic cancer. *Cancer Epidemiol. Biomark. Prev.*, **3**, 209–12.

Ferraris, A.M., Racchi, O., Rapezzi, D., Gaetani, G.F. & Boffetta, P. (1997). Familial Hodgkin's disease: a disease of young adulthood? *Ann. Hematol.*, **74**, 131–4.

Ferris, M.K., Pround, V.K., Narva, S.F. et al. (1987). Neurocutaneous melanosis syndrome. *Clin. Genet.*, **41**, A57.

Figueiredo, B.C., Sandrini, R., Zambetti, G.P. et al. (2006). Penetrance of adrenocortical tumour associated with the germline TP53 R337H mutation. *J. Med. Genet.*, **43**(1), 91–6.

Filling-Katz, M.R., Choyke, P., Patronas, N. et al. (1991). Central nervous involvement in von Hippel–Lindau disease. *Neurology*, **41**, 41–6.

Fine, J.M., Muller, J.Y., Rochu, D. et al. (1986). Waldenstrom's macroglobulinaemia in monozygotic twins. *Acta Med. Scand.*, **220**, 369–73.

Finlay, A.Y. & Marks, R. (1979). Familial Kaposi's sarcoma. *Br. J. Dermatol.*, **100**, 323–5.

Fiorentino, D.F., Nguyen, J.C., Egbert, B.M. & Swetter, S.M. (2004). Muir–Torre syndrome: confirmation of diagnosis by immunohistochemical analysis of cutaneous lesions. *J. Am. Acad. Dermatol.*, **50**(3), 476–8.

Fisch, R.O., McCabe, E.R. & Dolden, D. (1978). Homotransplantation in a patient with hepatoma and hereditary tyrosinaemia. *J. Pediatr.*, **93**, 592–6.

Fischer, S. (1978). La genodermatose scleroatrophiante et keratodermique des extremities. *Ann. Dermatol. Venereol.*, **105**, 1079–82.

Fitzgerald, M.G., Bean, J.M., Hedge, S.R. et al. (1997). Hetreozygous ATM mutations do not contribute to early onset of breast cancer. *Nat. Genet.*, **15**, 307–10.

Flanders, T.Y. & Foulkes, W.D. (1996). Pancreatic adenocarcinoma: epidemiology and genetics. *J. Med. Genet.*, **33**, 889–98.

Fletcher, O., Easton, D., Anderson, K., Gilham, C., Jay, M. & Peto, J. (2004). Lifetime risks of common cancers among retinoblastoma survivors. *Natl. Cancer Inst.*, **96**(5), 357–63.

Floy, K.M., Hess, R.O. & Meisner, L.F. (1990). DNA polymerase alpha defect in the N syndrome. *Am. J. Med. Genet.*, **35**, 301–5.

Fodde, R. (2003). The multiple functions of tumour suppressors: it's all in APC. *Nature Cell Biol.*, **5**, 190–2.

Fodde, R., Kuipers, J., Smits, R. et al. (2001). Mutations in the APC tumour suppressor gene cause chromosome instability. *Nat. Cell Biol.*, **3**, 433–8.

Fogarty, P.F., Yamaguchi, H., Wiestner, A., et al. (2003). Late presentation of dyskeratosis congenita as apparently acquired aplastic anaemia due to mutations in telomerase RNA. *Lancet*, **362**, 1628–30.

Fong, L.Y., Fidanza,V., Zanesi, N., Lock, L.F., Siracusa, L.D., Mancini, R., Siprashvili, Z., Ottey, M., Martin, S.E., Druck, T., McCue, P.A., Croce, C.M. & Huebner, K. (2000). Muir–Torre-like syndrome in Fhit-deficient mice. *Proc. Natl. Acad. Sci. USA*, **97**(9), 4742–7.

Ford, A.M., Ridge, S.A., Cabrera, M.E., Mahmoud, H., Steel, C.M., Chan, L.C. & Greaves, M. (1993). In utero rearrangements in the trithorax-related oncogene in infant leukaemias. *Nature*, **363**, 358–60.

Ford, D., Easton, D.F., Bishop, D.T. et al. & Breast Cancer Linkage Consortium (2004). Risks of cancer in BRCA1 mutation carriers. *Lancet*, **343**, 692–5.

Ford, D., Easton, D.F. & Peto, J. (1995). Estimates of the gene frequency of BRCA1 and its contribution to breast and ovarian cancer incidence. *Am. J. Hum. Genet.*, **57**, 1457–62.

Ford, D., Easton, D.F., Stratton, M., et al. (1998). Genetic heterogeneity and penetrance analysis of the BRCA1 and BRCA2 genes in breast cancer families. *Am. J. Hum. Genet.*, **62**, 676–89.

Forman, D., Oliver, R.T.D., Brett, A.R. et al. (1992). Familial testicular cancer: a report of the UK register, estimation of risk and HLA class I sib pair analysis. *Br. J. Cancer*, **65**, 255–62.

Forrest, P. (1990). *Breast Cancer The Decision to Screen.* Nuffield Provincial Hospitals Trust Fourth HM Queen Elizabeth the Queen Mother Fellowship, London.

Foster, J.H., Donogue, T.A. & Berman, M.M. (1978). Familial liver cell adenomas and diabetes mellitus. *New Engl. J. Med.*, **299**, 239–41.

Foster, K.A., Harrington, P., Kerr, J., Russell, P., DiCioccio, R.A., Scott, I.V., Jacobs, I., Chenevix-Trench, G., Ponder, B.A. & Gayther, S.A. (1996). Somatic and germline mutations of the BRCA2 gene in sporadic ovarian cancer. *Cancer Res.*, **56**, 3622–5.

Foulkes, W.D. (1995). Review: a tale of four syndromes: familial adenomatous polyposis, Gardner syndrome, attenuated APC and Turcot syndrome. *Q. J. Med.*, **88**, 853–63.

Foulkes, W.D. (2006). BRCA1 and BRCA2: chemosensitivity, treatment outcomes and prognosis. *Fam. Cancer*, in press.

Foulkes, W.D., Brunet, J.-S., Sieh, W., Black, M.J., Shenouda, G. & Narod, S.A. (1996). Familial risks of squamous cell carcinoma of the head and neck: retrospective case–control study. *Br. Med. J.*, **313**, 716–21.

Foulkes, W.D., Thiffault, I., Gruber, S.B. et al. (2002). The founder mutation MSH2* 1906G-->C is an important cause of hereditary nonpolyposis colorectal cancer in the Ashkenazi Jewish population. *Am. J. Hum. Genet.* **71**, 1395–412.

Foulkes, W.D., Stefansson, I.M., Chappuis, P.O., Begin, L.R., Goffin, J.R., Wong, N., Trudel, M. & Akslen, L.A. (2003). Germline BRCA1 mutations and a basal epithelial phenotype in breast cancer. *J. Natl. Cancer Inst.*, **95**, 1482–5.

Foulkes, W.D., Brunet, J.-S., Stefansson, I.M., Straume, O., Chappuis, P.O., Begin, L.R., Hamel, N., Goffin, J.R., Wong, N., Trudel, M., Kapusta, L., Porter, P. & Akslen, L.A. (2004). The prognostic implication of the basal-like (cyclin E high/p27 low/p53 +/glomeruloid-microvascular-proliferation +) phenotype of BRCA1-related breast cancer. *Cancer Res.*, **64**, 830–5.

Fox, H., Emery, J.L., Goodbody, R.A. et al. (1964). Neurocutaneous melanosis. *Arch. Dis. Child.*, **39**, 508.

Fraumeni, J.F. & Thomas, L.B. (1967). Malignant bladder tumors in a man and his three sons. *J. Am. Med. Assoc.*, **201**, 507–9.

Fraumeni Jr, J.F., Grundy, G.W., Creagan, E.T. et al. (1975). Six families prone to ovarian cancer. *Cancer*, **36**, 364–9.

Frebourg, T., Barbier, N., Yan, Y.X. et al. (1995). Germline p53 mutations in 15 families with Li–Fraumeni syndrome. *Am. J. Hum. Genet.*, **56**, 608–15.

Freedman, M.H., Bonilla, M.A., Fier, C., Bolyard, A.A., Scarlata, D., Boxer, L.A., Brown, S., Cham, B., Kannourakis, G., Kinsey, S.E., Mori, P.G., Cottle, T., Welte, K. & Dale, D.C. (2000). Myelodysplasia syndrome and acute myeloid leukemia in patients with congenital neutropenia receiving G-CSF therapy. *Blood*, **96**, 429–36.

Frenk, E. & Tapernoux, B. (1974). Hyperkeratosis lenticularis perstans (Flegel). *Humangenetik*, **24**, 151–3.

Fresko, D., Lazarus, S.S., Dotan, J. & Reingold, M. (1982). Early presentation of carcinoma of the small bowel in Crohn's disease ('Crohn's carcinoma'). Case reports and review of the literature. *Gastroenterology*, **82**, 783–9.

Friborg, J. et al. (2003). Cancer in Greenlandic Inuit 1973–1997: a cohort study. *Int. J. Cancer*, **107**(6), 1017–22.

Friedl, W., Kruse, R., Uhlhaas, S. et al. (1999). Frequent 4-bp deletion in exon 9 of the *SMAD4/ MADH4* gene in familial juvenile polyposis patients. *Gene. Chrom. Cancer*, **25**, 403–6.

Friedl, W., Uhlhaas, S., Schulmann, K. et al. (2002). Juvenile polyposis: massive gastric polyposis is more common in MADH4 mutation carriers than in BMPR1A mutation carriers. *Hum. Genet.*, **111**, 108–11.

Friedland, M.L., Wittels, E.G. & Robinson, R.J. (1981). Polycythemia vera in identical twins. *Am. J. Hematol.*, **10**, 101–3.

Friedman, E., deMarco, L., Gejman, P.V. et al. (1992). Allelic loss from chromosome 11 in parathyroid tumors. *Cancer Res.*, **52**, 6804–9.

Friedman, J.M. & Fialklow, P.J. (1976). Familial carcinoma of the pancreas. *Clin. Genet.*, **9**, 463–9.

Friedman, L.S., Szabo, C.I., Ostermeyer, E.A., Dowd, P., Butler, L., Park, T., Lee, M.K., Goode, E.L., Rowell, S.E. & King, M.C. (1995). Novel inherited mutations and variable expressivity of BRCA1 alleles, including the founder mutation 185delAG in Ashkenazi Jewish families. *Am. J. Hum. Genet.*, **57**, 1284–97.

Friedrich Jr, E.G. & MacLaren, N.K. (1984). Genetic aspects of vulvar Lichen Sclerosus. *Am. J. Obstet. Gynecol.*, **150**, 161–6.

Frieling, T., Berges, W., Borchard, F. et al. (1988). Family occurrence of achalasia and diffuse spasm of the oesophagus. *Gut*, **29**, 1595–602.

Friend, S.H. (1996). Breast cancer susceptibility testing: realities in the post-genomic era. *Nat. Genet.*, **13**, 16–17.

Friend, S.H., Bernards, R., Rogelj, S. et al. (1986). A human DNA segment with properties of the gene that predisposes to retinoblastoma and osteosarcoma. *Nature*, **323**, 643–6.

Fritsch-Polanz, R., Jordan, J.H., Eeli, X.A. et al. (2001). Mutation analysis of C-Kit in patients with myelodysplastic syndrome without mastocytosis and cases of systemic mastocytosis. *Br. J. Haematol.*, **13**, 357–64.

Fryns, J.P. & Chrzanowska, K. (1988). Mucosal neuromata syndrome (MEN type Ilb(III)). *J. Med. Genet.*, **25**, 703–6.

Fryns, J.P., Haspeslagh, M., de Muelenaere, A. & van den Berghe, H. (1985). 9p trisomy and 18p distal monosomy and multiple cutaneous leiomyomata. *Hum. Genet.*, **70**, 284–6.

Fuchs, B. & Pritchard, D.J. (2002). Etiology of osteosarcomas. *Clin. Orthop. Relat. Res.*, **397**, 40–52.

Fuchs, E. (1996). The cytoskeleton and disease: genetic disorders of intermediate filaments. *Ann. Rev. Genet.*, **30**, 197–231.

Fujita, M., Enanoto, T., Yoshinok, K. et al. (1993). Microsatellite instability and alterations in the LMSH2 gene in human ovarian cancer. *Int. J. Cancer*, **64**, 361–6.

Fukhro, et al. (2002). Blue rubber bleb naevus syndrome and gastrointestinal haemorrhage: which treatment? *Eur. J. Paed. Surg.*, **12**, 129–33.

Fusaro, R.M. & Lynch, H.T. (1982). Cutaneous signs of cancer-associated genodermatoses. In *Cancer-Associated Genodermatoses*, eds. Lynch, H.T. & Fusaro, R.M. Van Norstrand Reinhold, New York, pp. 104–44.

Futreal, P.A., Liu, Q., Shattuk Eidens, D. et al. (1994). BRCA1 mutations in primary breast and ovarian carcinomas. *Science*, **266**, 120–2.

Gadelha, M.R., Une, K.N., Rohde, K., Vaisman, M., Kineman, R.D. & Frohman, L.A. (2000). Isolated familial somatotropinomas: establishment of linkage to chromosome 11q13.1–11q13.3 and evidence for a potential second locus at chromosome 2p16–12. *J. Clin. Endocrinol. Metab.*, **85**, 707–14.

Gaglia, P., Atkin, W.S., Whitelaw, S. et al. (1995). Variables associated with the risk of colorectal adenomas in asymptomatic patients with a family history of colorectal cancer. *Gut*, **36**, 385–90.

Gail, M.H., Brinton, L.A. & Byar, D.P. (1989). Projecting individualized probabilities of developing breast cancer for white females who are being examined annually. *J. Natl. Cancer Inst.*, **84**, 1879–86.

Gallione, C.J., Pasyk, K.A., Boon, L.N. et al. (1995). A gene for familial venous malformation maps to chromosome 9p in a second large kindred. *J. Med. Genet.*, **32**, 197–9.

Gamez, J., Playan, A., Andreu, A.L. et al. (1998). Familial multiple symmetric lipomatosis associated with the A8344G mutation of mitochondrial DNA. *Neurology*, **51**, 258–60.

Ganslandt, O., Buchfelder, M. & Grabenauer, G.G. (2000). Primary spinal germinoma in a patient with concomitant Klinefelter's syndrome. *Br. J. Neurosurg.*, **14**, 252–5.

Garber, J.E. & Offit, K. (2005). Hereditary cancer predisposition syndromes. *J. Clin. Oncol.*, **23**, 276–92.

Garber, J.E., Li, P.P., Kingston, J.E. et al. (1988). Hepatoblastoma and familial adenomatous polyposis. *J. Natl. Cancer Inst.*, **80**, 1626–8.

Garber, J.E., Burke, E.M., Lavally, B.L. et al. (1990). Choroid plexus tumors in the breast cancer-sarcoma syndrome. *Cancer*, **66**, 2658–60.

Garber, J.E., Goldstein, A.M., Kantor, A.F. et al. (1991). Follow-up study of twenty-four families with Li–Fraumeni syndrome. *Cancer Res.*, **51**, 6094–7.

Gardner, E., Papi, L., Easton, D.F. et al. (1993). Genetic linkage studies map the multiple endocrine neoplasia type 2 loci to a small interval on chromosome 10q11.2. *Hum. Mol. Genet.*, **2**, 241–6.

Garman, M.E., Blumberg, M.A., Ernst, R. & Rainer, S.S. (2003). Familial leiomyomatosis: a review and discussion of pathogenesis. *Dermatology*, **207**, 210–3.

Gatti, R.A., Berkel, I., Boder, E. et al. (1988). Localization of an ataxia telangiectasia gene to chromosome 11q22–23. *Nature*, **336**, 577–80.

Gatti, R.A., Tward, A. & Concannon, P. (1999). Cancer risk in ATM heterozygotes: a model of phenotypic and mechanistic differences between missense and truncating mutations. *Mol. Genet. Metab.*, **68**, 419–23.

Gatto, N.M., Frucht, H., Sundararajan, V., Jacobson, J.S., Grann, V.R. & Neugut, A.I. (2003). Risk of perforation after colonoscopy and sigmoidoscopy: a population-based study. *J. Natl. Cancer Inst.*, **95**, 230–6.

Gayther, S.A., Warren, W., Mazoyer, S. et al. (1995). Germline mutations of the BRCA1 gene in breast and ovarian cancer families provide evidence for genotype/phenotype correlation. *Nat. Genet.*, **11**, 428–33.

Gayther, S.A., Mangion, J., Russel, P. et al. (1997a). Variation of risks of breast and ovarian cancer associated with different germline mutations of the BRCA2 gene. *Nat. Genet.*, **15**, 101–5.

Gayther, S.A., Harrington, P., Russell, P., Kharkevich, G., Garkavtseva, R.F. & Ponder, B.A. (1997b). Frequently occurring germ-line mutations of the BRCA1 gene in ovarian cancer families from Russia [letter]. *Am. J. Hum. Genet.*, **60**, 1239–42.

Gayther, S.A., Gorringe, K.L., Ramus, S.J. et al. (1998). Identification of germ-line E-cadherin mutations in gastric cancer families of European origin. *Cancer Res.*, **58**, 4086–9.

Gayther, S.A., de Foy, K.A., Harrington, P. et al. (2000). The frequency of germ-line mutations in the breast cancer predisposition genes BRCA1 and BRCA2 in familial prostate cancer. The Cancer Research Campaign/British Prostate Group United Kingdom Familial Prostate Cancer Study Collaborators. *Cancer Res.*, **60**, 4513–18.

Gazda, H., Lipton, J.M., Willig, T.N., Ball, S., Niemeyer, C.M., Tchernia, G., Mohandas, N., Daly, M.J., Ploszynska, A., Orfali, K.A., Vlachos, A., Glader, B.E., Rokicka-Milewska, R., Ohara, A., Baker, D., Pospisilova, D., Webber, A., Viskochil, D.H., Nathan, D.G., Beggs, A.H., Sieff, C.A. (2001). Evidence for linkage of familial Diamond–Blackfan anemia to chromosome 8p23.3–p22 and for non-19q non-8p disease. *Blood*, **97**(7), 2145–50.

Gelberg, K.H., Fitzgerald, E.F., Hwang, S. et al. (1997). Growth and development and other risk factors for osteosarcoma in children and young adults. *Int. J. Epidemiol.*, **26**, 272–8.

Gentry Jr, W.C., Eskritt, N.R. & Gorlin, R.J. (1978). Multiple hamartomata syndrome (Cowden disease). *Arch. Dermatol.*, **114**, 743–6.

Genuardi, M., Klutz, M., Devriendt, K. et al. (2001). Multiple lipomas linked to an RBI gene mutation in a large pedigree with low penetrance retinoblastoma. *Eur. J. Hum. Genet.*, **9**(9), 690–4.

Ghadirian, P., Liu, G., Gallinger, S., Schmocker, B., Paradis, A.J., Lal, G., Brunet, J.S., Foulkes, W.D. & Narod, S.A. (2002). Risk of pancreatic cancer among individuals with a family history of cancer of the pancreas. *Int. J. Cancer*, **97**, 807–10.

Ghimenti, C., Sensi, E., Presciuttini, S., Brunetti, I.M., Conte, P., Bevilacqua, G. & Caligo, M.A. (2002). Germline mutations of the BRCA1-associated ring domain (BARD1) gene in breast and breast/ovarian families negative for BRCA1 and BRCA2 alterations. *Gene. Chromosome. Cancer*, **33**, 235–42.

Ghiorzo, P., Ciotti, P., Mantelli, M., Heouaine, A., Queirolo, P., Rainero, M.L., Ferrari, C., Santi, P.L., De Marchi, R., Farris, A., Ajmar, F., Bruzzi, P. & Bianchi-Scarra, G. (1999). Characterization of ligurian melanoma families and risk of occurrence of other neoplasia. *Int. J. Cancer*, **83**, 441–8.

Ghiorzo, P., Pastorino, L., Bonelli, L. et al. (2004). INK4/ARF germline alterations in pancreatic cancer patients. *Ann. Oncol.*, **15**(1), 70–8.

Giannelli, F. (1986). DNA maintenance and its relation to human pathology. *J. Cell. Sci. Suppl.*, **4**, 383–416.

Giardiello, F.M., Welsh, S.B., Hamilton, S.R. et al. (1987). Increased risk of cancer in the Peutz–Jeghers syndrome. *New Engl. J. Med.*, **316**, 1511–14.

Giardiello, F.M., Petersen, G.M., Piantadosi, S. et al. (1997). APC gene mutations and extraintestinal phenotype of familial adenomatous polyposis. *Gut*, **40**, 521–5.

Gibril, F., Chen, Y.J., Schrump, D.S., Vortmeyer, A., Zhuang, Z., Lubensky, I.A., Reynolds, J.C., Louie, A., Entsuah, L.K., Huang, K., Asgharian, B. & Jensen, R.T. (2003). Prospective study of thymic carcinoids in patients with multiple endocrine neoplasia type 1. *J. Clin. Endocrinol. Metab.*, **88**, 1066–81.

Gicquel, C., Gaston, V., Mandelbaum, J., Siffro, J.-P., Flahault, A. & Le Bouc, Y. (2003). In vitro fertilization may increase the risk of Beckwith–Wiedemann syndrome related to abnormal imprinting of the KCNQ1OT gene. *Am. J. Hum. Genet.*, **72**, 1338–41.

Giebel, L.B., Tripathi, R.K., Strunk, K.M. et al. (1991). Tyrosine gene mutations associated with type 1B ('yellow') oculocutaneous albinism. *Am. J. Hum. Genet.*, **48**, 1159–67.

Gilchrist, D.M. & Savard, M.L. (1989). Ependymomas in two sisters and a maternal male cousin. *Am. J. Med. Genet.*, **45**, A22.

Gilgenkrantz, S., Mujica, P., Chery, M. et al. (1989). Mapping the breakpoint at 11 p11.2 in synovial sarcoma. *Cytogenet. Cell Genet.*, **51**, 1004 [Abstract].

Gillanders, E., Hank Juo, S.H., Holland, E.A. et al. (2003). Localization of a novel melanoma susceptibility locus to 1p22. *Am. J. Hum. Genet.*, **73**(2), 301–13.

Gimm, O., Marsh, D.J., Andrew, S.D. et al. (1997). Germline dinucleotide mutation in codon 883 of the *RET* proto-oncogene in multiple endocrine neoplasia type 2B without codon 918 mutation. *J. Clin. Endocrinol. Metab.*, **82**, 3902–4.

Gimm, O., Armanios, M., Dziema, H., Neumann, H.P.H. & Eng, C. (2000). Somatic and occult germline mutations in *SDHD*, a mitochondrial complex II gene, in non-familial pheochromocytomas. *Cancer Res.*, **60**, 6822–5.

Giraud, S., Zhang, C.X., Serova-Sinilnikova, O., et al. (1998). Germ-line mutation analysis in patients with multiple endocrine neoplasia type 1 and related disorders. *Am. J. Hum. Genet.*, **63**, 455–67.

Gisbert, J.P., Garcia-Buey, L. & Alonso, A. (2004). Hepatocellular carcinoma risk in patients with porphyria cutanea tarda. *Eur. J. Gastroenterol. Hepatol* **16**, 689–92.

Gismondi, V., Bonelli, L., Sciallero, S. et al. (2002). Prevalence of the E1317Q variant of the APC gene in Italian patients with colorectal adenomas. *Genet. Test.*, **6**, 313–17.

Godard, B., Foulkes, W.D., Provencher, D., Brunet, J.S., Tonin, P.N., Mes-Masson, A.M, Narod, S.A. & Ghadirian, P. (1998). Risk factors for familial and sporadic ovarian cancer among French Canadians: a case–control study. *Am. J. Obstet. Gynecol.*, **179**, 403–10.

Goerttler, E.A. & Jung, E.G. (1975). Porokeratosis of Mibelli and skin carcinoma: a critical review. *Humangenetik*, **26**, 291–6.

Goffin, J., Chappuis, P.O., Wong, N. & Foulkes, W.D. (2001). Re: Magnetic resonance imaging and mammography in women with a hereditary risk of breast cancer. *J. Natl. Cancer Inst.*, **93**, 1754–5.

Gold, B., Kalush, F., Bergeron, J., Scott, K., Mitra, N., Wilson, K., Ellis, N., Huang, H., Chen, M., Lippert, R., Halldorsson, B.V., Woodworth, B., White, T., Clark, A.G., Parl, F.F., Broder, S., Dean, M. & Offit, K. (2004). Estrogen receptor genotypes and haplotypes associated with breast cancer risk. *Cancer Res.*, **64**, 8891–900.

Gold, E.B., Leviton, A., Lopez, R., Austin, D.F., Gilles, F.H., Hedley-Whyte, E.T., Kolonel, L.N., Lyon, J.L., Swanson, G.M. & Weiss, N.S. (1994). The role of family history in risk of childhood brain tumors. *Cancer*, **73**, 1302–11.

Goldberg, G.I., Eisen, A.Z. & Bauer, E.A. (1988). Tissue stress and tumour promotion. *Arch. Dermatol.*, **124**, 737–41.

Goldfarb, D.A., Neumann, H.P.H., Penn, I., Novick, A.C. (1998). Results of renal transplantation in patients with renal cell carcinoma in Von Hippel–Lindau disease. *Transplantation*, **64**, 1726–9.

Goldgar, D.E., Easton, D.F., Cannon-Albright, L.A. & Skolnick, M.H. (1994). Systematic population-based assessment of cancer risk in first-degree relatives of cancer probands. *J. Natl. Cancer Inst.*, **86**, 1600–8.

Goldstein, A.M., Dracopoli, N.C., Engelstein, M., Fraser, M.C., Clark Jr, W.H. & Tucker, M.A. (1994). Linkage of cutaneous malignant melanoma dysplastic nevi to chromosome 9p, and evidence for genetic heterogeneity. *Am. J. Hum. Genet.*, **54**, 489–96.

Goldstein, A.M., Fraser, M.C., Struwing, J.R. et al. (1995). Increased risk of pancreatic cancer in melanoma-prone kindreds with p16INK4 mutations. *New Engl. J. Med.*, **333**, 970–4.

Goldstein, A.M., Struewing, J.P., Fraser, M.C., Smith, M.W. & Tucker, M.A. (2004). Prospective risk of cancer in CDKN2A germline mutation carriers. *J. Med. Genet.*, **41**, 421–4.

Gomez, M.R. (ed.). (1988). *Tuberous Sclerosis.* Raven Press, New York.

Goodman, S.N. (2002). The mammography dilemma: a crisis for evidence-based medicine? *Ann. Int. Med.*, **137**, 363–5.

Goodman, R.M., Caren, J., Ziprkowski, M. et al. (1971). Genetic consideration in giant pigmented hairy naevus. *Br. J. Dermatol.*, **85**, 150–7.

Goodship, J., Redfearn, A., Milligan, D. et al. (1991). Transmission of proteus syndrome from father to son? *J. Med. Genet.*, **28**, 781–6.

Goorin, A.M., Abelson, H.T. & Frei, E. (1985). Osteosarcoma: fifteen years later. *New Engl. J. Med.*, **313**, 1637–43.

Goransdotter Ericson, K., Fadeel, B., Nilsson-Ardnor, S. et al. (2001). Spectrum of perforin gene mutations in familial hemophagocytic lymphohistiocytosis. *Am. J. Hum. Genet.*, **68**, 590–7.

Gorlin, R.J. (1976). Some soft tissue heritable tumours. *Birth Defect.*, **XII**, 7–14.

Gorlin, R.J. (1984). Proteus syndrome. *J. Clin. Dysmorphol.*, **2**, 8–9.

Gorlin, R.J. (1987). Nevoid basal-cell carcinoma syndrome. *Medicine*, **66**, 98–113.

Gorlin, R.J. (1995). Nevoid basal cell carcinoma syndrome. *Dermatol. Clin.*, **13**, 113–25.

Gorlin, R.J. & Koutlas, I.G. (1998). Multiple schwannomas, multiple naevi, and multiple vaginal leiomyomas: a new dominant syndrome. *Am. J. Med. Genet.*, **78**, 76–81.

Gorlin, R.J., Sedano, H.O., Vickers, R.A. & Cervenka, J. (1968). Multiple mucosal neuromas, phaeochromocytoma and medullary carcinoma of the thyroid – a syndrome. *Cancer*, **22**, 293–9.

Gorlin, R.J., Cohen, M.M., Condon, L.M. & Burke, B.A. (1992). Bannayan-Riley-Ruvalcaba syndrome. *Am. J. Med. Genet.*, **44**, 307–14.

Gorski, B., Byrski, T., Huzarski, T., Jakubowska, A., Menkiszak, J., Gronwald, J., Pluzanska, A., Bebenek, M., Fischer-Maliszewska, L., Grzybowska, E., Narod, S.A. & Lubinski, J. (2000). Founder mutations in the BRCA1 gene in Polish families with breast-ovarian cancer. *Am. J. Hum. Genet.*, **66**, 1963–8.

Goss, K.H., Risinger, M.A., Kordich, J.J., Snaz, M.M., Straughen, L.E., Capobianco, A.J., German, J., Boivin, G.P. & Groden, J. (2002). Enhanced tumor formation in mice heterozygous for Blm mutation. *Science*, **297**(5589), 2051–3.

Goss, P.E. & Bulbul, M.A. (1990). Familial testicular cancer in five members of a cancer-prone kindred. *Cancer*, **66**, 2044–6.

Gotlieb, W.H., Friedman, E., Bar-Sade, R.B., Kruglikova, A., Hirsh-Yechezkel, G., Modan, B., Inbar, M., Davidson, B., Kopolovic, J., Novikov, I. & Ben-Baruch, G. (1998). Rates of Jewish ancestral mutations in BRCA1 and BRCA2 in borderline ovarian tumors. *J. Natl. Cancer Inst.*, **90**, 995–1000.

Goto, M., Miller, R.W., Ishikawa, Y. & Sugano, H. (1996). Excess of rare cancers in Werner syndrome (adult progeria). *Cancer Epidemiol. Biomark. Prev.*, **5**(4), 239–46.

Gotz, A., Kopera, D., Wach, F. et al. (1999). Porokeratosis Mibelli; case report and literature review. *Hantarz*, **50**, 435–8.

Goudie, D.R., Yuille, M.A.R., Affara, N.A. & Ferguson-Smith, M.A. (1991). Localisation of the gene for multiple self healing squamous epithelioma (Ferguson–Smith type) to the long arm of chromosome 9. *Cytogenet. Cell Genet.*, **58**, 1939.

Gould, D.J. & Barker, D.J. (1978). Follicular atrophoderma with multiple basal cell carcinomas. *Br. J. Dermatol.*, **99**, 431–5.

Gould, S.R., Stewart, J.B. & Temple, D.N. (1990). Rectal polyposis in tuberose sclerosis. *J. Ment. Defic. Res.*, **34**, 465–73.

Graham Jr, J.M., Anayne-Yeboa, K., Raams, A. et al. (2001). Cerebro-oculo-facio-skeletal syndrome with a nucleotide excision repair defect and a mutated XPD gene, with prenatal diagnosis in a triplet pregnancy. *Am. J. Hum. Genet.*, **69**, 291–300.

Granwetter, L. (1995). Ewing's sarcoma and extracranial peripheral neuroectodermal tumours. *Curr. Opin. Oncol.*, **7**, 355–60.

Gravholt, C.H., Fedder, J., Naeraa, R.W. & Muller, J. (2000). Occurrence of gonadoblastoma in females with Turner syndrome and Y chromosome material: a population study. *J. Clin. Endocrinol. Metab.*, **85**, 3199–202.

Green, J.S., Bowmer, M.I. & Johnson, G.J. (1986). Von Hippel–Lindau disease in a Newfoundland kindred. *Can. Med. Assoc. J.*, **134**, 133–46.

Greenberg, F., Stein, F., Gresnik, M.V. et al. (1986). The Perlman nephroblastomatosis syndrome. *Am. J. Med. Genet.*, **24**, 101–10.

Greenblatt, M.S., Chappuis, P.O., Bond, J.P., Hamel, N. & Foulkes, W.D. (2001). TP53 mutations in breast cancer associated with BRCA1 or BRCA2 germ-line mutations: distinctive spectrum and structural distribution. *Cancer Res.*, **61**, 4092–7.

Greene, M.H., Tucker, M.A., Clark Jr, W.H., Kraemer, K.H., Elder, D.E. & Fraser, M.C. (1987). Hereditary melanoma and the dysplastic nevus syndrome: the risk of cancers other than melanoma. *J. Am. Acad. Dermatol.*, **16**, 792–7.

Griffin, C.A., McKeon, C., Israel, M.A. et al. (1986). Comparison of constitutional and tumour-associated 11;22 translocations: nonidentical breakpoints on chromosomes 11 and 22. *Proc. Natl. Acad. Sci. USA*, **83**, 6122–6.

Griffiths, D.F.R., Williams, G.T. & Wilhaus, E.D. (1987). Duodenal carcinoid tumours, phaeochromocytoma and neurofibromatosis. Islet cell tumour, phaeochromocytoma and von Hippel–Lindau complex: two distinctive neuroendocrine syndromes. *Q. J. Med.*, **64**, 769–82.

Griffiths, G.M. (2002). Albinism & immunity: what's the link? *Curr. Mol. Med.*, **2**, 479–83.

Grignon, D.J., Shum, D.T. & Bruckschwaiger, O. (1987). Transitional cell carcinoma in the Muir–Torre syndrome. *J. Urol.*, **38**, 406–8.

Gripp, K.W., Scott Jr, C.I., Nicholson, L. et al. (2002). Five additional Costello patients with rhabdomyosarcoma: proposal for a tumour screening protocol. *Am. J. Med. Genet.*, **108**, 80–7.

Grob, J.J., Bretton, A., Bonafe, J.L. et al. (1987). Keratitis, icthyosis and deafness (KID) syndrome. *Arch. Dermatol.*, **123**, 777–82.

Groden, J., Thlivens, A. & Samowitz, W. (1991). Identification and characterisation of the familial adenomatous polyposis coli gene. *Cell*, **66**, 589–600.

Groet, J., McElwain, S., Spinelli, M. et al. (2003). Acquired mutations in GATA1 in neonates with Downs syndrome with transient myeloid disorders. *Lancet*, **361**, 1617–20.

Gronskov, K. et al. (2001). Population-based risk estimates of Wilms tumor in sporadic aniridia. A comprehensive mutation screening procedure of PAX6 identifies 80% of mutations in aniridia. *Hum. Genet.*, **109**(1), 11–18.

Groves, C.J., Saunders, B.P., Spigelman, A.D. & Phillips, R.K. (2002). Duodenal cancer in patients with familial adenomatous polyposis (FAP); results of a 10 year prospective study. Gut, **50**, 636–41.

Gruber, S.B., Ellis, N.A., Rennert, G., Offit, K., Scott, K.K., Almog, R., Kolachana, P., Bonner, J.D., Kirchhoff, T., Tomsho, L.P., Nafa, K., Pierce, H., Low, M., Satagopan, J., Rennert, H., Huang, H., Greenson, J.K., Groden, J., Rapaport, B., Shia, J., Johnson, S., Gregersen, P.K., Harris, C.C. & Boyd, J. (2002). BLM heterozygosity and the risk of colorectal cancer. *Science*, **297**(5589), 2013.

Grufferman, S., Cole, P., Smith, P.G. & Lukes, R.J. (1977). Hodgkin's disease in siblings. *New Engl. J. Med.*, **296**, 248–50.

Grufferman, S., Gillman, M.W., Pasternak, L.R., Peterson, C.L. & Young, W.G. (1980). Familial carotid body tumors: case report and epidemiologic review. *Cancer*, **46**: 2116–22.

Grundbacher, F.J. (1972). Genetic aspects of selective IgA deficiency. *J. Med. Genet.*, **9**, 344–7.

Grundy, P., Telzerow, P., Paterson, M.C. et al. (1991). Chromosome 11 uniparental disomy predisposing to embryonal neoplasms. *Lancet*, **338**, 1079–80.

Gryfe, R., Di Nicola, N., Lal, G., Gallinger, S. & Redston, M. (1999). Inherited colorectal polyposis and cancer risk of the APC I1307K polymorphism. *Am. J. Hum. Genet.*, **64**, 378–84.

Gryfe, R., Kim, H., Hsieh, E.T.K., Aronson, M.D., Holowaty, E.J., Bull, S.B., Redston, M. and Gallinger, S. (2000). Tumor microsatellite instability and clinical outcome in young patients with colorectal cancer. *New Engl. J. Med.*, **342**(2), 69–77.

Guarneri, B., Borgia, F., Cannaro, S.P. et al. (2000). Multiple familial BCCs and a case of segmental manifestations. *Dermatol.*, **200**, 299–302.

Gubler, J.G., Bargetzi, M.J. & Meyer, U.A. (1990). Primary liver carcinoma in two sisters with acute intermittent porphyria. *Am. J. Med.*, **89**, 540–1.

Guilford, P., Hopkins, J., Harraway, J. et al. (1998). E-cadherin germline mutations in familial gastric cancer. *Nature*, **392**, 402–5.

Gul, D. et al. (2002). Third case of WAGR syndrome with severe obesity and constitutional deletion of chromosome (11)(p12p14). *Am. J. Med. Genet.*, **107**(1), 70–1.

Gunel, M., Awad, I.A., Finberg, K. et al. (1996). Genetic heterogeneity of inherited cerebral cavernous malformation. *Neurosurgery*, **38**, 1265–71.

Gunz, F.W., Gunz, J.P., Veale, A.M.O., Chapman, C.J. & Houston, I.E. (1975). Familial leukaemia: a study of 909 families. *Scand. J. Haematol.*, **15**, 117–31.

Gustavson, K.H., Garmstorp, I. & Meurling, S. (1975). Bilateral teratoma of testis in two brothers with 47XXY Klinefelter's syndrome. *Clin. Genet.*, **8**, 5–10.

Gustavsson, P., Willig, T.-N., van Hareingen, A. et al. (1997). Diamond–Blackfan anaemia: genetic homogeneity for a gene on chromosome 19q13 restricted to 1.8Mb. *Nat. Genet.*, **16**, 368–71.

Gutierrez, P.P., Eggenmena, T., Holler, D. et al. (2002). Phenotype diversity in familial cylindromatosis: a frameshift mutation in the tumour expressor gene CYLD underlies different tumours of skin. *J. Invest. Dermatol.*, **119**, 527–31.

Habdous, M. et al. (2004). Glutathione S-transferases genetic polymorphisms and human diseases: overview of epidemiological studies. *Ann. Biol. Clin. (Paris).*, **62**(1), 15–24.

Haber, R.M. & Hanna, W.M. (1996). Kindler syndrome. Clinical and ultrastructural findings. *Arch. Dermatol.*, **132**, 1487–90.

Haerer, A.F., Jackson, J.F. & Evers, C.G. (1969). Ataxia telangiectasia with gastric adenocarcinoma. *J. Am. Med. Assoc.*, **210**, 1884–7.

Hahn, H., Wickling, C., Zaphiropoulous, P.G. et al. (1996). Mutations of the human homologue of *Drosophila* patched in the nevoid basal cell carcinoma syndrome. *Cell*, **85**, 841–51.

Hahn, S.A., Greenhalf, B., Ellis, I., Sina-Frey, M., Rieder, H., Korte, B., Gerdes, B., Kress, R., Ziegler, A., Raeburn, J.A., Campra, D., Grutzmann, R., Rehder, H., Rothmund, M., Schmiegel, W., Neoptolemos, J.P. & Bartsch, D.K. (2003). BRCA2 germline mutations in familial pancreatic carcinoma. *J. Natl. Cancer Inst.*, **95**, 214–21.

Hahnloser, D., Petersen, G.M., Rabe, K. et al. (2003). The APC E1317Q variant in adenomatous polyps and colorectal cancers. *Cancer Epidemiol. Biomark. Prev.*, **12**, 1023–8.

Halford, S.E., Rowan, R.J., Lipton, L. et al. (2003). Germline mutations but not somatic changes at the MYH locus contributes to the pathogenesis of unselected colorectal cancer. *Am. J. path.*, **162**, 1545–8.

Hall, B.D. (1985). Leukaemia and Prader–Willi syndrome. *Lancet*, **i**, 46.

Hamel, N., Wong, N., Alpert, L. et al. (2006). Mixed ovarian germ cell tumor in a *BRCA2* mutation carrier. *Int. J. Gynecol. Pathol.* (in press).

Hamilton, S.R., Liu, B., Parsons, R.E. et al. (1995). The molecular basis of Turcot's syndrome. *New Engl. J. Med.*, **332**, 839–47.

Hamm, H. (1999). Cutaneous mosaics of lethal mutations. *Am. J. Med. Genet.*, **85**, 342–5.

Hamm, J., Traupe, H., Brocker, E.B. et al. (1996). The scleroatrophic syndrome of Huriez: a cancer-prone genodermatosis. *Br. J. Dermatol.*, **134**, 512–18.

Hammami, M.M., al-Zahrani, A., Butt, A., Vencer, L.J. & Hussain, S.S. (1997). Primary hyperparathyroidism-associated polyostotic fibrous dysplasia: absence of McCune–Albright syndrome mutations. *J. Endocrinol. Invest.*, **20**, 552–8.

Hampel, H., Sweet, K., Westman, J.A. et al. (2004). *J. Med. Genet.*, **41**, 81–91.

Haneke, E. & Gutschmidt, E. (1979). Premature multiple Bowen's disease in poikiloderma congenitale with warty hyperkeratoses. *Dermatologica*, **158**, 384–8.

Hanks, S., Coleman, K., Reid, S., Plaja, A., Firth, H., Fitzpatrick, D., Kidd, A., Mehes, K., Nash, R., Robin, N., Shannon, N., Tolmie, J., Swansbury, J., Irrthum, A., Douglas, J. & Rahman, N. (2004). Constitutional aneuploidy and cancer predisposition caused by biallelic mutations in BUB1B. *Nat. Genet.*, **36**(11), 1159–61.

Hanssen, A.M.N. & Fryns, J.P. (1995). Cowden syndrome. *J. Med. Genet.*, **32**, 117–19.

Happle, R. (1989). The McCune Albright syndrome: a lethal gene surviving by mosaicism. *Clin. Genet.*, **29**, 321–4.

Happle, R. (2000). Nonsyndromic type of hereditary multiple basal cell carcinoma. *Am. J. Med. Genet.*, **95**, 161–3.

Harach, H.R., Williams, G.T. & Williams, E.D. (1994). Familial adenomatous polyposis associated thyroid carcinoma: a distinct type of follicular cell neoplasm. *Histopathology*, **25**, 549–61.

Harach, H.R., Soubeyran, I., Brown, A., Bonneau, D. & Longy, M. (1999). Thyroid pathologic findings in patients with Cowden disease. *Ann. Diagn. Pathol.*, **3**, 331–40.

Harada, H., Hashimoto, K. & Ko, M.S.H. (1996). The gene for multiple familial trichoepithelioma maps to chromosome 9p21. *J. Invest. Dermatol.*, **107**, 41–3.

Harland, M., Meloni, R., Gruis, N. et al. (1997). Germline mutations of the CDKN2 gene in UK melanoma families. *Hum. Mol. Genet.*, **6**, 2061–7.

Harland, M., Holland, E.A., Ghiorzo, P. et al. (2000). Mutation screening of the CDKN2A promoter in melanoma families. *Gene. Chromosome. Cancer*, **28**(1), 45–57.

Harland, M., Mistry, S., Bishop, D.T. & Bishop, J.A. (2001). A deep intronic mutation in CDKN2A is associated with disease in a subset of melanoma pedigrees. *Hum. Mol. Genet.*, **10**(23), 2679–86.

Harnden, D.G., Maclean, N. & Langlands, A.O. (1971). Carcinoma of the breast and Klinefelter syndrome. *J. Med. Genet.*, **8**, 460–1.

Harper, P.S. (1972). Calcifying epithelioma of Malherbe. Association with myotonic muscular dystrophy. *Arch. Dermatol.*, **106**, 41–4.

Harper, P.S. (1973). Heredity and gastrointestinal tumours. *Clin. Gastroenterol.*, **2**, 695–701.

Harper, P.S., Harper, R.M.J. & Howel-Evans, A.W. (1970). Carcinoma of the oesophagus with tylosis. *Q. J. Med.*, **39**, 317–33.

Harris, A.L. (1991). Telling changes of base. *Nature*, **350**, 377–8.

Harris, O.D., Cook, W.T., Thompson, H. & Waterhouse II, J.A. (1967). Malignancy in adult coeliac disease and ideopathic steatorrhoea. *Am. J. Med.*, **42**, 895–912.

Harris, W.R. (1990). Chondrosarcoma complicating total hip arthroplasty in Maffucci's syndrome. *Clin. Orthop.*, **260**, 212–14.

Harrison, S.A. & Bacon, B.R. (2005). Relation of hemochromatosis with hepatocellular carcinoma: epidemiology, natural history, pathophysiology, screening, treatment, and prevention. *Med. Clin. North Am.*, **89**(2), 391–409.

Hartge, P., Schiffman, M.H., Hoover, R., McGowan, L., Lesher, L. & Norris, H.J. (1989). A case–control study of epithelial ovarian cancer. *Am. J. Obstetr. Gynecol.*, **161**, 10–16.

Hartley, A.L., Birch, J.M., Marsden, H.B. et al. (1986). Breast cancer risk in mothers of children with osteosarcoma and chondrosarcoma. *Br. J. Cancer*, **54**, 819–23.

Hartley, A.L., Birch, J.M., Marsden, H.B., Harris, M. & Blair, V. (1988). Neurofibromatosis in children with soft tissue sarcoma. *Pediatr. Hematol. Oncol.*, **5**, 7–16.

Hartley, A.L., Birch, J.M., Kelsey, A.M. et al. (1990). Epidemiological and familial aspects of hepatoblastoma. *Med. Pediatr. Oncol.*, **18**, 103–9.

Hartley, A.L., Birch, J.M., Blair, V. et al. (1993). Patterns of cancer in the families of children with soft tissue sarcomas. *Cancer*, **72**, 923–30.

Hartmann, A. et al. (2002). Frequent microsatellite instability in sporadic tumors of the upper urinary tract. *Cancer Res.* **62**(23), 6796–802.

Hartman, A.R. & Ford, J.M. (2002). BRCA1 induces DNA damage recognition factors and enhances nucleotide excision repair. *Nat. Genet.*, **32**, 180–4.

Harwood, C.A., McGregor, J.M., Swale, V.J., Proby, C.M., Leigh, I.M., Newton, R., Khorshid, S.M. & Cerio, R. (2003). High frequency and diversity of cutaneous appendageal tumors in organ transplant recipients. *J. Am. Acad. Dermatol.*, **48**(3), 401–8.

Hashibe, M., Brennan, P., Strange, R.C., Bhiseym, R., Cascorbi, I., Lazarus, P., Oude Ophuis, M.B., Benhamou, S., Foulkes, W.D., Katoh, T., Coutelle, C., Romkes, M., Gaspari, L., Taioli, E. & Boffetta, P. (2003). Meta- and pooled analyses of GSTM1, GSTT1, GSTP1, and CYP1A1 genotypes and risk of head and neck cancer. *Cancer Epidemiol. Biomark. Prev.*, **12**, 1509–17.

Hashizume, R., Fukuda, M., Maeda, I., Nishikawa, H., Oyake, D., Yabuki, Y., Ogata, H. & Ohta, T. (2001). The RING heterodimer BRCA1-BARD1 is a ubiquitin ligase inactivated by a breast cancer-derived mutation. *J. Biol. Chem.*, **276**, 14537–40.

Hasle, H. (2001). Pattern of malignant disorders in individuals with Downs syndrome. *Lancet Oncol.*, **2**, 429–36.

Hasle, H., Mellengaard, A., Nielson, J. & Hanses, J. (1995). Cancer incidence in men with Klinefelter syndrome. *Br. J. Cancer*, **71**, 416–20.

Hasle, H., Hammerstrup Clemensau, I. & Mikkelson, M. (2000). Risks of leukaemia and other tumours in individuals with Downs syndrome. *Lancet*, **355**, 165–9.

Hatada, I., Ohashi, H., Fukushima, Y. et al. (1996). An imprinted gene p57^{KIP2} is mutated in Beckwith–Wiedemann syndrome. *Nat. Genet.*, **14**, 171–3.

Hauben, E.I. et al. (2003). Multiple primary malignancies in osteosarcoma patients. Incidence and predictive value of osteosarcoma subtype for cancer syndromes related with osteosarcoma. *Eur. J. Hum. Genet.*, **11**(8), 611–18.

Hayoz, D., Extermann, M., Odermatt, B.F. et al. (1993). Familial primary gastric lymphoma. *Gut*, **34**, 136–40.

Hayward, B.E., De Vos, M., Sheridan, E. & Bonthron, D.T. (2004). PMS2 mutations in HNPCC. *Clin. Genet.*, **66**(6), 566–7.

Hayward, N.K. (2003). Genetics of melanoma predisposition. *Oncogene*, **22**, 3053–62.

Hearle, N., Damato, B.E., Humphreys, J., Wixey, J., Green, H., Stone, J., Easton, D.F., Houlston, R.S. (2003). Contribution of germline mutations in BRCA2, P16(INK4A), P14(ARF) and P15 to uveal melanoma. *Invest. Ophthalmol. Vis. Sci.*, **44**(2), 458–62.

Hecht, J.T., Hogue, D., Strong, L.C. et al. (1995). Hereditary multiple exostosis and chondrosarcoma: linkage to chromosome 11 and loss of heterozygosity for EXT-linked markers on chromosomes 11 and 8. *Am. J. Hum. Genet.*, **56**, 1125–31.

Hecht, J.T., Hogue, D., Wang, Y. et al. (1997). Hereditary multiple exostoses (EXT): mutational studies of familial EXT1 cases and EXR-associated malignancies. *Am. J. Hum. Genet.*, **60**, 80–6.

Hedenfalk, I., Duggan, D., Chen, Y., Radmacher, M., Bittner, M., Simon, R., Meltzer, P., Gusterson, B., Esteller, M., Kallioniemi, O.P., Wilfond, B., Borg, A. & Trent, J. (2001). Gene-expression profiles in hereditary breast cancer. *New Engl. J. Med.*, **344**, 539–48.

Heim, S. & Mitelman, F. (1987). *Cancer Cytogenetics*. Alan Liss Inc., New York.

Heim, S., Nilbert, M., Vanni, R. et al. (1988). A specific translocation (t(12:14) (q14–15;q23–24) characterises a subgroup of uterine leiomyomas. *Cancer Genet. Cytogenet.*, **32**, 13–17.

Heiman, R., Verhest, A., Verschraegen, J., Grosjean, W., Draps, J.P. & Hecht, F. (1988). Hereditary intestinal neurofibromatosis. *Neurofibromatosis*, **1**, 26–32.

Heimdal, K., Olsson, H., Tretli, S., Fossa, S.D., Borresen, A.L. & Bishop, D.T. (1997). A segregation analysis of testicular cancer based on Norwegian and Swedish families. *Br. J. Cancer*, **75**, 1084–7.

Heiskanen, I., Luostarinen, T. & Jarvinen, H.J. (2000). Impact of screening examinations on survival in familial adenomatous polyposis. *Scand. J. Gastroenterol.*, **35**(12), 1284–7.

Hemminki, A., Tomlinson, I., Markie, D. et al. (1997). Localisation of a susceptibility locus for Peutz-Jeghers syndrome to 19p using comparative genomic hybridization and targeted linkage analysis. *Nat. Genet.*, **15**, 87–90.

Hemminki, A., Markie, D., Tomlinson, I. et al. (1998). A serine/threonine kinase gene defective in Peutz–Jeghers syndrome. *Nature*, **391**, 184–7.

Hemminki, K. (2002). Re: Familial multiple myeloma: a family study and review of the literature. *J. Natl. Cancer Inst.*, **94**(6), 462–3.

Hemminki, K. & Li, X. (2004). Familial renal cell cancer appears to have a recessive component. *J. Med. Genet.*, **41**(5), e58.

Hemminki, K., Vaittinen, P. & Kyyronen, P. (1998). Age-specific familial risks in common cancers of the offspring. *Int. J. Cancer*, **78**, 172–5.

Hennekam, R.C.M. (1991). Hereditary multiple exostoses. *J. Med. Genet.*, **28**, 262–6.

Henneveld, H.T., van Lingen, R.A., Hamel, B.C.J., Stolte-Dijkstra, I. & van Essen, A.J. (1999). Perlman syndrome: four additional cases and review. *Am. J. Med. Genet.*, **86**, 439–46.

Hennies, H.-C., Hagedorn, M. & Rais, A. (1995). Palmoplantar keratoderma in association with carcinoma of the esophagus maps to chromosome 17q distal to the keratin gene cluster. *Genomics*, **29**, 537–40.

Herera, L., Kakatis, S. & Gibas, L. (1986). Gardner syndrome in a man with an interstitial deletion of 5q. *Am. J. Med. Genet.*, **25**, 473–6.

Herzog, C.E., Andrassy, R.J. & Eftekhari, F. (2000). Childhood cancers: hepatoblastoma. *Oncologist.*, **5**(6), 445–53.

Hes, F.J., McKee, S., Taphoorn, M.J.B., Rehal, P., van der Luijt, R.B., McMahon, R., van der Smagt, J.J., Dow, D., Zewald, R.A., Whittaker, J., Lips, C.J.M., MacDonald, F., Pearson, P.L. & Maher, E.R. (2000). Cryptic von Hippel–Lindau disease: germline mutations in patients with haemangioblastoma only. *J. Med. Gen.*, **37**, 939–43.

Heutink, P., van der Mey, A.G.L., Sandkuijl, L.A. et al. (1992). A gene subject to genomic imprinting and responsible for hereditary paragangliomas maps to 11q23-qter. *Hum. Mol. Genet.*, **1**, 7–10.

Heutink, P., van Schothorst, E.M. & van der Mey, A.G.L. (1994). Further localization of the gene for hereditary paragangliomas and evidence for linkage in unrelated families. *Eur. J. Hum. Genet.*, **2**, 148–58.

Hewitt, C., Lee Wu, C., Evans, G. et al. (2002). Germline mutation of ARF in a melanoma kindred. *Hum. Mol. Genet.*, **11**(11), 1273–9.

Hibi, K., Kondo, K., Akiyama, S. et al. (1997). Frequent genetic instability in small intestinal carcinomas. *Jpn. J. Cancer Res.*, **86**, 357–60.

Hildesheim, A., Apple, R.J., Chen, C.J., Wang, S.S., Cheng, Y.J., Klitz, W., Mack, S.J., Chen, I.H., Hsu, M.M., Yang, C.S., Brinton, L.A., Levine, P.H. & Erlich, H.A. (2002). Association of HLA class I and II alleles and extended haplotypes with nasopharyngeal carcinoma in Taiwan. *J. Natl. Cancer Inst.*, **94**, 1780–9.

Hildreth, N.G., Kelsey, J.L., LiVolsi, V.A., Fischer, D.B., Holford, T.R., Mostow, E.D., Schwartz, P.E. & White, C. (1981). An epidemiologic study of epithelial carcinoma of the ovary. *Am. J. Epidemiol.*, **114**, 398–405.

Hillmann, A., Ozaki, T. & Winkelmann, W. (2000). Familial occurrence of osteosarcoma. A case report and review of the literature. *J. Cancer Res. Clin. Oncol.*, **126**, 497–502.

Hirsch, B., Shimamura, A., Moreau, L., Baldinger, S., Hag-alshiekh, M., Bostrom, B., Sencer, S. & D'Andrea, A.D. (2004). Association of biallelic BRCA2/FANCD1 mutations with spontaneous chromosomal instability and solid tumors of childhood. *Blood*, **103**, 2554–9.

Hirschman, B.A., Pollack, B.H., Tomlinson, G.E. et al. (2005). The spectrum of APC mutations in children with hepatoblastoma from familial adenomatous polyposis kindreds. *J. Paediatrics*, **147**, 263–6.

Hirvonen, A. (1995). Genetic factors in individual responses to environmental exposures. *J. Occup. Environ. Med.*, **37**, 37–43.

Hitzler, J.K. & Zipursky, A. (2005). Origins of leukaemia in children with Down syndrome. *Nat. Rev. Cancer.*, **5**(1), 11–20.

Hjalgrim, H., Rasmussen, S., Rostgaard, K., Nielsen, N.M., Koch-Henriksen, N., Munksgaard, L., Storm, H.H. & Melbye, M. (2004). Familial clustering of Hodgkin lymphoma and multiple sclerosis. *J. Natl. Cancer Inst.*, **96**(10), 780–4.

Ho, C.Y., Otterud, B., Legare, R.D. et al. (1996). Linkage of a familial platelet disorder with a propensity to develop myeloid malignancies to human chromosome 21q22.1–22.2. *Blood*, **87**, 5218–24.

Hoanq, M.P., Sinkre, P. & Albores-Savedras, J. (2002). Rhabdomyosarcoma arising in a congenital melanogotic naevus. *Am. J. Dermatopath.*, **24**, 26–9.

Hochberg, F.H., Dasilva, A.B., Galdabini, J. & Richardson Jr, E.P. (1974). Gastrointestinal involvement in Von Recklinghausen's neurofibromatosis. *Neurology*, **24**, 1144–51.

Hodes, M.E. & Norins, A.L. (1977). Pachonychia congenita and steatocystoma multiplex. *Clin. Genet.*, **11**, 359–64.

Hodges, A.K., Li, S., Maynard, J., Parry, L., Braverman, R., Cheadle, J.P., DeClue, J.E. & Sampson, J.R. (2001). Pathological mutations in TSC1 and TSC2 disrupt the interaction between hamartin and tuberin. *Hum Mol Genet.*, **10**, 2899–905.

Hodgson, S.V. & Murday, V. (1994). Other genetic conditions associated with gastrointestinal polyps. In *Familial Adenomatous Polyposis and Other Polyposis Syndromes*, eds.

Phillips, R.K.S., Spigelman, A.D. & Thomson, J.P.S. Edward Arnold, London, pp. 215–27.

Hodgson, S.V., Coonar, A.S., Hanson, P.J.V. et al. (1993). Two cases of 5q deletions in patients with familial adenomatous polyposis: possible link with Caroli's disease. *J. Med. Genet.*, **30**, 369–75.

Hodgson, S.V., Bishop, D.T. & Jay, B. (1994). Genetic heterogeneity of congenital hypertrophy of the retinal pigment epithelium (CHRPE) in families with familial adenomatous polyposis. *J. Med. Genet.*, **31**, 55–8.

Hodgson, S.V., Bishop, D.T., Dunlop, M.G. et al. (1995). Suggested screening guidelines for familial colorectal cancer. *J. Med. Screening*, **2**, 45–51.

Hodgson, S.V., Heap, E., Cameron, J. et al. (1999). Risk factors for detecting germline BRCA1 and BRCA2 founder mutations in Ashkenazi Jewish women with breast or ovarian cancer. *J. Med. Genet.*, **36**, 369–73.

Hodgson, S.V., Haiter, N.E., Caligo, M. et al. (2000). A survey of the cement clinical facilities for the management of familial cancer in Europe. European Union BIOHED II, *J. Med. Genet.*, **37**, 600–7.

Hofstra, R.M., Cheng, N.C., Hansen, C. et al. (1996). No mutations found by RET mutationscanning in sporadic and hereditary neuroblastoma. *Hum. Genet.*, **97**, 362–4.

Hofstra, R.M.W., Landsvater, R.M., Ceccherini, I., et al. (1994). A mutation in the *RET* proto-oncogene associated with multiple endocrine neoplasia type 2B and sporadic medullary thyroid carcinoma. *Nature*, **367**, 375–6.

Hogg, R. & Friedlander, M. (2004). Biology of epithelial ovarian cancer: implications for screening women at high genetic risk. *J. Clin. Oncol.*, **22**, 1315–27.

Holbach, L.M., von Moller, A., Decker, C., Junemann, A.G., Rummelt-Hofmann, C. & Ballhausen, W.G. (2002). Loss of fragile histidine triad (FHIT) expression and microsatellite instability in periocular sebaceous gland carcinoma in patients with Muir–Torre syndrome. *Am. J. Ophthalmol.*, **134**(1), 147–8.

Holland, E., Beaton, S., Becker, T. et al. (1995). Analysis of the p1 6 gene, CDKN2, in 17 Australian melanoma kindreds. *Oncogene*, **11**, 2289–94.

Holland, E.A., Schmid, H., Kefford, R.F. & Mann, G.J. (1999). CDKN2A (P16(INK4a)) and CDK4 mutation analysis in 131 Australian melanoma probands: effect of family history and multiple primary melanomas. *Gene. Chromosome. Cancer*, **25**(4), 339–48.

Holmes, G.K., Prior, P., Lane, M.R. et al. (1989). Malignancy in coeliac disease: effect of a gluten-free diet. *Gut*, **30**, 333–8.

Holmes, G.K.T., Dunn, G.I., Cockel, R. & Brookes, V.C. (1980). Adenocarcinoma of the upper small bowel complicating coeliac disease. *Gut*, **21**, 1010–15.

Hopyan, S., Gokgoz, N., Poon, R. et al. (2002). A mutant PTH/PTHrP type I receptor in enchondromatosis. *Nat. Genet.*, **30**, 306–10.

Horn, L.C., Raptis, G. & Fischer, U. (2002). Familial cancer history in patients with carcinoma of the cervix uteri. *Eur. J. Obstet. Gynecol. Reprod. Biol.*, **101**, 54–7.

Horwitz, L.J., Levy, R.N. & Rosner, F. (1985). Multiple myeloma in three siblings. *Arch. Int. Med.*, **145**, 1449–50.

Horwitz, M., Goode, E.L. & Jarvik, G.P. (1996). Anticipation in familial leukemia. *Am. J. Hum. Genet.*, **59**, 990–8.

Horwitz, M., Benson, K.F., Li, F.Q., Wolff, J., Leppert, M.F., Hobson, L., Mangelsdorf, M., Yu, S., Hewett, D., Richards, R.I. & Raskind, W.H. (1997). Genetic heterogeneity in familial acute myelogenous leukemia: evidence for a second locus at chromosome 16q21–23.2. *Am. J. Hum. Genetic.*, **61**, 873–81.

Houdayer, C., Gauthier-Villars, M., Lange, A. et al. (2004). Comprehensive screening for constitutional RBI mutations by DHPLC and QMPSF. *Hum. Mutat.*, **23**, 193–202.

Houlston, R. et al. (1998). Mutations in DPC4 (SMAD4) cause juvenile polyposis syndrome but only account for a minority of cases. *Hum. Mol. Genet.*, **7**, 1907–12.

Houlston, R.S. & Ford, D. (1996). Genetics of coeliac disease. *Q. J. Med.*, **89**, 737–43.

Houlston, R.S., Murday, V., Haracopos, C. et al. (1990). Screening and genetic counselling for relatives of patients with colorectal cancer in a family cancer clinic. *Br. Med. J.*, **301**, 366–8.

Houlston, R.S., Sellick, G., Yuille, M., Matutes, E., Catovsky, D. (2003). Causation of chronic lymphocytic leukemia – insights from familial disease. *Leukemia Res.*, **27**, 871–6.

Howdle, P.D., Jalal, P.K., Holmes, G.K. & Houlston, R.S. (2003). Primary small-bowel malignancy in the UK and its association with coeliac disease. *QJM.*, **96**, 345–53.

Howe, J.R., Norton, J.A. & Wells, S.A. (1993). Prevalence of pheochromocytoma and hyper-parathyroidism in multiple endocrine neoplasia type 2A: results of long-term follow-up. *Surgery*, **114**, 1070–7.

Howe, J.R., Roth, S., Ringold, J.C. et al. (1998b). Mutations in the *SMAD4/DPC4* gene in juvenile polyposis. *Science*, **280**, 1086–8.

Howe, J.R., Blair, J.A., Sayed, M.G. et al. (2001). Germline mutations of *BMPR1A* in juvenile polyposis. *Nat. Genet.*, **28**, 184–7.

Howell, V.M., Haven, C.J., Kahnoski, K. et al. (2003). *HRPT2* mutations are associated with malignancy in sporadic parathyroid tumours. *J. Med. Genet.*, **40**, 657–63.

Howes, N., Lerch, M.M., Greenhalf, W., Stocken, D.D., Ellis, I., Simon, P., Truninger, K., Ammann, R., Cavallini, G., Charnley, R.M., Uomo, G., Delhaye, M., Spicak, J., Drumm, B., Jansen, J., Mountford, R., Whitcomb, D.C. & Neoptolemos, J.P. (2004). Clinical and genetic characteristics of hereditary pancreatitis in Europe. *Clin. Gastroenterol. Hepatol.*, **2**, 252–61.

Howlett, N.G., Taniguchi, T., Olson, S., Cox, B., Waisfisz, Q., De Die-Smulders, C., Persky, N., Grompe, M., Joenje, H., Pals, G., Ikeda, H., Fox, E.A. & D'Andrea, A.D. (2002). Biallelic inactivation of BRCA2 in Fanconi anemia. *Science*, **297**, 606–9.

Hu, M., Zhang, G.Y., Arbuckle, S., Graf, N., Shun, A., Silink, M., Lewis, D., Alexander, S.I. (2004). Prophylactic bilateral nephrectomies in two paediatric patients with missense mutations in the WT1 gene. *Nephrol. Dial. Transplant.*, **19**(1), 223–6.

Hu, N., Li, G., Li, W.J., Wang, C., Goldstein, A.M., Tang, Z.Z., Roth, M.J., Dawsey, S.M., Huang, J., Wang, Q.H., Ding, T., Giffen, C., Taylor, P.R. & Emmert-Buck, M.R. (2002). Infrequent mutation in the BRCA2 gene in esophageal squamous cell carcinoma. *Clin. Cancer Res.*, **8**, 1121–6.

Hu, N., Wang, C., Han, X.Y., He, L.J., Tang, Z.Z., Giffen, C., Emmert-Buck, M.R., Goldstein, A.M. & Taylor, P.R. (2004). Evaluation of BRCA2 in the genetic susceptibility of familial esophageal cancer. *Oncogene*, **23**, 852–8.

Huang, D.P., Lo, K.-W., Choi, P.H.K. et al. (1991). Loss of heterozygosity on the short arm of chromosome 3 in nasopharyngeal carcinoma. *Cancer Genet. Cytogenet.*, **54**, 91–9.

Huang, H.S., Yeo, J., Shaw, Y. et al. (1988). Suppression of neoplastic phenotype by replacement of the RB gene in human cancer cells. *Science*, **242**, 1563–6.

Huang, R.L., Chao, C.F., Ding, D.C. et al. (2004). Multiple epithelial and non-epithelial tumours in hereditary non-polyposis colorectal cancer: characterisation of germline and somatic mutations of the MSH2 gene and heterogeneity of replication error phenotypes. *Cancer Genet. Cytogenet.*, **153**, 108–14.

Huang, S.C., Koch, C.A., Vortmeyer, A.O. et al. (2000). Duplication of the mutant *RET* allele in trisomy 10 or loss of the wild-type allele in multiple endocrine neoplasia type 2-associated pheochromocytoma. *Cancer Res.*, **60**, 6223–6.

Hubbard, V.G. & Whittaker, S.J. (2004). Multiple familial pilomatrixomas: an unusual case. *J. Cutan. Pathol.*, **31**, 281–3.

Huff, V., Amos, C.I., Douglass, E.G. et al. (1997). Evidence for genetic heterogeneity in familial Wilms' tumor. *Cancer Res.*, **57**, 1859–62.

Hughes-Benzie, R.M., Pilia, G., Xuan, J.Y. et al. (1996). Simpson–Golabi–Behmel syndrome: genotype/phenotype analysis of 18 affected males from 7 unrelated families. *Am. J. Med. Genet.*, **66**, 227–34.

Hughes-Davies, L., Huntsman, D., Ruas, M. et al. (2003). EMSY links the BRCA2 pathway to sporadic breast and ovarian cancer. *Cell*, **115**, 523–35.

Hung, K.L., Wu, C.M., Huang, J.S. & How, S.W. (1990). Familial medulloblastoma in siblings: report in one family and review of the literature. *Surg. Neurol.*, **33**, 341–6.

Huntsman, D.G., Carneiro, F., Lewis, F.R., MacLeod, P.M., Hayashi, A., Monaghan, K.G., Maung, R., Seruca, R., Jackson, C.E. & Caldas, C. (2001). Early gastric cancer in young, asymptomatic carriers of germ-line E-cadherin mutations. *New Engl. J. Med.*, **344**(25), 1904–9.

Huson, S.M., Harper, P.S. & Compston, D.A.S. (1988). Von Recklinghausen neurofibromatosis. *Brain*, **111**, 1355–81.

Huson, S.M., Compston, D.A.S. & Harper, P.S. (1989). A genetic study of von Recklinghausen neurofibromatosis in south east Wales. II. Guidelines for genetic counselling. *J. Med. Genet.*, **26**, 712–21.

Hwang, S.L., Lozano, G., Amos, C.L. & Strong, L.C. (2003). Germline *p53* mutations in a cohort with childhood sarcoma: sex differences in cancer risk. *Am. J. Hum. Genet.*, **72**, 975–83.

Hyer, N., Beveridge, I., Domizio, P. & Phillips, R. (2000). Clinical management of gastrointestimal polyps in children. *J. Paed. Gastro. Nutrit.*, **21**, 469–72.

Hyer, W. & Fell, J.M. (2001). Screening for familial adenomatous polyposis. *Arch. Dis. Child*, **84**, 377–80.

Iannello, S., Fabbri, G., Bosco, P. et al. (2003). A clinical variant of familial Hermansky–Pudlak syndrome. *Medscape. Gen. Med.*, **5**, 3.

Ilyas, M. & Tomlinson, I. (1997). The interactions of APC, E-cadherin and beta-catenin in tumour development and progression. *J. Pathol.*, **182**(2), 128–32.

Imai, K., Morio, T., Zhu, Y., Jin, Y., Itoh, S., Kajiwara, M., Yata, J., Mizutani, S., Ochs, H.D. & Nonoyama, S. (2004). Clinical course of patients with WASP gene mutations. *Blood*, **103**, 456–64.

Inoki, K., Corradetti, M.N. & Guan, K.L. (2005). Dysregulation of the TSC-mTOR pathway in human disease. *Nat. Genet.*, **37**, 19–24.

Irving, R.M., Moffatt, D., Hardy, D. et al. (1994). Somatic NF2 gene mutations in familial and non-familial vestibular schwannoma. *Hum. Mol. Genet.*, **3**, 347–50.

Ishibe, N., Sgambati, M.T., Fontaine, L., et al. (2001). Clinical characteristics of familial B-CLL in the National Cancer Institute Familial Registry. *Leuk. Lymphoma*, **42**, 99–108.

Ishitobi, M., Miyoshi, Y., Hasegawa, S., Egawa, C., Tamaki, Y., Monden, M. & Noguchi, S. (2003). Mutational analysis of BARD1 in familial breast cancer patients in Japan. *Cancer Lett.*, **200**, 1–7.

Ismail, S.M.I. & Walker, S.M. (1990). Bilateral virilising sclerosing stromal tumours of the ovary in a pregnant woman with Gorlin's syndrome: implications for pathogenesis of ovarian stromal neoplasms. *Histopathology*, **17**, 159–63.

Ito, E., Sato, Y., Kawauchi, K. et al. (1987). Type 1a glycogen storage disease with hepatoblastoma in siblings. *Cancer*, **59**, 1776–80.

Itoh, H. & Ohsato, K. (1985). Turcot syndrome and its characteristic colonic manifestations. *Dis. Colon Rectum*, **28**, 399–402.

Itoh, H., Houlston, R.S., Haracopos, C. et al. (1990). Risk of cancer death in first-degree relatives of patients with hereditary non-polyposis cancer syndrome (Lynch type II): a study of 130 kindreds in the United Kingdom. *Br. J. Surg.*, **77**, 1367–70.

Izatt, L., Hodgson, S.V. & Solomon, E. (1997). A study of germline mutations in ataxia telangiectasia mutated in young breast cancer patients. *J. Med. Genet.*, **34**, s32.

Jablonska, S., Orth, G., Jarzabek-Chorzelska, M. et al. (1979). Twenty-one years of follow up studies of familial epidermodysplasia verruciformis. *Cancer Res.*, **39**, 1074–82.

Jackson, A.W., Muldal, S. & Ockey, C.H. (1965). Carcinoma of the male breast in association with Klinefelter's syndrome. *Br. Med. J.*, **i**, 223–7.

Jacobs, A. (1989). Benzene and leukaemia. *Br. J. Haematol.*, **12**, 119–21.

Jacobs, I. & Lancaster, J. (1996). The molecular genetics of sporadic and familial epithelial ovarian cancer. *Int. J. Gynaecol. Cancer*, **6**, 337–55.

Jacobs, I., Davies, A.P., Bridges, J., Stabile, I., Fay, T., Lower, A., Grudzinskas, J.G. & Oram, D. (1993). Prevalence screening for ovarian cancer in postmenopausal women by CA 125 measurement and ultrasonography [see comments]. *Br. Med. J.*, **306**, 1030–4.

Jacobs, I.J, Skates, S.J., MacDonald, N., Menon, U., Rosenthal, A.N., Davies, A.P., Woolas, R., Jeyarajah, A.R., Sibley, K., Lowe, D.G. & Oram, D.H. (1999). Screening for ovarian cancer: a pilot randomised controlled trial [see comments]. *Lancet*, **353**, 1207–10.

Jacquemont, S., Boceno, M., Rival, J.M., Mechinaud, F. & David, A. (2002). High risk of malignancy in mosaic variegated aneuploidy syndrome. *Am. J. Med. Genet.*, **109**(1), 17–21.

Jadresic, L., Wadey, R.B., Buckle, B., Barratt, T.M., Mitchell, C.D. & Cowell, J.K. (1991). Molecular analysis of chromosome region 11p13 in patients with Drash syndrome. *Hum. Genet.*, **86**, 497–501.

Jaeger, E.E., Woodford-Richens, K.L., Lockett, M., Rowan, A.J., Sawyer, E.J., Heinimann, K., Rozen, P., Murday, V.A., Whitelaw, S.C., Ginsberg, A. et al. (2003). An ancestral Ashkenazi haplotype at the HMPS/CRAC1 locus on 15q13–q14 is associated with hereditary mixed polyposis syndrome. *Am. J. Hum. Genet.*, **72**, 1261–7.

Jain, D., Hui, P., McNamara, J., Schwartz, D., German, J. & Reyes-Mugica, M. (2001). Bloom syndrome in sibs: first reports of hepatocellular carcinoma and Wilms tumor with documented anaplasia and nephrogenic rests. *Pediatr. Dev. Pathol.*, **4**(6), 585–9.

Jagelman, D.G., DeCosse, J.J., Bussey, H.J.R. & The Leeds Castle Polyposis Group (1988). Upper gastrointestinal cancer in familial polyposis coli. *Lancet*, **i**, 1149–51.

Jakubowska, A., Nej, K., Huzarski, T. et al. (2002). BRCA2 gene mutations in families with aggregations of breast and stomach cancers. *Br. J. Cancer*, **87**, 888–91.

Janecke, A.R., Hennies, H.C., Gunther, B. et al. (2005). GJB2 mutations in keratitisichthyosis-deafness syndrome including its fatal form. *Am. J. Med. Genet.*, **133**, 128–131.

Janezic, S.A., Ziogas, A., Krumroy, L.M., Krasner, M., Plummer, S.J., Cohen, P., Gildea, M., Barker, D., Haile, R., Casey, G. & Anton-Culver, H. (1999). Germline BRCA1 alterations in a population-based series of ovarian cancer cases. *Hum. Mol. Genet.*, **8**, 889–97.

Jarvinen, H.J., Mecklin, J.P. & Sistonen, P. (1995). Screening reduces colorectal cancer rate in families with hereditary nonpolyposis colorectal cancer. *Gastroenterology*, **108**, 1405–11.

Jarvinen, H.J., Aarnio, M., Mustonen, H., Aktan-Collan, K., Aaltonen, L.A., Peltomaki, P., de La, C.A. & Mecklin, J.P. (2000). Controlled 15-year trial on screening for colorectal cancer in families with hereditary nonpolyposis colorectal cancer. *Gastroenterol.*, **118**, 829–34.

Jarvinen, J. & Franssila, K.O. (1984). Familial juvenile polyposis coli: increased risk of colorectal cancer. *Gut*, **25**, 792–800.

Jass, J.R. (1995a). Colorectal adenomas in surgical specimens from subjects with hereditary non-polyposis colorectal cancer. *Histopathology*, **27**, 263–7.

Jass, J.R. (1995b). Colorectal adenoma progression and genetic change: is there a link? *Ann. Med.*, **27**, 301–6.

Jass, J.R. (2004). HNPCC and sporadic colorectal cancer: a review of the morphological similarities and differences. *Fam Cancer*, **3**(2), 93–100.

Jass, J.R., Williams, C.B., Bussey, H.J.R. & Morson, B.C. (1988). Juvenile polyposis – a precancerous condition. *Histopathology*, **13**, 619–30.

Jass, J.R., Whitehall, V.L., Young, J. & Leggett, B.A. (2002). Emerging concepts in colorectal neoplasia. *Gastroenterol.*, **123**, 862–76.

Jedlickova, K., Stockton, D.W. & Prchal, J.T. (2003). Possible primary familial and congenital polycythemia locus at 7q22.1–7q22.2. *Blood Cell. Mol. Dis.*, **31**, 327–31.

Jeevaratnam, P., Cottier, D.S., Browett, P.J. et al. (1996). Familial giant hyperplastic polyposis predisposing to colorectal cancer: a new hereditary bowel cancer syndrome. *J. Pathol.*, **179**, 20–5.

Jeghers, H., McKusick, V.A. & Katz, K.H. (1949). Generalised intestinal polyposis and melanin spots of the oral mucosa, lips and digits. *New Engl. J. Med.*, **241**, 31–6, 993–1005.

Jenne, D.E., Reimann, H., Nezu, J.-I. et al. (1998). Peutz–Jeghers syndrome is caused by mutations in a novel serine threonine kinase. *Nat. Genet.*, **18**, 38–44.

Jensen, D.A., Warburg, M. & Dupont, A. (1976). Ocular pathology in the elfin face syndrome (the Fanconi–Schlesinger type of idiopathic hypercalcaemia of infancy). *Ophthalmologica*, **172**, 434–4.

Jia, W.H., Feng, B.J., Xu, Z.L., Zhang, X.S., Huang, P., Huang, L.X., Yu, X.J., Feng, Q.S., Yao, M.H., Shugart, Y.Y. & Zeng, Y.X. (2004). Familial risk and clustering of nasopharyngeal carcinoma in Guangdong, China. *Cancer*, **101**, 363–9.

Jin, Y., Mazza, C., Christie, J.R., Giliani, S., Fiorini, M., Mella, P., Gandellini, F., Stewart, D.M., Zhu, Q., Nelson, D.L., Notarangelo, L.D. & Ochs, H.D. (2004). Mutations of the Wiskott–Aldrich Syndrome Protein (WASP): hotspots, effect on transcription, and translation and phenotype/genotype correlation. *Blood*, **104**, 4010–19.

Johannesdottir, G., Gudmundsson, J., Bergthorsson, J.T., Arason, A., Agnarsson, B.A., Eiriksdottir, G., Johannsson, O.T., Borg, A., Ingvarsson, S., Easton, D.F., Egilsson, V. & Barkardottir, R.B. (1996). High prevalence of the 999del5 mutation in icelandic breast and ovarian cancer patients. *Cancer Res.*, **56**, 3663–5.

Johannsson, O., Ostermeyer, E.A., Hakansson, S., Friedman, L.S., Johansson, U., Sellberg, G., Brondum-Nielsen, K., Sele, V., Olsson, H., King, M.C. & Borg, A. (1996). Founding BRCA1 mutations in hereditary breast and ovarian cancer in southern Sweden. *Am. J. Hum. Genet.*, **58**, 441–50.

Johns, L.E. & Houlston, R.S. (2000). N-acetyl transferase-2 and bladder cancer risk: a meta-analysis. *Environ. Mol. Mutagen.*, **36**(3), 221–7.

Johns, L.E. & Houlston, R.S. (2003). A systematic review and meta-analysis of familial prostate cancer risk. *BJU Int.*, **91**, 789–94.

Johnson, J.A. (1989). Ataxia telangiectasia and other α-fetoprotein-associated disorders. In *Genetic Epidemiology of Cancer*, eds. Lynch, H.T. & Hirayama, T. CRC Press, Boca Raton, pp. 145–57.

Johnson, R.L., Rothman, A.L., Xie, J. et al. (1996). Human homolog of patched, a candidate gene for the basal cell nevus syndrome. *Science*, **272**, 1668–71.

Johnson, S.R. & Tattersfield, A.E. (2002). Lymphangioleiomyomatosis. *Semin. Respir. Crit. Care Med.*, **23**(2), 85–92.

Joishy, S.K., Cooper, R.A. & Rowley, P.J. (1977). Alveolar cell carcinoma in identical twins. Similarity in time of onset, histochemistry, and site of metastasis. *Ann. Int. Med.*, **87**, 447–50.

Jolly, K.W., Malkin, D., Douglass, E.C., Brown, T.F., Sinclair, A.E. & Look, A.T. (1994). Splice-site mutation of the p53 gene in a family with hereditary breast-ovarian cancer. *Oncogene*, **9**, 97–102.

Jonasdottir, T.J., Mellersh, C.S., Moe, L., Heggebo, R., Gamlem, H., Ostrander, E.A. & Lingaas, F. (2000). Genetic mapping of a naturally occurring hereditary renal cancer syndrome in dogs. *Proc. Natl. Acad. Sci. USA*, **97**(8), 4132–7.

Jones, A.C., Shyamsundar, M.M., Thomas, M.W., Maynard, J., Idziaszczyk, S., Tomkins, S., Sampson, J.R. & Cheadle, J.P. (1999). Comprehensive mutation analysis of TSC1 and TSC2- and phenotypic correlations in 150 families with tuberous sclerosis. *Am. J. Hum. Genet.*, **64**, 1305–15.

Jones, W., Harman, C., Ng, A. & Shaw, J. (1999). The incidence of malignant melanoma in Auckland, New Zealand: highest rates in the world. *World J. Surg.*, **23**, 732–5.

Jonkman, M.F., Rulo, H.F. & Duipmans, J.C. (2003). From gene to disease: epidermiolysis bullosa due to mutations in or around the hemidesmosome. *Ned. Tijschr. Geneeskd.*, **147**, 1108–13.

Jonsson, G., Bendahl, P.O., Sandberg, T. et al. (2005). Mapping of a novel ocular and cutaneous malignant melanoma susceptibility locus to chromosome 9q 21–32, *J. Nat. Cancer Inst.*, **97**, 1377–82.

Judge, T.A., Lewis, J.D. & Lichtenstein, G.R. (2002). Colonic dysplasia and cancer in inflammatory bowel disease. *Gastrointest. Endosc. Clin. N. Am.*, **12**, 495–523.

Judson, I.R., Wiltshaw, E. & Newland, A.C. (1985). Multiple myeloma in a pair of monozygotic twins: the first reported case. *Br. J. Haematol.*, **60**, 551–4.

Kaelin, W.G. & Maher, E.R. (1998). The VHL tumour suppressor gene paradigm. *Trend. Genet.*, **14**, 423–5.

Kahraman, M.M. & Prieur, D.J. (1991). Prenatal diagnosis of Chediak–Higashi syndrome in the cat by evaluation of cultured chorionic cells. *Am. J. Med. Genet.*, **40**, 311–15.

Kalff, M.W. & Hijmans, W. (1969). Immunoglobulin analysis in families of macroglobulinaemia patients. *Clin. Exp. Immunol.*, **5**, 479–98.

Kamb, A., Gruis, N., Weaver-Feldhaus, J. et al. (1994). A cell cycle regulator potentially involved in genesis of many tumor types. *Science*, **264**, 436–40.

Kaneko, H., Isogai, K., Fukao, T., Matzui, E., Kasahara, K., Yachie, A., Seki, H., Koizumi, S., Arai, M., Utunomiya, J., Miki, Y. & Kando, N. (2004). Relatively common mutations of the Bloom syndrome gene in the Japanese population. *Int. J. Mol. Med.*, **14**(3), 439–42.

Kanter, W.R., Eldridge, R., Fabricant, R., Allen, J.C. & Koerber, T. (1980). Central neurofibromatosis with bilateral acoustic neuroma: genetic, clinical and biochemical distinctions from peripheral neurofibromatosis. *Neurology*, **30**, 851–9.

Karim, M.A., Suzuki, K., Fukai, K. et al. (2002). Apparent genotype–phenotype correlation in childhood, adolescent and adult Chegiac; Higashi syndrome. *Am. J. Med. Genet.*, **108**, 16–22.

Karlan, B.Y., Baldwin, R.L., Lopez-Luevanos, E., Raffel, L.J., Barbuto, D., Narod, S. & Platt, L.D. (1999). Peritoneal serous papillary carcinoma, a phenotypic variant of familial ovarian cancer: implications for ovarian cancer screening. *Am. J. Obstet. Gynecol.*, **180**, 917–28.

Kas, K., Voz, M.L., Roijer, E. et al. (1997). Promoter swapping between genes for a novel zinc finger protein and beta-catenin pleiomorphic adenomas with t(3:8)(p21;q12) translocations. *Nat. Genet.*, **15**, 170–4.

Kasirga, E., Ozkinay, F., Tutuncuoglu, S. et al. (1996). Four siblings with achalasia, alacrimia and neurological abnormalities in a consanguineous family. *Clin. Genet.*, **49**, 296–9.

Kasprzak, L., Mesurolle, B., Tremblay, F. et al. (2005). Invasive breast cancer following bilateral subcutaneous mastectomy in a *BRCA2* mutation carrier: a case report and review of the literature. *World J. Surg. Oncol.*, **3**, 52.

Kassem, M., Kruse, T.A., Wong, F.K., Larsson, C. & Teh, B.T. (2000). Familial isolated hyperparathyroidism as a variant of multiple endocrine neoplasia type 1 in a large Danish kindred. *J. Clin. Endocrinol. Metab.*, **85**, 165–7.

Katagiri, K., Takasaki, S., Fujiwara, S. et al. (1996). Purification and structural analysis of extracellular matrix of a skin tumour from a patient with juvenile hyaline fibromatosis. *J. Dermatol. Sci.*, **13**, 37–8.

Kattwinkel, J., Lapey, A., Di Sant Agnese, P.A. et al. (1973). Hereditary pancreatitis: 3 new kindreds and a critical review of the literature. *Pediatrics*, **51**, 55–69.

Kaufman, D.K., Kimmel, D.W., Parisi, J.E. & Michels, V.V. (1993). A familial syndrome with cutaneous malignant melanoma and cerebral astrocytoma. *Neurology*, **43**, 1728–31.

Kauppinen, R. (2005). Porphyrias. *Lancet*, **365**, 241–52.

Kauppinen, R., Mutzajoki, S., Pihlaja, H. et al. (1995). Acute intermittent porphyria in Finland: 19 mutations in the porphobilinogen deaminase gene. *Hum. Mol. Genet.*, **4**, 215–22.

Kawaguchi, K., Sakamaki, H., Onozawa, Y. et al. (1990). Dyskeratosis congenita (Zissner–Cole–Engman syndrome). *Virchows Arch. A. Pathol. Anat. Histopathol.*, **417**, 247–53.

Kefford, R., Bishop, J.N., Tucker, M. et al. (2002). Genetic testing for melanoma. *Lancet Oncol.*, **3**(11), 653–4.

Kekki, M., Siurala, M., Varis, K. et al. (1987). Classification principles and genetics of chronic gastritis. *Scand. J. Gastroenterol.*, **22**(Suppl 141), 1–28.

Kelsell, D.P., Risk, J.M., Leigh, I.M. et al. (1996). Close mapping of the focal non-epidermolytic palmoplantar keratoderma (PPK) locus associated with oesophageal cancer (TOC). *Hum. Mol. Genet.*, **5**, 857–60.

Kelsell, D.P., Wilgoss, A.L., Richard, G. et al. (2000). Connexin mutations associated with palmoplantar keratoderma and profound deafness in a single family. *Eur. J. Hum. Genet.*, **8**, 141–4.

Kerber, R.A. & Slattery, M.L. (1995). The impact of family history on ovarian cancer risk. The Utah Population Database. *Arch. Int. Med.*, **155**, 905–12.

Kerr, N.J., Chun, Y.H., Yun, K., Heathcott, R.W., Reeve, A.E. & Sullivan, M.J. (2002). Pancreatoblastoma is associated with chromosome 11p loss of heterozygosity and IGF2 overexpression. *Med. Pediatr. Oncol.*, **39**, 52–4.

Kersey, J.H., Shapiro, R.S. & Filipovich, A.H. (1988). Relationship of immunodeficiency to lymphoid malignancy. *Pediatr. Infect. Dis. J.*, **7**, 510–12.

Keung, Y.-K., Buss, D., Chauvenet, A. & Pettenati, M. (2002). Haematologic malignancy and Klinefelter syndrome: a chance association?

Khanna, K.K. (2000). Cancer risk and the ATM gene; a continuing debate. *J. Nat. Cancer Inst.*, **92**, 795–802.

Kibirige, M.S., Birch, J.M., Campbell, R.H., Cattamaneni, H.R. & Blair, V.A. (1989). Review of astrocytoma in childhood. *Pediatr. Hematol. Oncol.*, **6**, 319–29.

Kidd, A., Carson, L. Gregory, D.W. et al. (1996). A Scottish family with Bazey—Dupre—Christol syndrome: follicular atrophoderma, congenital hypotrichosis, and basal cell carcinoma. *J. Med. Genet.*, **33**, 493–7.

Kiemeney, L.A. & Schoenberg, M. (1996). Familial transitional cell carcinoma. *J. Urol.*, **156**, 867–72.

Kikuchi, M., Tayama, T., Hayakawa, H., Takahashi, I., Hoshino, H. & Ohsaka, A. (1995). Familial thrombocytosis. *Br. J. Haematol.*, **89**, 900–2.

Kim, H., Lee, J.E., Cho, E.J., Liu, J.O. & Youn, H.D. (2003). Menin, a tumor suppressor, represses JunD-Mediated Transcriptional Activity by Association with an mSin3A-Histone Deacetylase Complex. *Cancer Res.*, **63**, 6135–9.

Kim, S.J. (2000). Blue rubber bleb naevus syndrome with central nervous syndrome involvement. *Ped. Neurol.*, **22**, 410–12.

Kimonis, V.E., Mehta, S.G., DiGiovanna, J.J., Bale, S.J. & Pastakia, B. (2004). Radiological features in 82 patients with nevoid basal cell carcinoma (NBCC or Gorlin) syndrome. *Genet. Med.*, **6**(6), 495–502.

Kimura, E.T., Nikiforova, M.N., Zhu, Z., Knauf, J.A., Nikiforov, Y.E. & Fagin, J.A. (2003). High prevalence of BRAF mutations in thyroid cancer: genetic evidence for constitutive activation of the RET/PTC-RAS-BRAF signaling pathway in papillary thyroid carcin-oma. *Cancer Res.*, **63**, 1454–7.

Kimyai-Asadi, A., Ketcher, L.B. & Ji, L.M.H. (2002). The molecular basis of hereditary pal-mar planter keratodermas. *J. Am. Acad. Demaltol.*, **47**(3), 327–43.

King, J.E., Dozois, R.R., Lindor, N.M. et al. (2000). Care of patients and their families with familial adenomatous polyposis. *Mayo Clin. Proc.*, **75**, 57–67.

Kinnear, P.E., Jay, B. & Witkop Jr, D.D.S. (1985). Albinism. *Surv. Ophthalmol.*, **30**, 75–101.

Kinzler, K., Nilbert, M.C., Su, L.-K. et al. (1991). Identification of FAP locus genes from chromosome 5q21. *Science*, **253**, 661–4.

Kinzler, K.W. & Vogelstein, B. (1987). Lessons from hereditary colorectal cancer. *Cell*, **95**, 159–70.

Kinzler, K.W. & Vogelstein, B. (1996). Lessons from hereditary colorectal cancer. *Cell*, **87**, 159–70.

Kinzler, K.W. & Vogelstein, B. (1997). Gatekeepers and caretakers. *Nature*, **386**, 761–2.

Kirchhoff, T., Satagopan, J.M., Kauff, N.D. et al. (2004). Frequency of BRCA1 and BRCA2 in unselected Ashkenazi Jewish patients with colorectal cancer. *J. Natl. Cancer Inst.*, **90**, 2–3.

Kirchhoff, T., Kauff, N.D., Mitra, N. et al. (2004). BRCA mutations and risk of prostate can-cer in Azhkenazi Jews Clin. *Cancer Res.*, **10**, 2918–21.

Kirkpatrick, C.H. (1994). Chronic mucocutaneous candidiasis. *J. Am. Acad. Dermatol.*, **31**, S14–17.

Kirschner, L.S., Carney, J.A., Pack, S.D. et al. (2000a). Mutations in the gene encoding the protein kinase A type 1-alpha regulatory subunit in patients with Carney complex. *Nat. Genet.*, **26**, 89–92.

Kirschner, L.S., Sandrini, F., Monbo, J., Lin, J.P., Carney, J.A. & Stratakis, C.A. (2000b). Genetic heterogeneity and spectrum of mutations of the *PRKAR1A* gene in patients with the Carney complex. *Hum. Mol. Genet.*, **9**, 3037–46.

Kitao, S., Shimamoto, A., Goto, M. et al. (1999). Mutations in RECQL4 cause a subset of Rothmund–Thomson syndrome. *Nat. Genet.*, **22**, 82–4.

Kiuru, M., Lehtonen, R., Arola, J. et al. (2002). Few *FH* mutations in sporadic counterparts of tumor types observed in hereditary leiomyomatosis and renal cell cancer families. *Cancer Res.*, **62**, 4554–7.

Klamt, B., Koziell, A., Poulat, F., Wieacker, P., Scambler, P., Berta, P. & Gessler, M. (1998). Frasier syndrome is caused by defective alternative splicing of WT1 leading to an altered ratio of WT1 +/− KTS splice isoforms. *Hum. Mol. Genet.*, **7**(4), 709–14.

Klausner, R.D. & Handler, S.D. (1994). Familial occurrence of pleomorphic adenoma. *Int. J. Pediatr. Otorhinolaryngol.*, **30**, 205–10.

Kleihues, P., Schauble, B., Zur, H.A., Esteve, J. & Ohgaki, H. (1997). Tumors associated with p53 germline mutations: a synopsis of 91 families. *Am. J. Pathol.*, **150**, 1–13.

Klemmer, S., Pascoe, L. & De Cosse, J. (1987). Occurrence of desmoids in patients with familial adenomatous polyposis of the colon. *Am. J. Med. Genet.*, **28**, 385–92.

Kligman, A.M. & Kirschbaum, J.D. (1964). Steatocystoma multiplex: a dermoid tumour. *J. Invest. Dermatol.*, **42**, 383–7.

Klitz, W., Aldrich, C.L., Fildes, N., Horning, S.J. & Begovich, A.B. (1994). Localization of pre-disposition to Hodgkin disease in the HLA class II region. *Am. J. Hum. Genet.*, **54**, 497–505.

Kluwe, L., Mautner, V., Heinrich, B., Dezube, R., Jacoby, L.B., Friedrich, R.E. & MacCollin, M. (2003). Molecular study of frequency of mosaicism in neurofibromatosis 2 patients with bilateral vestibular schwannomas. *J. Med. Genet.*, **40**, 109–14.

Knudson, A.G. (1971). Mutation and cancer: statistical study of retinoblastoma. *Proc. Natl. Acad. Sci. USA*, **68**, 820–3.

Knudson, A.G. & Strong, L.C. (1972). Mutation and cancer: neuroblastoma and phaeochromocytoma. *Am. J. Hum. Genet.*, **24**, 514–32.

Kobayashi, T., Hirayama, Y., Kobayashi, E., Kubo, Y. & Hino, O. (1995). A germline insertion in the tuberous sclerosis (Tsc2) gene gives rise to the Eker rat model of dominantly inherited cancer. *Nat. Genet.*, **9**, 70–4.

Koch, C.A., Huang, S.C., Moley, J.F. et al. (2001). Allelic imbalance of the mutant and wild-type *RET* allele in MEN 2A-associated medullary thyroid carcinoma. *Oncogene*, **20**, 7809–11.

Koch, M., Gaedke, H. & Jenkins, H. (1989). Family history of ovarian cancer patients: a case–control study. *Int. J. Epidemiol.*, **18**, 782–5.

Koh, T.H.H.G., Cooper, J.E., Newman, C.L. et al. (1986). Pancreatoblastoma in a neonate with Wiedemann–Beckwith syndrome. *Eur. J. Pediatr.*, **145**, 435–8.

Koinuma, K., Shitoh, K., Miyakura, Y., Furukawa, T., Yamashita, Y., Ota, J., Ohki, R., Choi, Y.L., Wada, T., Konishi, F., Nagai, H. & Mano, H. (2004). Mutations of BRAF are associated with extensive hMLH1 promoter methylation in sporadic colorectal carcinomas. *Int. J. Cancer*, **108**, 237–42.

Kolodner, R.D., Hall, N.R. & Lipford, J. (1994). Structure of the human MSH2 locus and analysis of two Muir–Torre kindreds for msh2 mutations. *Genomics*, **24**, 516–26.

Kondo, T., Okabe, M. et al. (1998). Familial essential thrombocythemia associated with one-base deletion in the 5'-untranslated region of the thrombopoietin gene. *Blood*, **92**, 1091–6.

Koopman, R.J.J. & Happle, R. (1991). Autosomal dominant transmission of the NAME syndrome (nevi, atrial myxoma, mucinosis of the skin and endocrine over activity). *Hum. Genet.*, **86**, 300–4.

Korge, B.P. & Krieg, T. (1996). The molecular basis for inherited bullous disease. *J. Mol. Med.*, **74**, 59–70.

Koufos, A., Grundy, P., Morgan, K. et al. (1989). Familial Wiedemann–Beckwith syndrome and a second Wilms' tumour locus both map to 11 p15.5. *Am. J. Hum. Genet.*, **44**, 711–19.

Kraemer, K.H. & Slor, H. (1985). Xeroderma pigmentosum. *Clin. Dermatol.*, **3**, 33–69.

Kralovics, R., Sokol, L. & Prchal, J.T. (1998). Absence of polycythemia in a child with a unique erythropoietin receptor mutation in a family with autosomal dominant primary polycythemia. *J. Clin. Invest.*, **102**(1), 124–9.

Kralovics, R., Stockton, D.W. & Prchal, J.T. (2003). Clonal hematopoiesis in familial polycythemia vera suggests the involvement of multiple mutational events in the early pathogenesis of the disease. *Blood*, **102**, 3793–6.

Kratzke, R.A., Otterson, G.A., Hogg, A. et al. (1994). Partial inactivation of the RB product in a family with incomplete penetrance of familial retinoblastoma and benign retinal tumors. *Oncogene*, **9**, 1321–6.

Kriege, M., Brekelmans, C.T., Boetes, C., Besnard, P.E., Zonderland, H.M., Obdeijn, I.M., Manoliu, R.A., Kok, T., Peterse, H., Tilanus-Linthorst, M.M., Muller, S.H., Meijer, S., Oosterwijk, J.C., Beex, L.V., Tollenaar, R.A., de Koning, H.J., Rutgers, E.J. & Klijn, J.G.

(2004). Efficacy of MRI and mammography for breast-cancer screening in women with a familial or genetic predisposition. *New Engl. J. Med.*, **351**, 427–37.

Kroll, T.G., Sarraf, P., Pecciarini, L. et al. (2000). PAX8-PPARgamma1 fusion oncogene in human thyroid carcinoma. *Science*, **289**, 1357–60.

Krontiris, T.G., Devlin, B., Karp, D.D. et al. (1993). An association between the risk of cancer and mutations in the HRAS1 minisatellite locus. *New Engl. J. Med.*, **329**, 517–23.

Kropilak, M., Jagleman, D.G., Fazio, V.W., Lavery, I.L. & McGannon, E. (1989). Brain tumours in familial adenomatous polyposis. *Dis. Colon Rectum*, **34**, 778–81.

Kruse, R., Rutten, A., Schweiger, N., Jakob, E., Mathiak, M., Propping, P., Mangold, E., Bisceglia, M. & Ruzicka, T. (2003). Frequency of microsatellite instability in unselected sebaceous gland neoplasias and hyperplasias. *J. Invest. Dermatol.*, **120**(5), 858–64.

Kuhl, C.K., Schmutzler, R.K., Leutner, C.C., Kempe, A., Wardelmann, E., Hocke, A., Maringa, M., Pfeifer, U., Krebs, D. & Schild, H.H. (2000). Breast MR imaging screening in 192 women proved or suspected to be carriers of a breast cancer susceptibility gene: preliminary results. *Radiology*, **215**, 267–79.

Kumar, D. (1984). Genetics of Indian childhood cirrhosis. *Trop. Geogr. Med.*, **36**, 313–16.

Kumar, D., Blank, C.E. & Ponder, B. (1989). A family with Turcot syndrome suggesting autosomal dominant inheritance. *J. Med. Genet.*, **26**, 592 [Abstract].

Kurjak, A. & Zalud, I. (1992). Transvaginal colour flow Doppler in the differentiation of benign and malignant ovarian masses. In *Ovarian Cancer 2*, eds. Sharp, F., Mason, P. & Creasman, W. Chapman and Hall, London.

Kurose, K., Araki, T., Matsunaka, T., Takada, Y. & Emi, M. (1999). Variant manifestation of Cowden disease in Japan: hamatomatous polyposis of the digestive tract with mutation of the *PTEN* gene. *Am. J. Hum. Genet.*, **64**, 308–10.

Kurtz, R.C., Sternberg, S.S., Miller, H.H. & Decosse, J.J. (1987). Upper gastrointestinal neoplasia in familial polyposis. *Dig. Dis. Sci.*, **32**, 459–65.

Kurzrock, R., Guterman, J.U. & Talpaz, M. (1988). The molecular genetics of Philadelphia chromosome-positive leukaemias. *New Engl. J. Med.*, **319**, 990–8.

Kurzrock, R., Ku, S. & Talpaz, M. (1995). Abnormalities in the PRAD1 (CYCLIN D1/BCL-1) oncogene are frequent in cervical and vulvar squamous cell carcinoma cell lines. *Cancer*, **75**, 584–90.

Kusafuka, T., Miao, J., Yoneda, A., Kuroda, S. & Fukuzawa, M. (2004). Novel germ-line deletion of SNF5/INI1/SMARCB1 gene in neonate presenting with congenital malignant rhabdoid tumor of kidney and brain primitive neuroectodermal tumor. *Gene. Chromosome. Cancer*, **40**, 133–9.

Kushner, B.H., Gilbert, F. & Helson, L. (1986). Familial neuroblastoma: case reports, literature review, and etiologic considerations. *Cancer*, **57**, 1887–93.

Kutler, D.I., Wreesmann, V.B. & Goberdhan, A. (2003). Human papillomavirus DNA and p53 polymorphisms in squamous cell carcinomas from Fanconi anaemia patients. *J. Natl. Cancer Inst.*, **19**, 1718–21.

Kwong, Y.L., Ng, M.H. & Ma, S.K. (2000). Familial acute myeloid leukemia with monosomy 7: late onset and involvement of a multipotential progenitor cell. *Cancer Genet. Cytogenet.*, **116**, 170–3.

La Nasa, G., Cottoni, E., Mulgaria, M. et al. (1995). HLA antigen distribution in different clinical subgroups demonstrates genetic heterogeneity in lichen planus. *Br. J. Dermatol.*, **132**, 897–900.

Laberge-le Couteulx, S., Jung, H.H., Labauge, P., Houtteville, J.P., Lescoat, C., Cecillon, M., Marechal, E., Joutel, A., Bach, J.F. & Tournier-Lasserve, E. (1999). Truncating mutations in CCM1, encoding KRIT1, cause hereditary cavernous angiomas. *Nat. Genet.*, **23**(2), 189–93.

Laberge-le Couteulx, S., Brezin, A.P., Fontaine, B., Tournier-Lasserve, E., Labauge, P. (2002). A novel KRIT1/CCM1 truncating mutation in a patient with cerebral and retinal cavernous angiomas. *Arch. Ophthalmol.*, **120**(2), 217–18.

Laiho, P., Launonen, V., Lahemo, P. et al. (2002). Low level MSI in most colorectal carcinomas. *Cancer Res.*, **62**, 1166–70.

Laken, S.J., Peterson, G.M. & Gruber, S.B. (1997). Familial colorectal cancer in Ashkenazim due to a hypermutable tract in APC. *Nat. Genet.*, **17**, 79–83.

Lakhani, S.R. (2004). Putting the brakes on cylindromatosis? *New Engl. J. Med.*, **350**, 187–8.

Lakhani, S.R., Jacquemier, J., Sloane, J.P. et al. (1998). Multifactorial analysis of differences between sporadic breast cancers and cancers involving BRCA1 and BRCA2 mutations. *J. Natl. Cancer Inst.*, **90**, 1138–45.

Lakhani, S.R., van de Vijver, M.J., Jacquemier, J., Anderson, T.J., Osin, P.P., McGuffog, L. & Easton, D.F. (2002). The pathology of familial breast cancer: predictive value of immunohistochemical markers estrogen receptor, progesterone receptor, HER-2, and p53 in patients with mutations in BRCA1 and BRCA2. *J. Clin. Oncol.*, **20**, 2310–18.

Lal, G., Liu, L., Hogg, D., Lassam, N.J., Redston, M.S. & Gallinger, S. (2000). Patients with both pancreatic adenocarcinoma and melanoma may harbor germline CDKN2A mutations. *Gene. Chromosome. Cancer*, **27**, 358–61.

Lalloo, F., Varley, J., Ellis, D. et al. (2003). Prediction of pathogenic mutations in patients with early onset breast cancer by family history. *Lancet*, **361**, 1101–2.

Lam, W.W. et al. (1999). Analysis of germline CDKN1C (p57KIP2) mutations in familial and sporadic Beckwith–Wiedemann syndrome (BWS) provides a novel genotype-phenotype correlation. *J. Med. Genet.*, **36**(7), 518–23.

Lamlum, H., AlTassan, N., Jaeger, E. et al. (2000). APC variants in patients with multiple colorectal adenomas, with evidence of the particular importance of E1317Q. *Hum. Mol. Genet.*, **9**, 2215–21.

Lammi, L. et al. (2004). Mutations in AXIN2 cause familial tooth agenisis and predispose to colorectal cancer. *Am. J. Hum. Genet.*, **74**, 1043–50.

Lampe, A.K., Hampton, P.J., Woodford-Richens, K., Tomlinson, I., Lawrence, C.M. & Douglas, F.S. (2003). Laugier–Hunziker syndrome: an important differential diagnosis for Peutz-Jeghers syndrome. *J. Med. Genet.*, **40**, E77.

Lamy, M., Aussannaire, M., Jammet, M.L. et al. (1954). Trois cas de maladie d'Ollier dans un fratrie. *Bull. Mem. Soc. Med. Hosp. Paris*, **70**, 62–70.

Lancaster, J.M., Wooster, R., Mangion, J., Phelan, C.M., Cochran, C., Gumbs, C., Seal, S., Barfoot, R., Collins, N., Bignell. G., Patel, S., Hamoudi, R., Larsson, C., Wiseman, R.W., Berchuck, A., Iglehart, J.D., Marks, J.R., Ashworth, A., Stratton, M.R. & Futreal, P.A.

(1996). BRCA2 mutations in primary breast and ovarian cancers. *Nat. Genet.*, **13**, 238–40.

Lane, J.E., Bowman, P.H. & Cohen, D.J. (2003). Epiderodysplasia verruciformis. *South Med. J.*, **96**, 613–5.

Langan, J.E., Cole, C.G., Huckle, E.J., Bryne, S., McRonald, F.E., Rowbottom, L., Ellis, A., Shaw, J.M., Leigh, I.M., Kelsell, D.P., Dunham, I., Field, J.K. & Risk, J.M. (2004). Novel microsatellite markers and single nucleotide polymorphisms refine the tylosis with oesophageal cancer t(TOC) minimal region on 17q25 to 42.5 kb: sequencing does not identify the causative gene. *Hum. Genet.*, **114**, 534–40.

Langer, K., Konrad, K. & Wolff, K. (1990). Keratitis, icthyosis and deafness (KID) syndrome: report of three cases and a review of the literature. *Br. J. Dermatol.*, **122**, 689–97.

Lanspa, S.J., Lynch, H.T., Smyrk, T.C. et al. (1990). Colorectal adenomas in the Lynch syndromes. Results of a colonoscopy screening program. *Gastroenterology*, **98**, 1117–22.

Lanzi, C., Borrello, M.G., Bongarzone, I. et al. (1992). Identification of the product of two oncogenic forms of the ret proto-oncogene in papillary thyroid carcinomas. *Oncogene*, **7**, 2189–94.

Larsson, C. & Friedman, E. (1994). Localization and identification of the multiple endocrine neoplasia type 1 disease gene. *Endocrinol. Metab. Clin. N. Am.*, **23**, 67–9.

Larsson, C., Skosgeid, B., Öberg, K., Nakamura, Y. & Nordenskjöld, M. (1988). Multiple endocrine neoplasia type 1 gene maps to chromosome 11 and is lost in insulinoma. *Nature*, **332**, 85–7.

Lasson, U., Harms, D. & Wiedemann, H.R. (1978). Osteogenic sarcoma complicating osteogenesis imperfecta tarda. *Eur. J. Paed.*, **129**, 215–18.

Latif, F., Tory, K., Gnarra, J. et al. (1993). Identification of the von Hippel–Lindau disease tumour suppressor gene. *Science*, **260**, 1317–20.

Lau, Y.F. (1999). Gonadoblastoma, testicular and prostate cancers, and the TSPY gene. *Am. J. Hum. Genetic.*, **64**, 921–7.

Le Couedic, J.P., Mitjavila, M.T., Villeval, J.L., Feger, F., Gobert S., Mayeux, P., Casadevall, N. & Vainchenker, W. (1996). Missense mutation of the erythropoietin receptor is a rare event in human erythroid malignancies. *Blood*, **87**, 1502–11.

Le Marchand, L., Doulou, T., Lum-Jones, A. et al. (2002). Association of the hOGG1 ser326cys polymorphism with lung cancer risk. *Cancer Epidemiol. Biomark. Prev.*, **11**, 409–12.

Leblanc, R., Melanson, D. & Wilkinson, R.D. (1996). Hereditary neurocutaneous angiomatosis. Report of four cases. *J. Neurosurg.*, **85**, 1135–42.

Lee, E.J., Schiffer, C.A., Misawa, S. & Testa, J.R. (1987). Clinical and cytogenetic features of familial erythroleukaemia. *Br. J. Haematol.*, **65**, 313–20.

Leeper, K., Garcia, R., Swisher, E., Goff, B., Greer, B. & Paley, P. (2002). Pathologic findings in prophylactic oophorectomy specimens in high-risk women. *Gynecol. Oncol.*, **87**, 52–6.

Leffell, D.J. & Braverman, J.M. (1986). Familial multiple lipomatosis. *J. Am. Acad. Dermatol.*, **15**, 275–9.

Laiho, P. et al. (2002). Low-level microsatellite instability in most colorectal carcinomas. *Cancer Res.*, **62**, 1166–7.

Lehmann, A.R. (2003). DNA repair-deficient diseases, xeroderma pigmentosum, Cockayne syndrome and trichothiodystrophy. *Biochimie*, **85**, 1101–11.

Lehtol, J. (1978). Family study of gastric carcinoma. *Scand. J. Gastroenterol.*, **13**(Suppl 50), 1–54.

Lehtonen, M., Dillner, J., Knekt, P. et al. (1996). Serologically diagnosed infection with human papillomavirus type 16 and risk for subsequent development of cervical carcinoma: nested case–control study. *Br. Med. J.*, **312**, 537–9.

Lehtonen, R., Kiuru, M.H., Vanharanta, S. et al. (2004). Biallelic inactivation of fumarate hydratase (FH) occurs in nonsyndromic uterine leiomyomas but is rare in other tumors. *Am. J. Pathol.*, **164**, 17–22.

Lendvay, T.S. & Marshall, F.F. (2003). The tuberous sclerosis complex and its highly variable manifestations. *J. Urol.*, **169**, 1635–42.

Lengauer, C., Kinzler, K.W. & Vogelstein, B. (1997). Genetic instability in colorectal cancers. *Nature*, **386**(6625), 623–7.

Leonard, A., Craft, A.W., Moss, C. & Malcolm, A.J. (1996). Osteogenic sarcoma in the Rothmund–Thomson syndrome. *Med. Pediatr. Oncol.*, **26**, 249–53.

Leppert, M., Burt, R., Hughes, J.P. et al. (1990). Genetic analysis of an inherited predisposition to colon cancer in a family with a variable number of adenomatous polyps. *New Engl. J. Med.*, **322**, 904–8.

Lerman, C., Narod, S., Schulman, K. et al. (1996). BRCA1 testing in families with hereditary breast-ovarian cancer. *J. Am. Med. Assoc.*, **275**, 1885–92.

Levanat, S., Gorlin, R.J., Fallet, S., Johnson, D.R., Fantasia, J.E. & Bale, A.E. (1996). A two-hit model for developmental defects in Gorlin syndrome. *Nat. Genet.*, **12**(1), 85–7.

Levitus, M., Rooimans, M.A., Steltenpool, J., Cool, N.F., Oostra, A.B., Mathew, C.G., Hoatlin, M.E., Waisfisz, Q., Arwert, F., De Winter, J.P. & Joenje, H. (2003). Heterogeneity in Fanconi anemia: evidence for two new genetic subtypes. *Blood*, **103**, 2498–503.

Levy-Lahad, E., Catane, R., Eisenberg, S., Kaufman, B., Hornreich, G., Lishinsky, E., Shohat, M., Weber, B.L., Beller, U., Lahad, A. & Halle, D. (1997). Founder BRCA1 and BRCA2 mutations in Ashkenazi Jews in Israel: frequency and differential penetrance in ovarian cancer and in breast–ovarian cancer families [see comments]. *Am. J. Hum. Genet.*, **60**, 1059–67.

Lewis, R.A. & Ketcham, A.S. (1973). Maffucci's syndrome: functional and neoplastic significance. *J. Bone Joint Surg.*, **55A**, 1465–79.

Lewis, R.A., Cohen, M.H. & Wise, G.N. (1975). Cavernous haemangioma of the retina and optic disc. *Br. J. Ophthalmol.*, **59**, 422–4.

Lewis, R.A., Riccardi, V.M., Gerson, L.P., Whitford, R. & Axelson, K.A. (1984). Von Recklinghausen neurofibromatosis: II. Incidence of optic-nerve gliomata. *Ophthalmology*, **91**, 929–35.

Li, C.K., Mang, O.W. & Foo, W. (1989). Epidemiology of paediatric cancer in Hong Kong 1982 to 1991. Hong Kong Cancer Registry. *Hong Kong Med. J.*, **5**, 128–34.

Li, F.P., Lokich, J., Lapey, J., Neptune, W.B. & Wilkins Jr, E.W. (1978). Familial mesothelioma after intense asbestos exposure at home. *J. Am. Med. Assoc.*, **240**, 467.

Li, F.P., Hecht, F., Kaiser-McCaw, B., Baranko, P.V. & Potter, N.U. (1981). Ataxia-pancytopenia: syndrome of cerebellar ataxia, hypoplastic anaemia, monosomy 7 and acute myelogenous leukaemia. *Cancer Genet. Cytogenet.*, **4**, 189–96.

Li, F.P., Fraumeni, J.F., Mulvihill, J.J. et al. (1988). A cancer family syndrome in 24 kindreds. *Cancer Res.*, **48**, 5358–62.

Li, F.P., Correa, P. & Fraumeni Jr, J.F. (1991). Testing for germline *p53* mutations in cancer families. *Cancer Epidemiol. Biomark. Prev.*, **1**, 91–4.

Li, M., Shuman, C., Fei, Y.L., Cutiongco, E., Bender, H.A., Stevens, C., Wilkins-Haug, L., Day-Salvatore, D., Yong, S.L., Geraghty, M.T., Squire, J. & Weksberg, R. (2001). GPC3 mutation analysis in a spectrum of patients with overgrowth expands the phenotype of Simpson–Golabi–Behmel syndrome. *Am. J. Med. Genet.*, **102**, 161–8.

Li, F.P. & Fraumeni, J.F. (1969). Soft tissue sarcomas, breast cancer, and other neoplasms: a familial syndrome? *Ann. Int. Med.*, **71**, 747–52.

Li, T.H., Hsu, C.K., Chiu, H.C. & Chang, C.H. (1997). Multiple asymptomatic hyperkeratotic papules on the lower part of the leg. Hyaline perstans (HLP) (Flegel disease). *Arch. Dermatol.*, **7**, 910–11, 913–14.

Li, X. & Hemminki, K. (2003). Familial and second lung cancer: a nation-wide epidemiological studying Sweden. *Lung Cancer*, **39**, 255–63.

Liaw, D., Marsh, D.J., Li, J. et al. (1997). Germline mutations of the PTEN gene in Cowden disease, an inherited breast and thyroid cancer syndrome. *Nat. Genet.*, **16**, 64–7.

Libutti, S.K., Choyke, P.L., Bartlett, D.L., Vargas, H., Walther, M., Lubensky, I., Glenn, G., Linehan, W.M. & Alexander, H.R. (1998). Pancreatic neuroendocrine tumors associated with von Hippel–Lindau disease: diagnostic and management recommendations. *Surgery*, **124**, 1153–9.

Lichtenstein, P., Holm, N.V., Verkasalo, P.K., Iliadou, A., Kaprio, J., Koskenvuo, M., Pukkala, E., Skytthe, A. & Hemminki, K. (2000). Environmental and heritable factors in the causation of cancer – analyses of cohorts of twins from Sweden, Denmark, and Finland. *New Engl. J. Med.*, **343**, 78–85.

Liede, A., Karlan, B.Y. & Narod, S.A. (2004). Cancer risks for male carriers of germline mutations in BRCA1 or BRCA2: a review of the literature. *J. Clin. Oncol.*, **22**(4), 735–42.

Lillicrap, D.A. & Sterndale, H. (1984). Familial chronic myeloid leukaemia. *Lancet*, **ii**, 699.

Lim, W., Hearle, N., Shah, B., Murday, V., Hodgson, S.V., Lucassen, A., Eccles, D., Talbot, I., Neale, K., Lim, A.G., O'Donohue, J., Donaldson, A., Macdonald, R.C., Young, I.D., Robinson, M.H., Lee, P.W., Stoodley, B.J., Tomlinson, I., Alderson, D., Holbrook, A.G., Vyas, S., Swarbrick, E.T., Lewis, A.A., Phillips, R.K. & Houlston, R.S. (2003). Further observations on LKB1/STK11 status and cancer risk in Peutz–Jeghers syndrome. *Br. J. Cancer*, **89**, 308–13.

Lim, W., Olschwang, S., Keller, J.J., Westerman, A.M., Menko, F.H., Boardman, L.A., Scott, R.J., Trimbath, J., Giardiello, F.M., Gruber, S.B., Gille, J.J., Offerhaus, G.J., de Rooij, F.W., Wilson, J.H., Spigelman, A.D., Phillips, R.K. & Houlston, R.S. (2004). Relative frequency and morphology of cancers in STK11 mutation carriers. *Gastroenterology*, **126**, 1788–94.

Lin, A.N. & Carter, D.M. (1989). Epidermolysis bullosa: when the skin falls apart. *J. Pediatr.*, **114**, 349–56.

Linder, D., McCaw, B.K. & Hecht, F. (1975). Parthenogenic origin of benign ovarian tera-tomas. *New Engl. J. Med.*, **292**, 63–6.

Lindor, N.M., Devries, E.M., Michels, V.V. et al. (1996). Rothmund–Thomson syndrome in siblings: evidence for acquired in vitro mosaicism. *Clin. Genet.*, **49**, 124–9.

Linet, M.S. et al. (1989). Familial cancer history and chronic lymphocytic leukemia. A case-control study. *Am. J. Epidemiol.*, **130**(4), 655–64.

Linos, D.A., Dozois, R.R., Dahlin, D.C. & Bartholomew, L.G. (1981). Does Peutz–Jeghers syndrome predispose to gastrointestinal malignancy? A later look. *Arch. Surg.*, **116**, 1182–4.

Lipton, L.R., Johnson, V., Cummings, C. et al. (2004). Refining the Amsterdam Criteria and Bethesda Guidelines: testing algorithms for the prediction of mismatch repair mutation status in the familial cancer clinic. *J. Clin. Oncol.*, **22**(24), 4934–43.

Liquori, C.L, Berg, M.J., Siegel, A.M. et al. (2003). Mutations in a gene encoding a novel protein containing a phosphotyrosine-binding domain cause type 2 cerebral cavernous malformations. *Am. J. Hum. Genetic.*, **73**(6), 1459–64.

Little, M.H., Williamson, K.A., Mannens, M. et al. (1993). Evidence that WT1 mutations in Denys–Drash syndrome patients may act in a dominant-negative fashion. *Hum. Mol. Genet.*, **2**, 259–64.

Liu, B., Nicolaides, N.C., Markowitz, S. et al. (1995). Mismatch repair gene defects in spor-adic colorectal cancers with microsatellite instability. *Nat. Genet.*, **9**, 48–55.

Liu, H.X., Zhou, X.L., Liu, T. et al. (2003). The role of hMLH3 in familial colorectal can-cer. *Cancer Res.*, **63**, 1894–9.

Liu, L., Dilworth, D., Gao, L., Monzon, J., Summers, A., Lassam, N. & Hogg, D. (1999). Mutation of the CDKN2A5'UTR creates an aberrant initiation codon and predisposes to melanoma. *Nat. Genet.*, **21**, 1–5.

Livadas, S., Mavrou, A., Sofocleous, C., van Vliet-Constantinidou, C., Dracopoulou, M. & Dacou-Voutetakis, C. (2003). Gonadoblastoma in a patient with del(9)(p22) and sex rever-sal: report of a case and review of the literature. *Cancer Genet. Cytogenet.*, **143**, 174–7.

Loewinger, R.J., Lichsteinstein, J.R., Dodson, W.E. & Eisen, A.Z. (1977). Maffucci's syndrome: a mesenchymal dysplasia and multiple tumour syndrome. *Br. J. Dermatol.*, **96**, 317–22.

Lohmann, D.R., Brandt, B., Hopping, W., Passarge, E. & Horsthemke, B. (1996). The spec-trum of RB1 germ-line mutations in hereditary retinoblastoma. *Am. J. Hum. Genet.*, **58**, 940–9.

Lohmann, D.R., Gerick, M., Brandt, B. et al. (1997). Constitutional RB1-gene mutations in patients with isolated unilateral retinoblastoma. *Am. J. Hum. Genet.*, **61**, 282–94.

Lohse, P. et al. (2002). Microsatellite instability, loss of heterozygosity and loss of hMLH1 and hMSH2 protein expression in endometrial carcinoma. *Hum. Pathol.*, **33**, 347–54.

Longy, M. & Lacombe, D. (1996). Cowden disease. Report of a family and review. *Ann. Génet.*, **39**, 35–42.

Lonn, U., Lonn, S., Nylen, U. et al. (1990). An abnormal profile of DNA replication inter-mediates in Bloom's syndrome. *Cancer Res.*, **50**, 3141–5.

Loo, J.C., Liu, L., Hao, A. et al. (2003). Germline splicing mutations of CDKN2A predis-pose to melanoma. *Oncogene*, **22**(41), 6387–94.

Look, A.T. (2003). A leukaemogenic twist for GATA1. *Nat. Genet.*, **32**, 83–4.

Lowy, A.M., Kordich, J.J., Gismondi, V., Varesco, L., Blough, R.I. & Groden, J. (2001). Numerous colonic adenomas in an individual with Bloom's syndrome. *Gastroenterol*, **121**(2), 435–9.

Loy, T.S., Diaz-Arias, A.A. & Perry, M.C. (1991). Familial erythrophagocytic lymphohistiocytosis. *Semin. Oncol.*, **18**, 34–9.

Lu, K.H., Cramer, D.W., Muto, M.G., Li, E.Y., Niloff, J. & Mok, S.C. (1999). A population-based study of BRCA1 and BRCA2 mutations in Jewish women with epithelial ovarian cancer. *Obstet. Gynecol.*, **93**, 34–7.

Lu, K.H., Garber, J.E., Cramer, D.W., Welch, W.R., Niloff, J., Schrag, D., Berkowitz, R. & Muto, M.G. (2000). Occult ovarian tumors in women with *BRCA1* or *BRCA2* mutations undergoing prophylactic oophorectomy. *J. Clin. Onc.*, **18**, 2728–32.

Lu, S., Day, N.E., Degos, L. et al. (1990). Linkage of a nasopharyngeal carcinoma susceptibility gene to the HLA locus. *Nature*, **346**, 470–1.

Lu, S.-L. et al. (1998). HNPCC associated with germline mutation in the TGF-beta type II receptor gene. *Nat. Genet.*, **19**, 17–18.

Lubensky, I.A. et al. (1999). Hereditary and sporadic papillary renal carcinomas with c-met mutations share a distinct morphological phenotype. *Am. J. Pathol.*, **155**(2), 517–26.

Lubs, M.-L., Bauer, M.S., Formas, M.E. & Djokic, B. (1991). Lisch nodules in neurofibromatosis type 1. *New Engl. J. Med.*, **324**, 1264–6.

Lucci-Cordisco, E., Zito, I., Gensini, F. & Genuardi, M. (2003). Hereditary nonpolyposis colorectal cancer and related conditions. *Am. J. Med. Genet.*, **122A**(4), 325–34.

Ludecke, H.J., Johnson, C., Wagner, M.J. et al. (1991). Molecular definition of the shortest region of deletion overlap in the Langer–Gideon syndrome. *Am. J. Hum. Genet.*, **49**, 1197–206.

Lumbroso, S., Paris, F., Sultan, C. et al. (2004). Activating 9Salpha mutations: analysis of 113 patients with signs of McCune—Albright syndrome—a European collaborative study. *J. Clin. Endocrinol. Metab.*, **89**, 2107–13.

Luo, G., Santoro, I.M., McDaniel, L.D., Nishijima, I., Mills, M., Youssoufian, H., Vogel, H., Schultz, R.A. & Bradley, A. (2000). Cancer predisposition caused by elevated mitotic recombination in Bloom mice. *Nat. Genet.*, **26**(4), 424–9.

Lynch, H.T. & de la Chapelle, A. (1999). Genetic susceptibility to nonpolyposis colorectal cancer. *J. Med. Genet.*, **36**, 801–18.

Lynch, H.T. & Fusaro, R.M. (1991). Pancreatic cancer and the familial atypical multiple mole melanoma (FAMMM) syndrome. *Pancreas*, **6**(2), 127–31.

Lynch, H.T. & Krush, A.J. (1971). Carcinoma of the breast and ovary in three families. *Surg. Gynecol. Obstet.*, **133**, 644–8.

Lynch, H.T. & Walzak, M.P. (1980). Genetics in urogenital cancer. *Urol. Clin. North Am.*, **7**(3), 815–29.

Lynch, H.T., Krush, A.J. & Larsen, A.L. (1967). Heredity and endometrial carcinoma. *South. Med. J.*, **60**, 231–5.

Lynch, H.T., Kaplan, A.R. & Lynch, J.F. (1974). Klinefelter syndrome and cancer: a family study. *J. Am. Med. Assoc.*, **229**, 809–11.

Lynch, H.T., Mulcahy, G.M., Harris, R.E. et al. (1978). Genetic and pathologic findings in a kindred with hereditary sarcoma, breast cancer, brain tumours, leukaemia, lung, laryngeal and adrenocortical carcinoma. *Cancer*, **41**, 2055–64.

Lynch, H.T., Walzak, M.P., Fried, R. et al. (1979). Familial factors in bladder cancer. *J. Urol.*, **122**, 458–61.

Lynch, H.T., Fusaro, R.M., Roberts, L., Voorhees, G.J. & Lynch, J.F. (1985). Muir–Torre syndrome in several members of family with a variant of the cancer family syndrome. *Br. J. Dermatol.*, **113**, 295–301.

Lynch, H.T., Marcus, J.N., Weisenburger, D.D. et al. (1989a). Genetic and immunopathological findings in a lymphoma family. *Br. J. Cancer*, **59**, 622–6.

Lynch, H.T., Smyrk, T.C., Lynch, P.M. et al. (1989b). Adenocarcinoma of the small bowel in Lynch syndrome II. *Cancer*, **64**, 2178–83.

Lynch, H.T., Ens, J.A. & Lynch, J.F. (1990a). The Lynch syndrome II and urological malignancies. *J. Urol.*, **143**, 24–8.

Lynch, H.T., Watson, P., Conway, T.A. et al. (1990b). Clinical/genetic features in hereditary breast cancer. *Breast Cancer Res. Treat.*, **15**, 63–71.

Lynch, H.T., Smyrk, T.C., Lanspa, S.J. et al. (1990c). Phenotypic variation in colorectal adenoma/cancer expression in 2 families with hereditary flat adenoma syndromem. *Cancer*, **60**, 909–15.

Lynch, H.T., Smyrk, T.C., Watson, P. et al. (1993). Genetics, natural history, tumour spectrum and pathology of hereditary non-polyposis colorectal cancer: an updated review. *Gastroenterology*, **104**, 1535–49.

Lynch, H.T., Smyrk, T. & Lynch, J.F. (1996a). Overview of natural history, pathology, molecular genetics and management of HNPCC (Lynch syndrome). *Int. J. Cancer*, **69**, 38–43.

Lynch, H.T., Smyrk, T., Kern, S.E. et al. (1996b). Familial pancreatic cancer: a review. *Semin. Oncol.*, **23**, 251–75.

Lynch, H.T., Sanger, W.G., Pirruccello, S., Quinn-Laquer, B. & Weisenburger, D.D. (2001). Familial multiple myeloma: a family study and review of the literature. *J. Natl. Cancer Inst.*, **93**(19), 1479–83.

Lynch, H.T., Brand, R.E., Hogg, D., Deters, C.A., Fusaro, R.M., Lynch, J.F., Liu, L., Knezetic, J., Lassam, N.J., Goggins, M. & Kern, S. (2002). Phenotypic variation in eight extended CDKN2A germline mutation familial atypical multiple mole melanoma-pancreatic carcinoma-prone families: the familial atypical mole melanoma-pancreatic carcinoma syndrome. *Cancer*, **94**, 84–96.

Lynch, H.T., Deters, C.A., Hogg, D. et al. (2003). Familial sarcoma: challenging pedigrees. Cancer, **98**, 1947–57.

Lyons, J., Landis, C.A., Harsh, G., et al. (1990). Two G protein oncogenes in human endocrine tumors. *Science*, **249**, 655–88.

MacCollin, M., Willett, C., Heinrich, B., Jacoby, L.B., Acierno Jr, J.S., Perry, A. & Louis, D.N. (2003). Familial schwannomatosis: exclusion of the NF2 locus as the germline event. *Neurology*, **60**(12), 1968–74.

MacDonald, C.E., Wicks, A.C. & Playford, R.J. (2000). Final results from 10 year cohort of patients undergoing surveillance for Barrett's oesophagus: observational study. *Br. Med. J.*, **321**, 1252–5.

MacGeoch, C., Newton Bishop, J., Bataille, V. et al. (1994). Genetic heterogeneity in familial malignant melanoma. *Hum. Mol. Genet.*, **3**, 2195–200.

Machatschek, J.N., Schrauder, A., Helm, F. et al. (2004). Acute lymphoblastic leukaemia and Klinefelter syndrome in children; two cases and review of the literature. *Paed. Haematol. Oncol.*, **21**, 621–6.

Mack, T.M., Cozen, W. & Shibata, D.K. (1995). Concordance for Hodgkin's Disease in identical twins suggesting genetic susceptibility to the young-adult form of the disease. *New Engl. J. Med.*, **332**, 413–8.

Mackey, S.E. & Creasman, W.T. (1995). Ovarian cancer screening [Review] [74 refs]. *J. Clin. Onc.*, **13**, 783–93.

Macklin, M.T. (1960). Inheritance of cancer of the stomach and large intestine in man. *J. Natl. Cancer Inst.*, **24**, 551–71.

MacPherson, G., Healey, C.S., Teare, M.D. et al. (2004). Association of a common variant of the CASP8 gene with reduced risk of breast cancer. *J. Natl. Cancer Inst.*, **96**, 1866–9.

Magenis, R.E., Tochen, M.L., Holahan, K.P., Carey, T., Allen, L. & Brown, M.G. (1984). Turner syndrome resulting from partial development of the Y chromosome short arm: localization of male determinants. *J. Pediatr.*, **105**, 916–19.

Magnusson, P.K., Lichtenstein, P. & Gyllensten, U.B. (2000). Heritability of cervical tumours. *Int. J. Cancer*, **88**, 698–701.

Mahaley, M.S., Mettlin, C., Natarajan, N., Laws, E.R. & Peace, B.B. (1989). National survey of patterns of care for brain-tumor patients. *J. Neurosurg.*, **71**, 826–36.

Maher, E.R. & Eng, C. (2002). The pressure rises: update on the genetics of phaeochromocytoma. *Hum. Mol. Genet.*, **11**: 2347–54.

Maher, E.R. & Reik, W. (2000). Beckwith–Wiedemann syndrome imprinting in clusters revisited. *J. Clin. Invest.* **105**, 247–52.

Maher, E.R. & Yates, J.R.W. (1991). Familial renal cell carcinoma – clinical and molecular genetic aspects. *Br. J. Cancer*, **63**, 176–9.

Maher, E.R., Yates, J.R.W. & Ferguson-Smith, M.A. (1990a). Statistical analysis of the two stage mutation model in von Hippel–Lindau disease and in sporadic cerebellar haemangioblastoma and renal cell carcinoma. *J. Med. Genet.*, **27**, 311–14.

Maher, E.R., Yates, J.R.W., Harries, R. et al. (1990b). Clinical features and natural history of von Hippel–Lindau disease. *Q. J. Med.*, **77**, 1151–63.

Maher, E.R., Bentley, E., Yates, J.R.W. et al. (1991). Mapping of the von Hippel–Lindau disease locus to a small region of chromosome 3p by genetic linkage analysis. *Genomics*, **10**, 957–60.

Maher, E.R., Morson, B., Beach, R. & Hodgson, S.V. (1992). Phenotypic variability ion hereditary non-polyposis colon cancer syndrome (HNPCC): association with infiltrative fibromatosis (desmoid tumor). *Cancer*, **69**, 2049–51.

Maher, E.R., Brueton, L.A., Bowdin, S.C., Luharia, A., Cooper, W., Cole, T.R., Macdonald, F., Sampson, J.R., Barratt, C.L., Reik, W. & Hawkins, M.M. (2003). Beckwith–Wiedemann syndrome and assisted reproduction technology (ART). *J. Med. Genet.*, **40**, 62–4.

Mahmoud, A.A.H., Yousef, G.M., Al-Hifzi, I. & Diamindos, E.P. (2002). Cockayne syndrome in three sisters with varying clinical presentation. *Am. J. Med. Genet.*, **111**, 81–5.

Mahood, J.M. (1983). Familial lichen planus. *Arch. Dermatol.*, **119**, 292–4.

Majewski, S. & Jablonska, S. (2004). Why epidermodysplasia verruciformis is a very rare disease and has raised such interest. *Int. J. Derm.*, **43**, 309–11.

Makkar, H.S. & Frieden, I.J. (2002). Congenital melanogtic naevi: an update for the pediatrician. *Curr. Opin. Paed.*, **14**, 397–403.

Malats, N., Casals, T., Porta, M., Guarner, L., Estivill, X. & Real, F.X. (2001). Cystic fibrosis transmembrane regulator (CFTR) DeltaF508 mutation and 5T allele in patients with chronic pancreatitis and exocrine pancreatic cancer. PANKRAS II Study Group. *Gut*, **48**, 70–4.

Malchoff, C.D. et al. (2000). Papillary thyroid carcinoma associated with papillary renal neoplasia: genetic linkage analysis of a distinct heritable tumor syndrome. *J. Clin. Endocrinol. Metab.*, **85**(5), 1758–64.

Malkin, D., Li, F.P., Strong, L.C. et al. (1990). Germline p53 mutations in a familial syndrome of breast cancer, sarcomas, and other neoplasms. *Science*, **250**, 1233–8.

Mallipeddi, R. (2002). Epidermolysis and cancer. *Clin. Exp. Dermatol.*, **27**, 616–23.

Mallory, S.B. (1995). Cowden Syndrome (Multiple hamartoma syndrome). *Dermatal. Clin.*, **13**, 27–31.

Mangold, E., Pagenstecher, C., Leister, M., Mathiak, M., Rutten, A., Friedl, W., Propping, P., Ruzicka, T. & Kruse, R. (2004). A genotype-phenotype correlation in HNPCC: strong predominance of msh2 mutations in 41 patients with Muir–Torre syndrome. *J. Med. Genet.*, **41**(7), 567–72.

Mann, J.R., Corkey, J.J., Fischer, H.J.W. et al. (1983). The X-linked recessive form of XY gonadal dysgenesis with a high incidence of gonadal germ cell tumours: clinical and genetic studies. *J. Med. Genet.*, **20**, 264–70.

Manski, T.J., Heffner, D.K., Glenn, G.M., Patronas, N.J., Pikus, A.T., Katz, D., Lebovics, R., Sledjeski, K., Choyke, P.L., Zbar, B., Linehan, W.M. & Oldfield, E.H. (1997). Endolymphatic sac tumors – a source of morbid hearing loss in von Hippel–Lindau disease. *J. Am. Med. Assoc.*, **277**, 1461–6.

Mansour, A.M., Barber, J.C., Reinecke, R.D. et al. (1989). Ocular choristomas. *Surv. Ophthalmol.*, **33**, 339–58.

Maraschio, P., Spadoni, E., Tanzarella, C., Antoccia, A., di Masi, A., Maghnie, M., Varon, R., Demuth, I., Tiepolo, L. & Danesino, C. (2003). Genetic heterogeneity for a Nijmegen breakage-like syndrome. *Clin. Genet.*, **63**, 283–90.

Marie, P.J., de Pollack, C., Chanson, P. & Lomri, A. (1997). Increased proliferation of osteoblastic cells expressing the activating Gs alpha mutation in monostotic and polyostotic fibrous dysplasia. *Am. J. Pathol.*, **150**, 1059–69.

Mariman, E.C.M., van Beersum, S.E.C., Cremers, C.W.R.J., Struycken, P.M. & Ropers, H.H. (1995). Fine mapping of a putatively imprinted gene for familial non-chromaffin paragangliomas to chromosome 11q13.1: evidence for genetic heterogeneity. *Hum. Genet.*, **95**, 56–62.

Marin, M.S., Lopez-Cima, M.F., Garcia-Castro, L., Pascual, T., Marron, M.G. & Tardon, A. (2004). Poly (AT) polymorphism in intron 11 of the XPC DNA repair gene enhances the risk of lung cancer. *Cancer Epidemiol. Biomark. Prev.*, **13**, 1788–93.

Maris, J.M., Kyemba, S.M., Rebbeck, T.R. et al. (1996). Familial predisposition to neuro-blastoma does not map to chromosome band 1p36. *Cancer Res.*, **56**, 3421–5.

Maris, J.M., Weiss, M.J., Mosse, Y., Hii, G., Guo, C., White, P.S., Hogarty, M.D., Mirensky, T., Brodeur, G.M., Rebbeck, T.R., Urbanek, M. & Shusterman, S. (2002). Evidence for a hered-itary neuroblastoma predisposition locus at chromosome 16p12–13. *Cancer Res.*, **62**, 6651–8.

Mark, J. & Dahlenfors, R. (1986). Cytogenetical observations in 100 human benign pleiomor-phic adenomas: specificity of the chromosomal aberrations and their relationship to sites of localised oncogenes. *Anticancer Res.*, **6**, 299–308.

Marsh, D.J., Andrew, S.D., Eng, C. et al. (1996a). Germline and somatic mutations in an onco-gene: *RET* mutations in inherited medullary thyroid carcinoma. *Cancer Res.*, **56**, 1241–3.

Marsh, D.J., Learoyd, D.L., Andrew, S.D. et al. (1996b). Somatic mutations in the *RET* proto-oncogene in sporadic medullary thyroid carcinoma. *Clin. Endocrinol.*, **44**, 249–57.

Marsh, D.J., Dahia, P.L.M., Zheng, Z. et al. (1997). Germline mutations in *PTEN* are pres-ent in Bannayan–Zonana syndrome. *Nat. Genet.*, **16**, 333–4.

Marsh, D.J., Coulon, V., Lunetta, K.L. et al. (1998). Mutation spectrum and genotype–phenotype analyses in Cowden disease and Bannayan–Zonana syndrome, two hamartoma syndromes with germline *PTEN* mutation. *Hum. Mol. Genet.*, **7**, 507–15.

Marsh, D.J., Kum, J.B., Lunetta, K.L. & et al. (1999). *PTEN* mutation spectrum and genotype-phenotype correlations in Bannayan–Riley–Ruvalcaba syndrome suggest a single entity with Cowden syndrome. *Hum. Mol. Genet.*, **8**, 1461–72.

Martasek, P., Nordamann, Y. & Grandchamp, B. (1994). Homozygous hereditary copor-phyria caused by arginine to tryptophane substitution in coporphyrin oxidase and common intragenic polymorphisms. *Hum. Mol. Genet.*, **3**, 477–80.

Martinez-Mir, A., Glaser, B., Chuang, G.S. et al. (2003). Germline fumarate hydratase mutations in families with multiple cutaneous and uterine myomata. *J. Invest. Dermatol.*, **121**, 741–4.

Martuza, R.L. & Eldridge, R.N. (1988). Neurofibromatosis 2 (bilateral acoustic neurofibro-matosis). *New Engl. J. Med.*, **318**, 684–8.

Marx, S.J., Simonds, W.F., Agarwal, S.K. et al. (2002). Hyerparathyroidism in hereditary syn-dromes: special expressions and special managements. *J. Bone Miner. Res.*, **17**(S2), 37–43.

Massague, J. (2000). How cells read TGF-beta signals. *Nat. Rev. Mol. Cell. Biol.*, **1**, 169–78.

Masuno, M., Imaizumir, K., Ishi, T. et al. (1998). Pilomatrixoma in Rubenstein–Taybi syn-drome. *Am. J. Med. Genet.*, **77**, 81–2.

Masutani, C., Kusumoto, R., Yamada, A., Dohmae, N., Yokoi, M., Yuasa, M., Araki, M., Iwai, S., Takio, K. & Hanaoka, F. (1999). The XPV (xeroderma pigmentosum variant) gene encodes human DNA polymerase eta. *Nature*, **399**, 700–4.

Matani, A. & Dritsas, C. (1973). Familial occurrence of thymoma. *Arch. Pathol.*, **95**, 90–1.

Mathers, J.C., Mickleburgh, I., Chapman, P.C., Bishop, D.T. & Burn, J. (2003). Concerted Action Polyp Prevention (CAPP) 1 Study. Can resistant starch and/or aspirin prevent the development of colonic neoplasia? The Concerted Action Polyp Prevention (CAPP) 1 Study. *Proc. Nutr. Soc.*, **62**, 51–7.

Mathew, C.G. & Lewis, C.M. (2004). Genetics of inflammatory bowel diesase: progress and prospects. *Hum. Mol. Genet.*, **13**(13 spec no **1**), R161–8.

Mathew, C.G.P., Chin, K.S., Easton, D.F. et al. (1987). A linked genetic marker for multiple endocrine neoplasia type 2A on chromosome 10. *Nature*, **328**, 527–8.

Matsushima, M., Kobayashi, K., Emi, M., Saito, H., Saito, J., Suzumori, K. & Nakamura, Y. (1995). Mutation analysis of the BRCA1 gene in 76 Japanese ovarian cancer patients: four germline mutations, but no evidence of somatic mutation. *Hum. Molec. Genet.*, **4**, 1953–6.

Matyakhina, L., Pack, S., Kirschner, L.S. et al. (2003). Xchromosome 2(2p16) abnormalities in Carney complex tumours. *J. Med. Genet.*, **40**, 268–77.

Mauro, J.A., Maslyn, R., Stein, A.A. et al. (1972). Squamous cell carcinoma of nail bed in hereditary ectodermal dysplasia. *NY State J. Med.*, **1**, 1065–6.

McCarthy, J.M., Rootman, J., Horsman, D. & White, V.A. (1993). Conjunctival and Uveal Melanoma in the Dysplastic Nevus syndrome. *Surv. Ophthalmol.*, **37**(5), 377–86.

McConnell, R.B. (1966). *The Genetics of Gastrointestinal Disorders.* Oxford University Press, Oxford.

McConville, C.M., Stankovic, T., Byrd, P.J. et al. (1996). Mutations associated with variant phenotypes in ataxia-telangiectasia. *Am. J. Hum. Genet.*, **59**, 320–30.

McCullough, D.L., Lamma, D.L., McLaughlin, A.P. et al. (1975). Familial transitional cell carcinoma of the bladder. *J. Urol.*, **113**, 629–35.

McDaniel, L.D., Chester, N., Watson, M., Borowsky, A.D., Leder, P. & Schultz, R.A. (2003). Chromosome instability and tumor predisposition inversely correlate with BLM protein levels. *DNA Repair (Amst)*, **2**(12), 1387–404.

McEwen, A.R., McConnell, D.T., Kenwright, D.N., Gaskell, D.J., Cherry, A. & Kidd, A.M. (2004). Occult cancer of the fallopian tube in a BRCA2 germline mutation carrier at prophylactic salpingo-oophorectomy. *Gynecol. Oncol.*, **92**, 992–4.

McGarrity, T.J., Mascari-Baker, M.J., Ruggiero, F.M. et al. (2003). Glycogenic acanthosis associated with germline PTEN mutation positive Cowden syndrome. *Am. J. Gastroenterol.*, **98**, 1429–34.

McGaughran, J.M., Harris, D.I., Donnai, D., Teare, D., MacLeod, R., Westerbeek, R., Kingston, H., Super, M., Harris, R. & Evans, D.G. (1999). Clinical study of type 1 eurofibromatosis in north west England. *J. Med. Genet.*, **36**(3), 197–203.

McGivern, A., Wynter, C.V. & Whitehall, V.L. (2004). Promoter hypermethylation frequency and BRAF mutation distinguish hereditary non-polyposis colon cancer from sporadic MSI-H colon cancer. *Fam. cancer*, **3**, 101–7.

McIntyre, J.F., Smith-Sorensen, B., Friend, S.H. et al. (1994). Germline mutations of the p53 tumour suppressor gene in children with osteosarcoma. *J. Clin. Oncol.*, **12**, 925–30.

McKeeby, J.K., Li, X., Zhuang, Z. et al. (2001). Multiple leiomyomas of the oesophagus, lung and uterus in multiple endocrine neoplasia type 1. *Am. J. Path.*, **159**, 1121–7.

McKeen, E.A., Bodurtha, J., Meadows, A.T., Douglas, E.G. & Mulvihill, J.J. (1978). Rhabdomyosarcoma complicating multiple neurofibromatosis. *J. Pediatr.*, **93**, 992–3.

McLaughlin, J.K., Mandel, J.S., Blot, W.J., Schuman, L.M., Mehl, E.S. & Fraumeni, J.F. (1984). A population-based case–control study of renal cell carcinoma. *J. Natl. Cancer Inst.*, **72**, 275–84.

McMaster, M.L. (2003). Familial Waldenstrom's macroglobulinaemia. *Semin. Oncol.*, **30**, 146–52.

Mecklin, J.P. (1987). Frequency of hereditary colorectal carcinoma. *Gastroenterology*, **93**, 1021–5.

Mecklin, J.P., Jarvinen, H.J. & Peltokalliop, P. (1986). Cancer family syndrome: genetic analysis of 22 Finnish kindreds. *Gastroenterology*, **90**, 328–33.

Meddeb, M., Valent, A., Danglot, G. et al. (1996). MDM2 amplification in a primary alveolar rhabdomyosarcoma displaying a t(2:13)(q35;q14). *Cytogenet. Cell Genet.*, **73**, 325–30.

Meetei, A.R., Levitus, M., Xue, Y., Medhurst, A.L., Zwaan, M., Ling, C., Rooimans, M.A., Bier, P., Hoatlin, M., Pals, G., de Winter, J.P., Wang, W. & Joenje, H. (2004). X-linked inheritance of Fanconi anemia complementation group B. *Nat. Genet.*, **36**, 1219–24.

Meijers-Heijboer, H., van Geel, B., van Putten, W.L., Henzen-Logmans, S.C., Seynaeve, C., Menke-Pluymers, M.B., Bartels, C.C., Verhoog, L.C., van den Ouweland, A.M., Niermeijer, M.F., Brekelmans, C.T. & Klijn, J.G. (2001). Breast cancer after prophylactic bilateral mastectomy in women with a BRCA1 or BRCA2 mutation. *New Engl. J. Med.*, **345**, 159–64.

Meijers-Heijboer, H., Wijnen, J., Vasen, H., Wasielewski, M., Wagner, A., Hollestelle, A., Elstrodt, F., van den, B.R., de Snoo, A., Fat, G.T., Brekelmans, C., Jagmohan, S., Franken, P., Verkuijlen, P., van den, O.A., Chapman, P., Tops, C., Moslein, G., Burn, J., Lynch, H., Klijn, J., Fodde, R. & Schutte, M. (2003). The CHEK2 1100delC mutation identifies families with a hereditary breast and colorectal cancer phenotype. *Am. J. Hum. Genet.*, **72**, 1308–14.

Meikle, A.W. & Smith, J.A. (1990). Epidemiology of prostate cancer. *Urol. Clin. North Am.*, **17**, 709–18.

Meissner, P.N., Dailey, T.A., Hift, R.J. et al. (1996). A R59W mutation in human protoporphyrinogen oxidase results in decreased enzyme activity and is prevalent in South Africans with variegate porphyria. *Nat. Genet.*, **13**, 95–7.

Menko, F.H. (1993). *Genetics of Colorectal Cancer for Clinical Practice.* Kluwer Academic, Dordrecht, pp. 58–82.

Menko, F.H., Kaspers, G.L., Meijer, G.A., Claes, K., van Hagen, J.M. & Gille, J.J. (2004). A homozygous MSH6 mutation in a child with cafe-au-lait spots, oligodendroglioma and rectal cancer. *Fam. Cancer*, **3**(2), 123–7.

Menon, A.G., Anderson, K.M., Riccardi, V.M. et al. (1990a). Chromosome 17p deletions and p53 gene mutations associated with the formation of malignant neurofibrosarcomas in von Recklinghausen neurofibromatosis. *Proc. Natl. Acad. Sci. USA*, **87**, 5433–9.

Merrick, Y. et al. (1986). Familial clustering of salivary gland carcinoma in Greenland. *Cancer*, **57**(10), 2097–102.

Mertens, W.C. & Bramwell, V. (1995). Osteosarcoma and other tumours of bone. *Curr. Opin. Oncol.*, **7**, 349–54.

Metcalfe, K., Lynch, H.T., Ghadirian, P., Tung, N., Olivotto, I., Warner, E., Olopade, O.I., Eisen, A., Weber, B., McLennan, J., Sun, P., Foulkes, W.D. & Narod, S.A. (2004). Contralateral breast cancer in BRCA1 and BRCA2 mutation carriers. *J. Clin. Oncol.*, **22**, 2328–35.

Mettlin, C., Croghan, I., Natarajan, N. & Lane, W. (1990). The association of age and familial risk in a case–control study of breast cancer. *Am. J. Epidemiol.*, **131**, 973–83.

Metze, D., Wigbes, B. & Hildebrand, A. (2001). Familial syringomas: a rare clinical variant. *Hantarzt*, **52**, 1045–8.

Meyn, M.S. (1999). Ataxia telangectasia, cancer and the pathobiology of the ATM gene. *Clin. Genet.*, **55**, 289–304.

Michaels, L. et al. (1999). Family with low-grade neuroendocrine carcinoma of salivary glands, severe sensorineural hearing loss, and enamel hypoplasia. *Am. J. Med. Genet.*, **83**(3), 183–6.

Michaelsson, G., Olsson, E. & Westermark, P. (1981). The Rombo syndrome: a familial disorder with vermiculate atrophodermia, milia, hypotrichosis, trichoepitheliomas, basal cell carcinoma and peripheral vasodilation with cyanosis. *Acta Derm. Venereol. (Stockh.)*, **61**, 497–503.

Michaely, P. & Bennett, V. (1993). The membrane binding-domain of ankyrin contains four independently folded subdomains, each comprised of six ankyrin repeats. *J. Biol. Chem.*, **268**, 22703–9.

Michels, V.V. & Stevens, J.C. (1982). Basal cell carcinoma in a patient with intestinal polyposis. *Clin. Genet.*, **22**, 80–2.

Miki, Y., Swensen, J., Shattuck Eidens, D. et al. (1994). A strong candidate for the breast and ovarian cancer susceptibility gene BRCA1. *Science*, **266**, 66–71.

Miki, Y., Katagiri, T., Kasumi, F. et al. (1996). Mutation analysis in the BRCA2 gene in primary breast cancer. *Nat. Genet.*, **13**, 238–40.

Miljkovic, J. (2004). An unusual generalised form of hyperkeratosis lenticularis perstans (Flegel's disease). *Wien. Klin. Wochenschr.*, **116**(Suppl 2), 78–80.

Miller, C.W., Aslo, A., Tsay, C. et al. (1990). Frequency and structure of p53 rearrangements in human osteosarcoma. *Cancer Res.*, **50**, 7950–4.

Miller, R.W. (1971). Deaths from childhood leukemia and solid tumours among twins and other sibs in the United States, 1960–67. *J. Natl. Cancer Inst.*, **46**, 203–9.

Milne, R.L., Knight, J.A., John, E.M. et al. (2005). Oral contraceptive use and risk of early–onset breast cancer in carriers and noncarriers of *BRCA1* and *BRCA2* mutations. *Cancer Epidemiol. Biomarkers Prev.*, **14**(2), 350–6.

Mitchell, R.J., Farrington, S.M., Dunlop, M.G. & Campbell, H. (2002). Mismatch repair genes hMLH1 and hMSH2 and colorectal cancer: a HuGE review. *Am. J. Epidemiol.*, **156**, 885–902.

Miyanaga, O., Miyamoto, Y., Shirahama, M. et al. (1989). A clinicopathological study of hepatocellular carcinoma patients with other primary malignancies. *Gan. No. Rinsho*, **35**, 1729–34.

Miyauchi, A., Futami, H., Hai, N. et al. (1999). Two germline missense mutations at codons 804 and 806 of the RET proto-oncogene in the same allele in a patient with multiple endocrine neoplasia type 2B without codon 918 mutation. *Jpn. J. Cancer Res.*, **90**(1), 1–5.

Miyaki, M., Nishio, J., Konishi, M. et al. (1997). Drastic genetic instability of tumours and normal tissues in Turcot syndrome. *Oncogene*, **15**, 2877–81.

Mizuta, R., Lasalle, J.M., Cheng, H.L., Shinohara, A., Ogawa, H., Copeland, N., Jenkins, N.A., Lalande, M. & Alt, F.W. (1997). RAB22 and RAB163/mouse BRCA2 – proteins that specifically interact with the RAD51 protein. *Proc. Natl. Acad. Sci. USA*, **94**, 6927–32.

Modan, B., Gak, E., Sade-Bruchim, R.B., Hirsh-Yechezkel, G., Theodor, L., Lubin, F., Ben-Baruch, G., Beller, U., Fishman, A., Dgani, R., Menczer, J., Papa, M. & Friedman, E.

(1996). High frequency of BRCA1 185delAG mutation in ovarian cancer in Israel. National Israel Study of Ovarian Cancer [see comments]. *J. Am. Med. Assoc.*, **276**, 1823–5.

Moglabey, Y.B., Kircheisen, R., Seoud, M., El Mogharbel, N., Van den Veyver, I. & Slim, R. (1999). Genetic mapping of a maternal locus responsible for familial hydatidiform moles. *Hum. Mol. Genet.*, **8**(4), 667–71.

Moll, A.C., Imhof, S.M., Bouter, L.M. et al. (1996). Second primary tumors in patients with hereditary retinoblastoma: a register-based follow-up study, 1945–1994. *Int. J. Cancer*, **67**, 15–19.

Mollica, F., Livolti, S. & Guarneri, B. (1984). New syndrome: exostoses, anetodermia, and brachydactyly. *Am. J. Med. Genet.*, **19**, 665–7.

Montalto, G., Cervello, M., Giannitrapani, L., Dantona, F., Terranova, A. & Castagnetta, L.A. (2002). Epidemiology, riskfactors, and natural history of hepatocellular carcinoma. *Ann. NY Acad. Sci.*, **963**, 13–20.

Montanaro, L., Tazzari, P.L. & Derenzini, M. (2003). Enhanced telomere shortening in transformed lymphoblasts from patients with X-linked dyskeratosis. *J. Clin. Path.*, **56**, 583–6.

Monzon, J., Liu, L., Brill, H. et al. (1998). CDKN2A mutations in multiple primary melanomas. *New Engl. J. Med.*, **338**(13), 879–87.

Moore, S.B. & Hoffman, D.L. (1988). Absence of HLA linkage in a family with osteitis deformans (Paget's disease of bone). *Tissue Antigens*, **31**, 69–70.

Moos, K.F. & Rennie, J.S. (1987). Squamous cell carcinoma arising in a mandibular keratocyst in a patient with Gorlin's syndrome. *Br. J. Oral Maxillofac. Surg.*, **25**(4), 280–4.

Mori, M., Harabuchi, I., Miyake, H., Casagrande, J.T., Henderson, B.E. & Ross, R.K. (1988). Reproductive, genetic, and dietary risk factors for ovarian cancer. *Am. J. Epidemiol.*, **128**, 771–7.

Morison, I.M., Becroft, D., Taniguchi, T. et al. (1996). Somatic overgrowth associated with over expression of insulin-like growth factor II. *Nat. Med.*, **2**, 311–16.

Morrell, D., Chase, C.L. & Swift, M. (1987). Cancer in families with severe combined immune deficiency. *J. Natl. Cancer Inst.*, **78**, 455–8.

Morrell, D., Chase, C.L. & Swift, M. (1990). Cancers in 44 families with ataxia telangiectasia. *Cancer Cell Cytogenet.*, **50**, 119–23.

Morrison, P.J. & Young, I.D. (1996). Syringomas, natal teeth and oligodontia: a new ectodermal dysplasia. *Clin. Dysmorphol.*, **5**, 63–6.

Morson, B. (1966). Factors influencing the prognosis of early cancer of the rectum. *Proc. R. Soc. Med.*, **59**, 607–12.

Mosbech, J. & Videbaek, A. (1955). On the aetiology of oesophageal carcinoma. *J. Natl. Cancer Inst.*, **15**, 1665–73.

Moser, M.J., Bigbee, W.L., Grant, S.G. et al. (2000). Genetic instability and hematologic disease risk in Werner syndrome patients and heterozygotes. *Cancer Res.*, **60**, 2492–6.

Moslehi, R., Chu, W., Karlan, B., Fishman, D., Risch, H., Fields, A., Smotkin, D., Ben-David, Y., Rosenblatt, J., Russo, D., Schwartz, P., Tung, N., Warner, E., Rosen, B., Friedman, J., Brunet, J.S. & Narod, S.A. (2000). BRCA1 and BRCA2 mutation analysis of 208 Ashkenazi Jewish women with ovarian cancer. *Am. J. Hum. Genet.*, **66**, 1259–72.

Moyhuddin, A., Baser, M.E., Watson, C., Purcell, S., Ramsden, R.T., Heiberg, A., Wallace, A.J. & Evans, D.G.R. (2003). Somatic mosaicism in neurofibromatosis 2: prevalence and risk of disease transmission to offspring. *J. Med. Genet.*, **40**, 459–63.

Moynahan, M.E., Cui, T.Y. & Jasin, M. (2001). Homology-directed DNA repair, mitomycin-c resistance, and chromosome stability is restored with correction of a Brca1 mutation. *Cancer Res.*, **61**, 4842–50.

Mueller, R.F. (1994). The Denys–Drash syndrome. *J. Med. Genet.*, **31**, 471–7.

Mugneret, F., Aurias, A., Lizard, S. et al. (1987). Der(16)t(1;16) (q11;all.1) is a consistent secondary chromosome change in Ewing's sarcoma. *Cytogenet. Cell Genet.*, **46**, 665.

Muir, E.G., Yates-Bell, A.J. & Barlow, K.A. (1967). Multiple primary carcinomata of colon, duodenum and larynx associated with keratokanthoma of the face. *Br. J. Surg.*, **54**, 191–5.

Muller, H. (1990). Recessively inherited deficiencies predisposing to cancer. *Anticancer Res.*, **10**, 513–18.

Muller, S., Gardner, H., Weber, B. et al. (1978). Wilm's tumour and adrenogenital carcinoma with hemihypertrophy and hamartomas. *Eur. J. Pediatr.*, **127**, 219.

Mulligan, L.M., Kwok, J.B.J., Healey, C.S. et al. (1993). Germline mutations of the *RET* proto-oncogene in multiple endocrine neoplasia type 2A. *Nature*, **363**, 458–60.

Mulligan, L.M., Eng, C., Healey, C.S. et al. (1994). Specific mutations of the *RET* proto-oncogene are related to disease phenotype in MEN 2A and FMTC. *Nat. Genet.*, **6**, 70–4.

Mulvihill, J.J., Ridolpi, R.L., Schultz, F.R. et al. (1975). Hepatic adenoma in Fanconi anaemia treated with oxymethalone. *J. Pediatr.*, **87**, 122–4.

Mulvihill, J.J., Cralnick, H.R., Whang-Peng, J. & Leventhal, B.C. (1977). Multiple childhood osteosarcomas in an American family with erythroid macrocytosis and skeletal abnormalities. *Cancer*, **40**, 3115–22.

Munemitsu, S., Albert, I., Souza, B. et al. (1995). Regulation of intracellular b catenin levels by the adenomatous polyposis coli (APC) tumour suppressor protein. *Proc. Natl. Acad. Sci. USA*, **92**, 3046–50.

Murdoch, S., Djuric, U., Mazhar, B. et al. (2006). Mutations in NALP7 cause recurrent hydatidiform moles and reproductive wastage in humans. *Nat. Genet.*, **38**(3), 300–2.

Murphy, K.M., Brune, K.A., Griffin, C., Sollenberger, J.E., Petersen, G.M., Bansal, R., Hruban, R.H. & Kern, S.E. (2002). Evaluation of candidate genes MAP2K4, MADH4, ACVR1B, and BRCA2 in familial pancreatic cancer: deleterious BRCA2 mutations in 17%. *Cancer Res.*, **62**, 3789–93.

Musarella, M.A. & Gallie, B.L. (1987). A simplified scheme for genetic counseling in retinoblastoma. *J. Pediatr. Ophthalmol. Strab.*, **24**, 124–5.

Muto, M.G., Cramer, D.W., Tangir, J., Berkowitz, R. & Mok, S. (1996). Frequency of the BRCA1 185delAG mutation among Jewish women with ovarian cancer and matched population controls. *Cancer Res.*, **56**, 1250–2.

Muto, R. et al. (2002). Prediction by FISH analysis of the occurrence of Wilms tumor in aniridia patients. *Am. J. Med. Genet.*, **108**(4), 285–9.

Mutter, G.L., Lin, M.-C., Fitzgerald, J.T. et al. (2000). Altered PTEN expression as a diagnostic marker for the earliest endometrial precancers. *J. Natl. Cancer Inst.*, **92**, 924–31.

Mutter, G.L., Ince, T., Baak, J.P.A., Kurst, G.A., Zhou, X.P. & Eng, C. (2001). Molecular identification of latent precancers in histologically normal endometrium. *Cancer Res.*, **61**, 4311–4.

Myhre, A.G., Stray-Pederson, A., Soangen, S. et al. (2004). Chronic mucocutaneous candidiasis and primary hypothyroidism in two families. *Eur. J. Paediatr*. e-publication.

Nadel, M. & Koss, L.G. (1967). Klinefelter's syndrome and male breast cancer. *Lancet*, **ii**, 366.

Nagase, H. & Nakamura, Y. (1993). Mutations of the APC (Adenomatous Polyposis Coli) gene. *Hum. Mutat.*, **2**, 425–34.

Nagase, S., Sato, S., Tezuka, F., Wada, Y., Yajima, A. & Horii, A. (1996). Deletion mapping on chromosome 10q25–26 in human endometrial cancer. *Br. J. Cancer*, **74**, 1979–83.

Nagata, H., Worobec, A.S., Oh, C.K. et al. (1995). Identification of a point mutation in the catalytic domain of the protooncogene c-kit in peripheral blood mononuclear cells of patients who have mastocytosis with an associated hematologic disorder. *Proc. Natl. Acad. Sci. USA*, **92**, 10560–4.

Nagle, D.L., Karim, M.A., Woolf, E.A. et al. (1996). Identification and mutation analysis of the complete gene for Chediak–Higashi syndrome. *Nat. Genet.*, **14**, 307–11.

Najean, Y. & Lecompte, T. (1990). Genetic thrombocytopenia with autosomal dominant transmission: a review of 54 cases. *Br. J. Haematol.*, **24**, 203–8.

Nakayama, Y., Takeno, Y., Tsugu, H. & Tomonanga, M. (1994). Maffucci's syndrome associated with intracranial chordoma: case report. *Neurosurgery*, **34**, 907–9.

Nancarrow, D., Mann, G., Holland, E. et al. (1993). Confirmation of chromosome 9p linkage in familial melanoma. *Am. J. Hum. Genet.*, **53**, 936–42.

Nancarrow, D.J., Palmer, J.M., Walters, M.K. et al. (1992). Exclusion of the familial melanoma locus (MLM) from the PND/D1S47 and MYCL1 regions of chromosome arm 1p in 7 Australian pedigrees. *Genomics*, **12**, 18–25.

Narod, S.A. & Foulkes, W.D. (2004). BRCA1 and BRCA2: 1994 and beyond. *Nat. Rev. Cancer*, **4**, 665–76.

Narod, S.A., Ford, D., Devilee, P., Barkardottir, R.B., Lynch, H.T., Smith, S.A., Ponder, B.A., Weber, B.L., Garber, J.E., Birch, J.M. et al. (1995a). An evaluation of genetic heterogeneity in 145 breast–ovarian cancer families. Breast Cancer Linkage Consortium. *Am. J. Hum. Genet.*, **56**, 254–64.

Narod, S.A., Goldgar, D., Cannon-Albright, L. et al. (1995b). Risk modifyers in carriers of BRCA1 mutations. *Int. J. Cancer*, **64**, 394–8.

Narod, S.A., Risch, H., Moslehi, R., Dorum, A., Neuhausen, S., Olsson, H., Provencher, D., Radice, P., Evans, G., Bishop, S., Brunet, J.S. & Ponder, B.A. (1998). Oral contraceptives and the risk of hereditary ovarian cancer. Hereditary Ovarian Cancer Clinical Study Group [see comments]. *New Engl. J. Med.*, **339**, 424–8.

Narod, S.A., Sun, P., Ghadirian, P., Lynch, H., Isaacs, C., Garber, J., Weber, B., Karlan, B., Fishman, D., Rosen, B., Tung, N. & Neuhausen, S.L. (2001). Tubal ligation and risk of ovarian cancer in carriers of BRCA1 or BRCA2 mutations: a case–control study. *Lancet*, **357**, 1467–70.

Narod, S.A., Dube, M.P., Klijn, J. et al. (2002). Oral contraceptives and the risk of breast cancer in BRCA1 and BRCA2 mutation carriers. *J. Natl. Cancer Inst.*, **94**, 1773–9.

Naryan, S., Fleming, C., Trainer, A.H. & Craig, J.A. (2001). Rothmund–Thomson syndrome with myelodysplasia. *Paed. Derm.*, **18**, 210–2.

Nathanson, K.L., Kanetsky, P.A., Hawes, R. et al. (2005). The Y deletion gr/gr and susceptibility to testicular germ cell tumor. *Am. J. Hum. Genet.*, **77**(6), 1034–43.

Naumova, A. & Sapienza, C. (1994). The genetics of retinoblastoma, revisited. *Am. J. Hum. Genet.*, **54**, 264–73.

NCCN (1999). NCCN practice guidelines: genetics/familial high risk cancer. *Oncology*, **13**(11A), 161–86.

Nelen, M.R., Padberg, G.W., Peeters, E.A.J. et al. (1996). Localization of the gene for Cowden disease to 10q22–23. *Nat. Genet.*, **13**, 114–6.

Nelen, M.R., van Staveren, C.G., Peeters, E.A.J. et al. (1997). Germline mutations in the *PTEN/MMAC1* gene in patients with Cowden disease. *Hum. Mol. Genet.*, **6**, 1383–7.

Nelen, M.R., Kremer, H., Konings, I.B.M. et al. (1999). Novel *PTEN* mutations in patients with Cowden disease: absence of clear genotype–phenotype correlations. *Eur. J. Hum. Genet.*, **7**, 267–73.

Neuhausen, S.L., Mazoyer, S., Friedman, L., Stratton, M., Offit, K., Caligo, A., Tomlinson, G., Cannon-Albright, L., Bishop, T., Kelsell, D., Solomon, E., Weber, B., Couch, F., Struewing, J., Tonin, P., Durocher, F., Narod, S., Skolnick, M.H., Lenoir, G., Serova, O., Ponder, B., Stoppa-Lyonnet, D., Easton, D., King, M.C. & Goldgar, D.E. (1996). Haplotype and phenotype analysis of six recurrent BRCA1 mutations in 61 families: results of an international study. *Am. J. Hum. Genet.*, **58**, 271–80.

Neuland, C.Y., Blattner, W.A., Mann, D.L., Fraser, M.C., Tsai, S. & Strong, D.M. (1983). Familial chronic lymphocytic leukemia. *J. Natl. Cancer Inst.*, **71**, 1143–50.

Neumann, H.P.H. & Wiestler, O.D. (1991). Clustering of features of von Hippel–Lindau syndrome: evidence for a complex genetic locus. *Lancet*, **337**, 1052–4.

Neumann, H.P.H., Bausch, B., McWhinney, S.R., Bender, B.U., Gimm, O., Franke, G., Schipper, J., Klisch, J., Altehoefer, C., Zerres, K., Januszewicz, A., Eng, C., Smith, W.M., Munk, R., Manz, T., Glaesker, S., Apel, T.W., Treier, M., Reineke, M., Walz, M.K., Hoang-Vu, C., Brauckhoff, M., Klein-Franke, A., Klose, P., Schmidt, H., Maier-Woelfle, M., Peczkowska, M., Szmigielski, C. & Eng, C. (2002). The Freiburg-Warsaw-Columbus Pheochromocytoma Study Group. Germ-line mutations in nonsyndromic pheochromocytoma. *N. Engl. J. Med.*, **346**, 1459–66.

Newschaffer, C.J., Topham, A., Herzberg, T., Weiner, S. & Weinberg, D.S. (2001). Risk of colorectal cancer after breast cancer. *Lancet*, **357**, 837–40.

Newton, J.A., Bataille, V., Griffiths, K. et al. (1993). How common is the atypical mole syndrome phenotype in apparently sporadic melanoma? *J. Am. Acad. Dermatol.*, **29**, 989–96.

Newton Bishop, J., Harland, M., Wachsmuth, R. et al. (2000). Genotype/phenotype and penetrance studies in melanoma families with germline CDKN2A mutations. *J. Invest. Dermatol.*, **114**, 28–33.

Newton Bishop, J.A., Bataille, V., Pinney, E. & Bishop, D.T. (1994). Family studies in melanoma: identification of the atypical mole syndrome (AMS) phenotype. *Melanoma Res.*, **4**(4), 199–206.

Nichols, C.R. (1992). Mediastinal germ cell tumours. *Semin. Thorac. Cardiovasc. Surg.*, **4**, 45–50.

Nicholson, P.W. & Harland, S.J. (1995). Inheritance and testicular cancer. *Br. J. Cancer*, **71**(2), 421–6.

Nickerson, M.L., Warren, M.B., Toro, J.R., Matrosova, V., Glenn, G., Turner, M.L., Duray, P., Merino, M., Choyke, P., Pavlovich, C.P., Sharma, N., Walther, M., Munroe, D., Hill, R., Maher, E., Greenberg, C., Lerman, M.I., Linehan, W.M., Zbar, B. & Schmidt, L.S. (2002). Mutations in a novel gene lead to kidney tumors, lung wall defects, and benign tumors of the hair follicle in patients with the Birt–Hogg–Dube syndrome. *Cancer Cell*, **2**(2), 157–64.

Nicoliades, N.C., Papadopoulos, N., Liu, B. et al. (1994). Mutations of two PMS homologues in hereditary non-polyposis colorectal cancer. *Nature*, **371**, 75–80.

Nieder, A.M., Taneja, S.S., Zeegers, M.P. & Ostre, H. (2003). Genetic counselling for prostate cancer risk. *Clin. Genet.* **63**, 169–76.

Niederau, C., Fischer, R., Sonnenberg, A. et al. (1985). Survival and cause of death in cirrhotic and non-cirrhotic patients with primary haemochromatosis. *New Engl. J. Med.*, **313**, 1256–63.

Niell, B.L., Long, J.C., Rennert, G. & Gruber. S.B. (2003). Genetic anthropology of the colorectal cancer-susceptibility allele APC I1307K: evidence of genetic drift within the Ashkenazim. *Am. J. Hum. Genet.*, **73**, 1250–60.

Niell, B.L., Rennert, G., Bonner, J.D. et al. (2004). BRCA1 and BRCA2 founder mutations and the risk of colorectal cancer. *J. Natl. Cancer Inst.*, **96**, 15–21.

Niell, B.L., Rennert, G., Bonner, J.D., Almog, R., Tomsho, L.P. & Gruber, S.B. (2004). BRCA1 and BRCA2 founder mutations and the risk of colorectal cancer. *J. Natl. Cancer Inst.*, **96**, 15–21.

Niemann, S. & Muller, U. (2000). Mutations in *SDHC* cause autosomal dominant paraganglioma. *Nat. Genet.*, **26**, 141–50.

Nijssen, P.C., Deprez, R.H., Tijssen, C.C. et al. (1994). Familial anaplastic ependymoma: evidence of loss of chromosome 22 in tumour cells. *J. Neurol. Neurosurg. Psychiat.*, **57**(10), 1245–8.

Nilsson, O., Tissell, L.-E., Jansson, S., Ahlman, H., Gimm, O. & Eng, C. (1999). Adrenal and extra-adrenal pheochromocytomas in a family with germline *RET* V804L mutation. *J. Am. Med. Aossc.*, **281**, 1587–8.

Nishijo, K. et al. (2004). Mutation analysis of the RECQL4 gene in sporadic osteosarcomas. *Int. J. Cancer*, **111**(3), 367–72.

Nishimoto, I.N., Pinheiro, N.A., Rogatto, S.R., Carvalho, A.L., de Moura, R.P., Caballero, O.L., Simpson, A. & Kowalski, L.P. (2004). Alcohol dehydrogenase 3 genotype as a risk factor for upper aerodigestive tract cancers. *Arch. Otolaryngol. Head Neck Surg.*, **130**, 78–82.

Nishimura, G. & Koslowski, K. (1990). Proteus syndrome. (Report of three cases.) *Australas. Radiol.*, **34**, 47–52.

Nisoli, E., Regianini, L., Briscini, L. et al. (2002). Multiple symmetric lipomatosis may be the consequence of defective noradrenergic modulation of proliferation and differentiation of brown fat cells. *J. Path.*, **198**, 378–87.

Noguchi, M., Yi, H., Rosenblatt, H.M. et al. (1993). Interleukin-2 receptor gamma chain mutation results in X-linked severe combined immunodeficiency in humans. *Cell*, **73**, 147–57.

Noguera-Irizarry, W.G., Hibshoosh, H. & Papadopoulos, K.P. (2003). Renal medullary carcinoma: case report and review of the literature. *Am. J. Clin. Oncol.*, **26**, 489–92.

Noorani, H.Z., Khan, H.N., Gallie, B.L. & Detsky, A.S. (1996). Cost comparison of molecular versus conventional screening of relatives at risk for retinoblastoma. *Am. J. Hum. Genet.*, **59**, 301–7.

Norris, W. (1820). A case of fungoid disease. *Edinb. Med. Surg. J.*, **16**, 562–5.

Norton, J.A., Fraker, D.L., Alexander, H.R. et al. (1999). Surgery to cure Zollinger–Ellison syndrome. *New Engl. J. Med.*, **341**, 635–44.

Nowell, P.C. & Hungerford, D.A. (1960). A minute chromosome in human chronic granulocytic leukaemia. *Science*, **132**, 1497.

Nugent, K.P., Phillips, R.K.S., Hodgson, S.V. et al. (1994). Phenotypic expression in familial adenomatous polyposis: partial prediction by mutation analysis. *Gut*, **35**, 1622–4.

Nystrom-Lahti, M., Kristo, P., Nicolaides, N.C., Chang, S.Y., Aaltonen, L.A., Moisio, A.L., Jarvinen, H.J., Mecklin, J.P., Kinzler, K.W. & Vogelstein, B. (1995). Founding mutations and Alu-mediated recombination in hereditary colon cancer. *Nat. Med.*, **1**(11), 1203–6.

O'Brien, P.K. & Wilansky, D.L. (1981). Familial thyroid nodulation and arrhenoblastoma. *Am. J. Clin. Pathol.*, **75**, 578–81.

Oddoux, C., Struewing, J.P., Clayton, C.M., Neuhausen, S., Brody, L.C., Kaback, M., Haas, B., Norton, L., Borgen, P., Jhanwar, S., Goldgar, D., Ostrer, H. & Offit, K. (1996). The carrier frequency of the BRCA2 6174delT mutation among Ashkenazi Jewish individuals is approximately 1-percent. *Nat. Genet.*, **14**, 188–90.

Odent, S., Atti-Bitach, T., Blayau, M., Mathieu, M., Aug, J., Delezo, d.A., Gall, J.Y., Le Marec, B., Munnich, A., David, V. & Vekemans, M. (1999). Expression of the Sonic hedgehog (SHH) gene during early human development and phenotypic expression of new mutations causing holoprosencephaly. *Hum. Mol. Genet.*, **8**(9), 1683–9.

Offit, K., Levran, O., Mullaney, B., Mah, K., Nafa, K., Batish, S.D., Diotti, R., Schneider, H., Deffenbaugh, A., Scholl, T., Proud, V.K., Robson, M., Norton, L., Ellis, N., Hanenberg, H. & Auerbach, A.D. (2003). Shared genetic susceptibility to breast cancer, brain tumors, and Fanconi anemia. *J. Natl. Cancer Inst.*, **95**, 1548–51.

Oh, J., Bailin, T., Fukai, K. et al. (1996). Positional cloning of a gene for Hermansy–Pudlak syndrome, a disorder of cytoplasmic organelles. *Nat. Genet.*, **14**, 300–6.

Ohne, M., Tomita, N., Monden, T. et al. (1996). Mutations of the transforming growth factor b type II receptor gene and microsatellite instability in gastric cancer. *Int. J. Cancer*, **68**, 203–6.

Oiso, N., Mizuno, N., Fukai, K. et al. (2004). Mild phenotype of familial cylindromatosis associated with an R758X nonsense mutation in the CYLD tumour suppressor gene. *B. J. Dermatol.*, **151**, 1084–6.

Okimoto, K., Sakurai, J., Kobayashi, T., Mitani, H., Hirayama, Y., Nickerson, M.L., Warren, M.B., Zbar, B., Schmidt, L.S. & Hino, O. (2004). A germ-line insertion in the

Birt–Hogg–Dube (BHD) gene gives rise to the Nihon rat model of inherited renal cancer. *Proc. Natl. Acad. Sci. USA*, **101**, 2023–7.

Olivier, M., Goldgar, D.E., Sodha, N. et al. (2003). Li–Fraumeni and related syndromes: correlation between tumor type, family structure and *TP53* genotype. *Cancer Res.*, **63**, 6643–50.

Olschwang, S., Laurent-Puig, P. et al. (1993). Germline mutations in the first 14 exons of the adenomatous polyposis coli (APC) gene. *Am. J. Hum. Genet.*, **52**, 273–9.

Olschwang, S., Serova-Sinilnikova, O.M., Lenoir, G.M. & Thomas, G. (1998). *PTEN* germline mutations in juvenile polyposis coli. *Nat. Genet.*, **18**, 12–14.

Olschwang, S., Eisinger, F. & Millat, B. (2005). An alternative to prophylactic colectomy for colon cancer prevention in HNPCC syndrome. *Gut*, **54**, 169–73.

Omura, N.E., Collison, D.W., Perry, A.E. & Myers, L.M. (2002). Sebaceous carcinoma in children. *J. Am. Acad. Dermatol.*, **47**(6), 950–3.

Ooi, W.L., Elston, R.C., Chen, V.W., Bailey-Wilson, J.E. & Rothschild, H. (1986). Increased family risk for lung cancer. *J. Natl. Cancer Inst.*, **16**, 217–20.

Orlow, S. (1997). Albinism: an update. *Semin. Cutan. Med. Surg.*, **16**, 24–9.

Orth, G., Jablonska, S., Jarzabek-Chorzetska, M. et al. (1979). Characteristics of the lesions and risk of malignant conversion associated with the type of human papillomavirus involved in epiderrnodysplasia verruciformis. *Dermatologica*, **158**, 309–27.

Oshima, M., Dinchuk, J.E., Kargman, S.L. et al. (1996). Suppression of intestinal polyposis in Apc delta knockout mice by inhibition of cyclooxygenase-2 (COX-2). *Cell*, **87**, 803–9.

Ostasiewicz, L.T., Huang, J.L., Wang, X. et al. (1995). Human protoporphyria genetic heterogeneity at the ferrochelatase locus. *Photodermatol. Photoimmunol. Photomed.*, **11**, 18–21.

Osterlind, A., Tucker, M.A., Hou-Jensen, K., Stone, B.J., Engholm, G. & Jensen, O.M. (1988a). The Danish case–control study of cutaneous malignant melanoma. I. Importance of host factors. *Int. J. Cancer*, **42**(2), 200–6.

Osterlind, A., Tucker, M.A., Stone, B.J. & Jensen, O.M. (1988b). The Danish case–control study of cutaneous malignant melanoma. II. Importance of UV-light exposure. *Int. J. Cancer*, **42**(3), 319–24.

Osterod, M. et al. (2002). A global DNA repair mechanism involving the Cockayne syndrome B (CSB) gene product can prevent the in vivo accumulation of endogenous oxidative DNA base damage. *Oncogene*, **21**(54), 8232–9.

Ottman, R., Pille, M.C., King, M.C. et al. (1986). Familial breast cancer in a population-based series. *Am. J. Epidemiol.*, **123**, 15–21.

Owen, L.N. (1967). Comparative aspects of bone tumours in man and dog. *Proc. R. Soc. Med.*, **60**, 1309–10.

Ozcelik, H., Schmocker, B., DiNicola, N. et al. (1997). Germline BRCA2 6174del T mutations in Ashkenazi Jewish pancreatic cancer patients. *Nat. Genet.*, **16**, 17–18.

Pack, K., Smith-Ravin, J., Phillips, R.K.S. & Hodgson, S.C. (1996). Exceptions to the rule: individuals with FAP-specific CHRPE and mutations in exon 6 of the APC gene. *Clin. Genet.*, **50**, 110–11.

Pal, T., Permuth-Wey, J., Betts, J.A. et al. (2005). *BRCA1* and *BRCA2* mutations account for a large proportion of ovarian carcinoma cases. *Cancer*, **104**(12), 2807–16.

Paller, A.S., Norton, K., Teevi, A. et al. (2003). Mutations in the capillary morphogenesis gene-2 result in the allelic disorder Juvenile hyaline fibromatosis and infantile systemic hyalinosis. *Am. J. Hum. Genet.*, **73**, 957–66.

Pannett, A.A., Kennedy, A.M., Turner, J.J. et al. (2003). Multiple endocrine neoplasia type 1 (MEN1) germline mutations in familial isolated primary hyperparathyroidism. *Clin. Endocrinol.*, **58**, 639–46.

Papi, L., Montali, E., Marconi, G., Guazzelli, R., Bigozzi, U., Maraschio, P. & Zuffardi, O. (1989). Evidence for a human mitotic mutant with pleiotropic effect. *Ann. Hum. Genet.*, **53**(Pt 3), 243–8.

Paraf, F., Sasseville, D., Watters, A.K., Narod, S., Ginsburg, O., Shibata, H. & Jothy, S. (1995). Clinicopathological relevance of the association between gastrointestinal and sebaceous neoplasms: the Muir–Torre syndrome [Review]. *Hum. Pathol.*, **26**(4), 422–7.

Paraf, F., Jothy, S. & Van Meir, E.G. (1997). Brain tumour–polyposis syndrome. Two genetic diseases? *J. Clin. Oncol.*, **15**, 2744–58.

Parazzini, F., Negri, E., La Vecchia, C., Restelli, C. & Franceschi, S. (1992). Family history of reproductive cancers and ovarian cancer risk: an Italian case–control study. *Am. J. Epidemiol.*, **135**, 35–40.

Park, Y.J., Shin, K.-H. & Park, J.-G. (2000). Risk of gastric cancer in hereditary nonpolyposis colorectal cancer in Korea. *Clin. Cancer Res.*, **6**, 2994–8.

Parker, J.A., Kalnins, V.I., Deck, J.H.N. et al. (1990). Histopathological features of congenital fundus lesions in familial adenomatous polyposis. *Can. J. Ophthalmol.*, **25**, 159–63.

Parkin, D., Whelan, S., Ferlay, J., Raymond, L. & Young, J. (1997). *Cancer Incidence in Five Continents*. IARC Scientific Publications No. 143. International Agency for Research on Cancer **II**, Lyon, France.

Parkin, D.M., Pisani, P. & Ferlay, J. (1993). Estimates of the worldwide incidence of eighteen major cancers in 1985. *Int. J. Cancer*, **55**, 891–903.

Parkin, D.M. et al. (1997). *Cancer Incidence in Five Continents*. 7th edn. IARC, Lyon.

Parry, D.M., Li, F.P., Strong, L.C. et al. (1982). Carotid body tumors in humans: genetics and epidemiology. *J. Natl. Cancer Inst.*, **68**, 573–8.

Parry, D.M., MacCollin, M.M., Kaiser-Kupfer, M.I. et al. (1996). Germ-line mutations in the neurofibromatosis 2 gene: correlations with disease severity and retinal abnormalities. *Am. J. Hum. Genet.*, **59**, 529–39.

Parsons, R., Li, G.-M., Langley, M.J. et al. (1993). Hypermutability and mismatch repair deficiency in RER tumour cells. *Cell*, **75**, 1227–36.

Patel, K.J., Yu, V.P., Lee, H., Corcoran, A., Thistlethwaite, F.C., Evans, M.J., Colledge, W.H., Friedman, L.S., Ponder, B.A. & Venkitaraman, A.R. (1998). Involvement of Brca2 in DNA repair. *Mol. Cell.*, **1**, 347–57.

Patel, S.R., Kvols, L.K. & Richardson, R.L. (1990). Familial testicular cancer: report of six cases and review of the literature. *Mayo Clin. Proc.*, **65**, 804–8.

Patrice, S.J., Sneed, P.K., Flickinger, J.C., Shrieve, D.C., Pollock, B.E., Alexander, E. III, Larson, D.A., Kondziolka, D.S., Gutin, P.H., Wara, W.M., McDermott, M.W., Lunsford, L.D. & Loeffler, J.S. (1996). Radiosurgery for hemangioblastoma: results of a multiinstitutional experience. *Int. J. Radiat. Oncol. Biol. Phys.*, **35**, 493–9.

Paul, S.M., Bacharach, B. & Goepp, C. (1987). A genetic influence on alveolar cell carcinoma. *J. Surg. Oncol.*, **36**, 249.

Pavlovich, C.P., Walther, M.M., Eyler, R.A., Hewitt, S.M., Zbar, B., Linehan, W.M. & Merino, M.J. (2002). Renal tumors in the Birt–Hogg–Dube syndrome. *Am. J. Surg. Pathol.*, **26**(12), 1542–52.

Peackocke, M. & Siminowitch, K.A. (1987). Linkage of the Wiscott–Aldrich syndrome with polymorphic DNA sequences from the human X chromosome. *Proc. Natl. Acad. Sci. USA*, **84**, 3430–3.

Pearson, R.W. (1988). Clinicopathologic types of epidermolysis bullosa and their non-dermatological complications. *Arch. Dermatol.*, **124**, 718–25.

Pearson, T., Jansen, S., Havenga, C., Stones, D.K. & Joubert, G. (2001). Fanconi anemia. A statistical evaluation of cytogenetic results obtained from South African families. *Cancer Genet. Cytogenet.*, **126**, 52–5.

Peel, D., Kolodner, R., Li, F. & Anton-Culver, H. (1997). Relationship between replication error (RER) and MSH2/MLH1 gene mutations in population-based HNPCC kindreds. *Am. J. Hum. Genet.*, **61S**, A208–1203.

Peel, D.J., Ziogas, A., Fox, E.A., Gildea, M., Laham, B., Clements, E., Kolodner, R.D. & Anton-Culver, H. (2000). Characterization of hereditary nonpolyposis colorectal cancer families from a population-based series of cases. *J. Natl. Cancer Inst.*, **92**, 1517–22.

Peelen, T., van Vliet, M., Petrij-Bosch, A., Mieremet, R., Szabo, C., van den Ouweland, A.M., Hogervorst, F., Brohet, R., Ligtenberg, M.J., Teugels, E., van der Luijt, R., van der Hout, A.H., Gille, J.J., Pals, G., Jedema, I., Olmer, R., van, L.I., Newman, B., Plandsoen, M., van der Est, M., Brink, G., Hageman, S., Arts, P.J., Bakker, M.M. & Devilee, P. (1997). A high proportion of novel mutations in BRCA1 with strong founder effects among Dutch and Belgian hereditary breast and ovarian cancer families [see comments]. *Am. J. Hum. Genet.*, **60**, 1041–9.

Pelletier, J., Bruening, W., Kashtan, C.E. et al. (1991a). Germline mutations in the Wilms' tumour suppressor gene are associated with abnormal urogenital development in Denys–Drash syndrome. *Cell*, **67**, 437–47.

Pelletier, J., Bruening, W., Li, F.P., Haber, D.A., Glaser, T. & Housman, D.E. (1991b). WT1 mutations contribute to abnormal genital system development and hereditary Wilms' tumour. *Nature*, **353**, 431–4.

Penrose, L.S., Mackenzie, H.J. & Karn, M.N. (1948). A genetic study of human mammary cancer. *Ann. Eugen.*, **14**, 234–66.

Perlmutter, D.H. (1995). Clinical manifestations of alpha 1-antitrypsin deficiency. *Gastroenterol. Clin. North Am.*, **24**, 27–43.

Perri, P., Longo, L., McConville, C., Cusano, R., Rees, S.A., Seri, M., Conte, M., Romeo, G., Devoto, M. & Tonini, G.P. (2002). Linkage analysis in families with recurrent neuroblastoma. *Ann. NY Acad. Sci.*, **963**, 74–84.

Peterson Jr, H.R., Bowlds, C.F. & Yam, L.T. (1984). Familial DiGuglielmo syndrome. *Cancer*, **54**, 932–8.

Peterson, R.D., Fuckhouser, J.D., Tuck-Muller, C.M. & Gatti, R.A. (1992). Cancer susceptibility in Ataxia Telangectasia. *Leukaemia*, **6**(Suppl 1), 8–13.

Peto, J., Easton, D.F., Matthews, F.E. et al. (1996). Cancer mortality in relatives of women with breast cancer: the OPCS study. *Int. J. Cancer*, **65**, 275–8.

Peto, J., Collins, N., Barfoot, R., Seal, S., Warren, W., Rahman, N., Easton, D.F., Evans, C., Deacon, J. & Stratton, M.R. (1999). Prevalence of BRCA1 and BRCA2 gene mutations in patients with early-onset breast cancer [see comments]. *J. Nat. Cancer Inst.*, **91**, 943–9.

Petrakis, N.L. (1977). Genetic factors in the aetiology of breast cancer. *Cancer*, **39**, 2709–15.

Peutz, J.L.A. (1921). Very remarkable case of familial polyposis of mucous membrane of intestinal tract and nasopharynx accompanied by peculiar pigmentations of skin and mucous membranes (Dutch). *Nederl. Maandschr. Geneesk.*, **10**, 134–46.

Peyster, R.G., Ginsberg, F. & Hoover, E.D. (1986). Computed tomography of familial pinealoblastoma. *J. Comput. Assist Tomogr.*, **10**, 32–3.

Pezzilli, R., Morselli-Labate, A.M., Mantovani, V., Romboli, E., Selva, P., Migliori, M., Corinaldesi, R. & Gullo, L. (2003). Mutations of the CFTR gene in pancreatic disease. *Pancreas*, **27**, 332–6.

Pharoah, P.D., Guilford, P. & Caldas, C. (2001). International Gastric Cancer Linkage Consortium. Incidence of gastric cancer and breast cancer in CDH1 (E-cadherin) mutation carriers from hereditary diffuse gastric cancer families. *Gastroenterology*, **121**(6), 1348–53.

Phelan, C.M., Rebbeck, T.R., Weber, B.L., Devilee, P., Ruttledge, M.H., Lynch, H.T., Lenoir, G.M., Stratton, M.R., Easton, D.F., Ponder, B.A., Cannon-Albright, L., Larsson, C., Goldgar, D.E. & Narod, S.A. (1996). Ovarian cancer risk in BRCA1 carriers is modified by the HRAS1 variable number of tandem repeat (VNTR) locus. *Nat. Genet.*, **12**, 309–11.

Phillips, R.K.S. & Spigelman, A.D. (1996). Can we safely delay or avoid prophylactic colectomy in familial adenomatous polyposis (FAP)? *Br. J. Surg.*, **83**, 769–70.

Phillips, R.K., Wallance, M.H., Lynch, P.M. et al. (2002). A randomised, double-blind placeto controlled study of celecoxib, a selective cyclo-oxygenase 2 inhibitor, on duodenal polyposis in familial adenomatous polyposis. *Gut*, **50**, 857–60.

Pilarski, R. & Eng, C. (2004). Will the real Cowden syndrome please stand up (again)? Expanding mutational and clinical spectra of the *PTEN* hamartoma tumour syndrome. *J. Med. Genet.*, **41**, 323–6.

Pilia, G., Hughes-Benzie, R.M., MacKenzie, A. et al. (1996). Mutations in GPC3, a glypican gene, cause the Simpson–Golabi–Behmel overgrowth syndrome. *Nat. Genet.*, **12**, 241–7.

Pinheiro, M. & Freire-Maia, N. (1994). Ectodermal dysplasias: a clinical classification and a causal review. *Am. J. Med. Genet.*, **53**, 153–62.

Pinto, E.M., Billerbeck, A.E., Villares, M.C. et al. (2004). Founder effect for the highly prevalent R337H mutation of tumor suppressor *p53* in Brazilian patients with adrenocortical tumors. *Arq. Bras. Endocrinal. Metabol.*, **48**(5), 647–50.

Piver, M.S., Jishi, M.F., Tsukada, Y. & Nava, G. (1993). Primary peritoneal carcinoma after prophylactic oophorectomy in women with a family history of ovarian cancer. A report to the Gilder Radner Familial Ovarian Cancer Registry. *Cancer*, **71**, 2751–5.

Plail, R.O., Bussey, H.J.R., Glazer, G. & Thomson, J.P.S. (1987). Adenomatous polyposis: an association with carcinoma of the thyroid. *Br. J. Surg.*, **74**, 377–80.

Polkinghorne, P.J., Ritchie, S., Neale, K., Schoeppener, G., Thomson, J.P.S. & Jay, B.S. (1990). Pigmented lesions of the retinal pigment epithelium and familial adenomatous polyposis. *Eye*, **4**, 216–21.

Pollak, M.R., Brown, E.M., Chou, Y.H. et al. (1993). Mutations in the human Ca(2+)-sensing receptor gene cause familial hypocalciuric hypercalcemia and neonatal severe hyperparathyroidism. *Cell*, **75**, 1297–303.

Polymeropoulos, M.H., Hurko, O., Hsu, F. et al. (1997). Linkage of the locus for cerebral cavernous hemangiomas to human chromosome 7q in four families of Mexican-American descent. *Neurology*, **48**, 752–7.

Ponder, B.A.J., Ponder, M.A., Coffey, R. et al. (1988). Risk estimation and screening in families of patients with medullary thyroid carcinoma. *Lancet*, **i**, 397–400.

Ponz de Leon, M. (1994). Familial tumors of other organs. *Recent Result. Cancer Res.*, **136**, 332–40.

Poppe, B., Van Limbergen, H., Van Roy, N., Vandecruys, E., De Paepe, A., Benoit, Y. & Speleman, F. (2001). Chromosomal aberrations in Bloom syndrome patients with myeloid malignancies. *Cancer Genet. Cytogenet.*, **128**(1), 39–42.

Porter, D.E., Lonie, L, Fraser, M. et al. (2004). Severity of disease and risk of malignant change in hereditary multiple exostoses. A genotype—phenotype study. *J. Bone Joint Surg. Br.*, **86**, 1041–6.

Porter, R.M. & Lane, E.B. (2003). Phenotypes, genotypes and their contribution to understanding keratin function. *Trend. Genet.*, **19**, 278–85.

Potter, D.D., Murray, J.A., Donohue, J.H., Burgart, L.J., Nagorney, D.M., van Heerden, J.A., Plevak, M.F., Zinsmeister, A.R. & Thibodeau, S.N. (2004). The role of defective mismatch repair in small bowel adenocarcinoma in celiac disease. *Cancer Res.*, **64**, 7073–7.

Potter, N.U., Sarmousakis, C. & Li, F.P. (1983). Cancer in relatives of patients with aplastic anemia. *Cancer Genet. Cytogenet.*, **9**, 61–5.

Pottern, L.M., Linet, M., Blair, A. et al. (1991). Familial cancers associated with subtypes of leukemia and non-Hodgkin's lymphoma. *Leuk. Res.*, **15**, 305–14.

Powell, S.M. (2002). Direct analysis for familial adenomatous polyposis mutations. Mol. *Biotechnol.*, **20**, 197–207.

Powell, S.M., Zilz, N., Beazer-Barclay, Y. et al. (1992). APC mutations occur early during colorectal tumorigenesis. *Nature*, **359**, 235–7.

Puck, J.M. et al. (1993). The interleukin-2 receptor gamma chain maps to Xq13.1 and is mutated in X-linked severe combined immunodeficiency, SCIDX1. *Hum. Mol. Genet.*, **2**(8), 1099–104.

Puck, J.M. et al. (1997). Mutation analysis of IL2RG in human X-linked severe combined immunodeficiency. *Blood.*, **89**(6), 1968–77.

Pulst, S.M., Rouleau, G.A., Marineau, C., Fain, P. & Sieb, J.P. (1993). Familial meningioma is not allelic to neurofibromatosis 2. *Neurology*, **43**(10), 2096–8.

Purdie, D., Green, A., Bain, C., Siskind, V., Ward, B., Hacker, N., Quinn, M., Wright, G., Russell, P. & Susil, B. (1995). Reproductive and other factors and risk of epithelial ovarian cancer: an Australian case–control study. Survey of Women's Health Study Group. *Int. J. Cancer*, **62**, 678–84.

Quinn, A.G. (1996). Molecular genetics of human non-melanoma skin cancer. *Cancer Surv.*, **26**, 89–114.

Rada, D.C., Koranda, F.C. & Kats, F.S. (1985). Resident's corner: chelitis glandularis – a disorder of ductal ectasia. *J. Dermatol. Surg. Oncol.*, **11**, 372–5.

Ragab, A.H., Abdel-Mageed, A., Shuster, J.J. et al. (1991). Clinical characteristics and treatment outcome of children with acute lymphoblastic leukaemia and Down's syndrome. *Cancer*, **67**, 1057–63.

Ragnarsson-Olding, B.K. (2004). Primary malignant melanoma of the vulva-an aggressive tumour for modelling the genesis of non-UV light-associated melanoma. *Acta oncol.*, **43**, 421–35.

Rahman, N., Arbour, L., Tonin, P. et al. (1996). Evidence for a familial Wilms' tumour gene (FWT1) on chromosome 17q12–q21. *Nat. Genet.*, **13**, 461–3.

Rahman, N. et al. (1998). Confirmation of FWT1 as a Wilms' tumour susceptibility gene and phenotypic characteristics of Wilms' tumour attributable to FWT1. *Hum. Genet.*, **103**(5), 547–56.

Rahman, N. et al. (2000). Penetrance of mutations in the familial Wilms tumor gene FWT1. *J. Natl. Cancer. Inst.*, **92**(8), 650–2.

Rahman, N., Dunstan, M., Tearc, M.D. et al. (2002). The gene for juvenile hyaline fibromatosis maps to chromosome 4q21. *Am. J. Hum. Genet.*, **71**, 975–80.

Rajagopalan, H., Nowak, M.A., Vogelstein, B. & Lengauer, C. (2003). The significance of unstable chromosomes in colorectal cancer. *Nat. Rev. Cancer*, **3**(9), 695–701.

Ramoz, N., Rueda, L.A., Bouadjar, B. et al. (2002). Mutations in two adjacent novel genes are associated with epidermodysplasia verruciformis. *Nat. Genet.*, **32**, 579–81.

Ramus, S.J., Kote-Jarai, Z., Friedman, L.S., Van der Looij, M., Gayther, S.A., Csokay, B., Ponder, B.A. & Olah, E. (1997). Analysis of BRCA1 and BRCA2 mutations in Hungarian families with breast or breast-ovarian cancer [letter]. *Am. J. Hum. Genet.*, **60**, 1242–6.

Randerson-Moor, J.A., Harland, M., Williams, S., Cuthbert-Heavens, D., Sheridan, E., Aveyard, J., Sibley, K., Whitaker, L., Knowles, M., Bishop, J.N. & Bishop, D.T. (2001). A germline deletion of p14(ARF) but not CDKN2A in a melanoma-neural system tumour syndrome family. *Hum. Mol. Genet.*, **10**, 55–62.

Rapin, I., Lindenbaum, Y., Dicson, D.W. et al. (2000). Cockayne syndrome and xeroderma pigmentosum. *Neurology*, **55**, 1442–9.

Rapley, E.A., Crockford, G.P., Teare, D. et al (2000). Localization to Xq27 of a susceptibility gene for testicular germ-cell tumours. *Nat. Genet.*, **24**, 197–200.

Ratnoff, W.D. & Gress, R.E. (1980). The familial occurrence of polycythemia rubra vera: report of a father and son, with consideration of the possible etiological role of exposure to organic solvents, including tetrachloroethylene. *Blood*, **56**, 233–6.

Rawstron, A.C., Yuille, M.R., Fuller, J., Cullen, M., Kennedy, B., Richards, S.J., Jack, A.S., Matutes, E., Catovsky, D., Hillmen, P. & Houlston, R.S. (2002). Inherited predisposition to CLL is detectable as subclinical monoclonal B-lymphocyte expansion. *Blood*, **100**(7), 2289–90.

Reardon, W., Harding, B., Winter, R. & Baraitser, M. (1996). Hemihypertrophy, hemimegalencephaly and polydactyly. *Am. J. Med. Genet.*, **66**, 144–9.

Reardon, W., Zhou, X.P. & Eng, C. (2001). A novel germline mutation of the *PTEN* gene in a patient with macrocephaly, ventricular dilatation and features of VATER association. *J. Med. Genet.*, **38**, 820–3.

Rebbeck, T.R., Levin, A.M., Eisen, A., Snyder, C., Watson, P., Cannon-Albright, L., Isaacs, C., Olopade, O., Garber, J.E., Godwin, A.K., Daly, M.B., Narod, S.A., Neuhausen, S.L., Lynch, H.T. & Weber, B.L. (1999). Breast cancer risk after bilateral prophylactic oophorectomy in BRCA1 mutation carriers [see comments]. *J. Natl. Cancer Inst.*, **91**, 1475–9.

Rebbeck, T.R., Lynch, H.T., Neuhausen, S.L., Narod, S.A., Van't Veer, L., Garber, J.E., Evans, G., Isaacs, C., Daly, M.B., Matloff, E., Olopade, O.I. & Weber, B.L. (2002). Prophylactic oophorectomy in carriers of BRCA1 or BRCA2 mutations. *New Engl. J. Med.*, **346**, 1616–22.

Rebbeck, T.R., Friebel, T., Lynch, H.T., Neuhausen, S.L., van, V., Garber, J.E., Evans, G.R., Narod, S.A., Isaacs, C., Matloff, E., Daly, M.B., Olopade, O.I. & Weber, B.L. (2004). Bilateral prophylactic mastectomy reduces breast cancer risk in BRCA1 and BRCA2 mutation carriers: the PROSE Study Group. *J. Clin. Oncol.*, **22**, 1055–62.

Rees, J.L. (2003). Genetics of hair and skin colour. *Ann. Rev. Genet.*, **37**, 67–90.

Renier, G., Ifrah, N., Chevailler, A., Saint-André, J.P., Boasson, M. & Hurez, D. (1989). Four brothers with Waldenstrom's macroglobulinaemia. *Cancer*, **64**, 1554–9.

Renkonen-Sinisalo, L., Aarnio, M., Mecklin, J.P. & Jarvinen, H.J. (2000). Surveillance improves survival of colorectal cancer in patients with HNPCC. *Cancer Detect. Prev.*, **24**, 137–42.

Reyes, C.M., Allen, B.A., Terdiman, J.P. et al. (2002). Comparison of selection strategies for genetic testing of patients with hereditary non-polyposis colorectal cancer: effectiveness and cost-effectiveness. *Cancer*, **95**, 1848–56.

Ribeiro, R.C., Sandrini, F., Figueiredo, B. et al. (2001). An inherited *p53* mutation that contributes in a tissue-specific manner to pediatric adrenal cortical carcinoma. *Proc. Natl. Acad. Sci. USA*, **98**, 9330–5.

Riccardi, V.M. & Eichner, J.E. (1986). *Neurofibromatosis: Phenotype, Natural History and Pathogenesis.* Johns Hopkins University Press, Baltimore.

Riccardi, V.M. & Lewis, R.A. (1988). Penetrance of von Recklinghausen neurofibromatosis: a distinction between predecessors and descendants. *Am. J. Hum. Genet.*, **42**, 284–9.

Ricciardone, M.D., Ozcelik, T., Cevher, B., Ozdag, H., Tuncer, M., Gurgey, A., Uzunalimoglu, O., Cetinkaya, H., Tanyeli, A., Erken, E. & Ozturk, M. (1999). Human MLH1 deficiency predisposes to hematological malignancy and neurofibromatosis type 1. *Cancer Res.*, **59**(2), 290–3.

Richards, C.S., Ward, P.A., Roa, B.B. et al. (1997). Screening for 185delAG in Ashkenazim. *Am. J. Hum. Genet.*, **60**, 1085–98.

Richards, F.M., Goudie, D.R., Cooper, W.N. et al. (1997). Mapping the multiple self-healing epithelioma (MSSE) gene and investigation of XP group A (XPA) and patched (PTCH) as candidate genes. *Hum. Genet.*, **101**, 317–22.

Richards, P.M., McKee, S.A. & Rajpar, M.H. (1999). Germline E-cadherin *(CDH1)* gene mutations predispose to familial gastric cancer and colorectal cancer. *Hum. Mol. Genet.*, **8**, 607–10.

Rickard, S.J. & Wilson, L.C. (2003). Analysis of *GNAS1* and overlapping transcripts identifies the parent-of-origin of mutations in patients with sporadic Albright hereditary

osteodystrophy and reveals a model system in which to observe the effects of splicing mutations on translated and untranslated messenger RNA. *Am. J. Hum. Genet.*, **72**, 961–74.

Ridley, M., Green, J. & Johnson, G. (1986). Retinal angiomatosis: the ocular manifestations
of von Hippel–Lindau disease. *Can. J. Ophthalmol.*, **21**, 276–83.

Risch, H.A., McLaughlin, J.R., Cole, D.E., Rosen, B., Bradley, L., Kwan, E., Jack, E.,
Vesprini, D.J., Kuperstein, G., Abrahamson, J.L., Fan, I., Wong, B. & Narod, S.A. (2001).
Prevalence and penetrance of germline BRCA1 and BRCA2 mutations in a population
series of 649 women with ovarian cancer. *Am. J. Hum. Genet.*, **68**, 700–10.

Risk, J.M., Evans, K.E., Jones, J., Langan, J.E., Rowbottom, L., McRonald, F.E., Mills, H.S.,
Ellis, A., Shaw, J.M., Leigh, I.M., Kelsell, D.P. & Field, J.K. (2002). Characterization of a
500 kb region on 17q25 and the exclusion of candidate genes as the familial tylosis
oesophageal cancer (TOC) locus. *Oncogene*, **21**, 6395–402.

Rizos, H., Puig, S., Badenas, C. et al. (2001). A melanoma-associated germline mutation in
exon 1beta inactivates p14ARF. *Oncogene*, **20**(39), 5543–7.

Roa, B.B., Boyd, A.A., Volcik, K. & Richards, C.S. (1996). Ashkenazi population frequencies
for common mutations in BRCA1 and BRCA2. *Nat. Genet.*, **14**, 185–7.

Robbins, T.O. & Bernstein, J. (1988). Renal involvement. In *Tuberous Sclerosis*, ed. Gomez,
M.R. Raven Press, New York, pp. 133–6.

Robboy, S.J., Noller, K.L., O'Brien, P. et al. (1984). Increased incidence of cervical and vaginal dysplasia in 3980 diethylstilbestrol-exposed young women. *J. Am. Med. Assoc.*, **252**,
2979–83.

Roberts, C.W., Leroux, M.M., Fleming, M.D. & Orkin, S.H. (2002). Highly penetrant,
rapid tumorigenesis through conditional inversion of the tumor suppressor gene Snf5.
Cancer Cell, **2**, 415–25.

Robertson, C.M., Tyrell, J.C. & Pritchard, J. (1991). Familial neural crest tumours. *Eur.
J. Pediatr.*, **150**, 789–92.

Robertson, D.M. (1988). Ophthalmic findings. In *Tuberous Sclerosis*, ed. Gomez, M.R. Raven
Press, New York, pp. 89–109.

Robinow, M., Johnson, G.F. & Minella, P.A. (1986). Aicardi syndrome, papilloma of the
choroid plexus, cleft lip and cleft posterior palate. *J. Pediatr.*, **104**, 404–5.

Robson, M.E., Glogowski, E., Sommer, G. et al. (2004). Pleomorphic characteristics of a
germline KIT mutation in a large kindred with gastrointestinal stromal tumours, hyperpigmentation, and dysphagia. *Clin. Cancer Res.*, **10**, 1250–4.

Rodriguez-Bigas, M.A., Boland, C.R., Hamilton, S.R. et al. (1997). A National Cancer
Institute workshop on hereditary non-polyposis colorectal cancer: meeting highlights and
Bethesda guidelines. *J. Nat. Cancer Inst.*, **89**, 1758–62.

Rodriguez-Sains, R.S. (1991). Ocular findings in patients with dysplastic nevus syndrome.
An update. *Dermatol. Clin.*, **9**(4), 723–8.

Roessler, E., Belloni, E., Gaudenz, K., Vargas, F., Schere, S.W., Tsui, L.C. & Muenke, M.
(1997). Mutations in the C-terminal domain of Sonic Hedgehog cause holoprosencephaly. *Hum. Mol. Genet.*, **6**(11), 1847–53.

Rogers, C.D., Couch, F.J., Brune, K. et al. (2004). Genetics of the FANCA gene in familial
pancreatic cancer. *J. Med. Genet.*, **41**(12), e126.

Rogers, L.F. (2003). Screening mammography: target of opportunity for the media. *Am. J. Roentgenol.*, **180**, 1.

Roggli, V.L., Kim, H.S. & Hawkins, E. (1980). Congenital generalized fibromatosis with viscera linvolvement. *Cancer*, **45**, 954–60.

Romania, A., Zakov, N., McGannon, E., Schroeder, T., Heyen, F. & Jagelman, G.D. (1989). Congenital hypertrophy of the retinal pigment epithelium in familial adenomatous polyposis. *Ophthalmology*, **96**, 879–84.

Rongioletti, F., Hazini, R., Gianotti, G. & Rebora A. (1989). Fibrofolliculomas, tricodiscomas and acrochordons (Birt–Hogg–Dube) associated with intestinal polyposis. *Clin. Exp. Dermatol.*, **14**(1), 72–4.

Rootwelt, H., Hoie, K., Berger, R. & Kvittinger, E.A. (1996). Fumarylacetoacetase mutations in tyrosinaemia type I. *Hum. Mutat.*, **7**, 239–3.

Rose, P.G. & Hunter, R.E. (1994). Advanced ovarian cancer in a woman with a family history of ovarian cancer, discovered at referral for prophylactic oophorectomy. A case report. *J. Repr. Med.*, **39**, 908–10.

Rosen, P.P., Lesser, M.L., Senie, R.T. et al. (1982). Epidemiology of breast carcinoma. III. Relationship of family history to tumour type. *Cancer*, **50**, 171–9.

Rosen, P.P., Holmes, G., Lesser, M.L. et al. (1985). Juvenile papillomatosis and breast carcinoma. *Cancer*, **55**, 1345–52.

Rosenberg, L., Palmer, J.R., Zauber, A.G., Warshauer, M.E., Lewis, J.L.J., Strom, B.L., Harlap, S. & Shapiro, S. (1994). A case–control study of oral contraceptive use and invasive epithelial ovarian cancer. *Am. J. Epidemiol.*, **139**, 654–61.

Rosenberg, P.S., Greene, M.H. & Alter, B.P. (2003). Cancer incidence in persons with Fanconi's anemia. *Blood*, **101**, 822–5.

Rossbach, H.C. Letson, D., Lacson, A. et al. (2005). Familial gigantiform cementoma with brittle bone disease, pathologic fractures and osteosarcoma: a possible explanation of an ancient mystery. *Paediat. Blood Cancer*, **44**, 390–6.

Roy, P.K., Venzon, D.J., Feigenbaum, K.M. et al. (2001). Gastric secretion in Zollinger–Ellison syndrome. Correlation with clinical expression, tumor extent and role in diagnosis – a prospective NIH study of 235 patients and a review of 984 cases in the literature. *Medicine*, **80**, 189–222.

Rozeman, L.B., Sangiorgi, L., Briaire-de Bruijn, I.H., Mainil-Varlet, P., Bertoni, F., Cleton-Jansen, A.M., Hogendoorn, P.C. & Bovee, J.V. (2004). Enchondromatosis (Ollier disease, Maffucci syndrome) is not caused by the PTHR1 mutation p.R150C. *Hum Mutat.*, **24**(6), 466–73.

Rozen, P., Naiman, T., Strul, H. et al. (2002). Clinical and screening implications of the I1307K APC gene variant in Israeli Ashkenazi Jews with familial colorectal neoplasia. Evidence for a founder effect. *Cancer*, **94**, 2561–8.

Rubie, H., Hartmann, O., Michon, J. et al. (1997). N-Myc gene amplification is a major prognostic factor in localized neuroblastoma: results of the French NBL 90 study. Neuroblastoma Study Group of the Societe Francaise d'Oncologie Pediatrique. *J. Clin. Oncol.*, **15**, 1171–82.

Rubin, S.C., Benjamin, I., Behbakht, K. et al. (1996). Clinical and pathological features of ovarian cancer in women with germline mutations of BRCA1. *New Engl. J. Med.*, **335**, 1413–16.

Rubin, S.C., Blackwood, M.A., Bandera, C., Behbakht, K., Benjamin, I., Rebbeck, T.R. & Boyd, J. (1998). BRCA1, BRCA2, and hereditary nonpolyposis colorectal cancer gene mutations in an unselected ovarian cancer population: relationship to family history and implications for genetic testing. *Am. J. Obstet. Gynecol.*, **178**, 670–7.

Ruiz-Maldonado, R., Tamayo, L., Laterza, A.M. & Duran, C. (1992). Giant pigmented nevi: clinical, histopathologic, and therapeutic considerations. *J. Pediatr.*, **120**, 906–11.

Rutherford, J., Chu, C.E., Duddy, P.M., Charlton, R.S., Chumas, P., Taylor, G.R., Lu, X., Barnes, D.M. & Camplejohn, R.S. (2002). Investigations on a clinically and functionally unusual and novel germline p53 mutation. *Br. J. Cancer*, **86**(10), 1592–6.

Rutter, J.L., Wacholder, S., Chetrit, A., Lubin, F., Menczer, J., Ebbers, S., Tucker, M.A., Struewing, J.P. & Hartge, P. (2003). Gynecologic surgeries and risk of ovarian cancer in women with BRCA1 and BRCA2 Ashkenazi founder mutations: an Israeli population-based case-control study. *J. Natl. Cancer Inst.*, **95**, 1072–8.

Ruttledge, M.H., Andermann, A.A., Phelan, C.M. et al. (1996). Type of mutation in the neurofibromatosis type 2 gene (NF2) frequently determines severity of disease. *Am. J. Hum. Genet.*, **59**, 331–42.

Ryynanen, M., Knowlton, R.G., Gabriela Parente, M. et al. (1991). Human type VII collagen: genetic linkage of the gene (COL7A1) on chromosome 3 to dominant dystrophic epidermolysis bullosa. *Am. J. Hum. Genet.*, **49**, 797–803.

Sahlin, P. & Stenman, G. (1995). Cytogenetics and molecular genetics of human solid tumours. *Scand. J. Plast. Reconstr. Surg. Hand Surg.*, **29**, 101–10.

Sahlin, P., Mark, J. & Stenman, G. (1994). Submicroscopic deletions of 3p sequences in pleiomorphic adenomas with t(3;8)(p21;q12). *Gene. Chromosom. Cancer*, **10**, 256–61.

Salmonsen, P.C., Ellsworth, R.M. & Kitchen, F.D. (1979). The occurrence of new retinoblastoma after treatment. *Ophthalmology*, **86**, 840–3.

Salovaara, R., Loukola, A., Kristo, P., Kaariainen, H., Ahtola, H., Eskelinen, M., Harkonen, N., Julkunen, R., Kangas, E., Ojala, S., Tulikoura, J., Valkamo, E., Jarvinen, H., Mecklin, J.P., Aaltonen, L.A. & de La, C.A. (2000). Population-based molecular detection of hereditary nonpolyposis colorectal cancer. *J. Clin. Oncol.*, **18**, 2193–200.

Sampson, J.R., Maheshwar, M.M., Aspinwall, R., Thompson, P., Cheadle, J.P., Ravine, D., Roy, S., Haan, E., Bernstein, J. & Harris, P.C. (1997). Renal cystic disease in tuberous sclerosis: role of the polycystic kidney disease 1 gene. *Am. J. Hum. Genet.*, **61**, 843–51.

Sampson, J.R., Dolwani, S., Jones, S., Eccles, D., Ellis, A., Evans, D.G., Frayling, I., Jordan, S., Maher, E.R., Mak, T., Maynard, J., Pigatto, F., Shaw, J. & Cheadle, J.P. (2003). Autosomal recessive colorectal adenomatous polyposis due to inherited mutations of MYH. *Lancet*, **362**(9377), 39–41.

Sanders, B.M., Draper, C.J. & Kingston, J.E. (1988). Retinoblastoma in Great Britain.

Sandhu, K., Handa, S. & Kanwar, A.J. (2003). Familial Lichen Planus. *Paed. Dermatol.*, **20**(2), 186.

Sandor, T., Srinya, M. & Monus, Z. (1976). Familial occurrence of giant cell hepatitis in infancy. *Acta Hepatogastroenterol.*, **23**, 101–4.

Sankila, R., Aaltonen, L.A. & Mecklin, J.-P. (1996). Better survival rates in patients with MLH1P1-associated hereditary colorectal cancer. *Gastroenterology*, **110**, 682–7.

Santoro, M., Dathan, N.A., Berlingieri, M.T. et al. (1990). Molecular characterisation of *RET/PTC3*, a novel rearranged verson of the *RET* proto-oncogene in a human thyroid papillary carcinoma. *Oncogene*, **9**, 509–16.

Santoro, M., Carlomagno, F., Romano, A. et al. (1995). Activation of *RET* as a dominant transforming gene by germline mutations of MEN 2A and MEN 2B. *Science*, **267**, 381–3.

Sarantaus, L., Vahteristo, P., Bloom, E., Tamminen, A., Unkila-Kallio, L., Butzow, R. & Nevanlinna, H. (2001). BRCA1 and BRCA2 mutations among 233 unselected Finnish ovarian carcinoma patients. *Eur. J. Hum. Genet.*, **9**, 424–30.

Sarraf, D., Payne, A.M., Kitchen, N.D. et al. (2000). Familial cavernous haemangioma: an expanding ocular spectrum. *Arch. Ophthalmol.*, **118**, 969–73.

Saviozzi, S., Saluto, A., Taylor, A.M. et al. (2002). A late-onset variant of Ataxia Telangectasia with a compound heterozygous genotype. *J. Med. Genet.*, **39**, 57–61.

Sato, K. & Nakajima, K. (2002). A novel missense mutation of AIRE gene in a patient with autoimmune polyendocrinopathy, candidiasis and ectodermal dystrophy (APECED) accompanied by progressive muscular atrophy; case report and review of the literature.

Satya-Murti, S., Navada, S. & Eames, F. (1986). Central nervous system involvement in blue rubber bleb nevus syndrome. *Arch. Neurol.*, **43**, 1184–6.

Savitsky, K., Bar-Shira, A., Gilad, S. et al. (1995). A single ataxia telangiectasia gene with a product similar to PI-3 kinase. *Science*, **268**, 1749–53.

Sayed, M.G. et al. (2002). Germline SMAD4 or BMPR1A mutations and phenotype of juvenile polyposis. *Ann. Surg. Oncol.*, **9**, 901–6.

Scheike, O., Visfeldt, J. & Petersen, B. (1973). Male breast cancer 3. Breast carcinoma in association with Klinefelter syndrome. *Acta. Path. Microbiol. Scand.* [A], **81**, 352–8.

Scheithauer, B.W., Laws, E.R., Kovacs, K., Horvath, E., Randall, R.V. & Carney, J.A. (1987). Pituitary adenomas of the multiple endocrine neoplasia type I syndrome. *Semin. Diagn. Pathol.*, **4**, 205–11.

Schildkraut, J.M. & Thompson, W.D. (1988). Familial ovarian cancer: a population based case–control study. *Am. J. Epidemiol.*, **128**, 456–66.

Schildkraut, J.M., Risch, N. & Thompson, W.D. (1989). Evaluating genetic association among ovarian, breast, and endometrial cancer: evidence for breast/ovarian cancer relationship. *Am. J. Hum. Genet.*, **45**, 521–9.

Schilling, T., Burck, J., Sinn, H.P. et al. (2001). Prognostic value of codon 918 (ATG->ACG) *RET* proto-oncogene mutations in sporadic medullary thyroid carcinoma. *Int. J. Cancer*, **95**, 62–6.

Schimke, R.N. (1984). Genetic aspects of multiple endocrine neoplasia. *Annu. Rev. Med.*, **35**, 25–31.

Schlemper, R.J., van der Maas, A.P.C. & Eikenboom, J.C.J. (1994). Familial essential thrombocythemia: clinical characteristics of 11 cases in one family. *Ann. Hematol.*, **68**, 153–8.

Schmidt, L., Duh, F.-M., Chen, F. et al. (1997). Germline and somatic mutations in the tyrosine kinase domain of the *MET* proto-oncogene in papillary renal carcinomas. *Nat. Genet.*, **16**, 68–73.

Schmidt, L.S. (2004). Birt–Hogg–Dube syndrome, a genodermatosis that increases risk for renal carcinoma. *Curr. Mol. Med.*, **4**, 877–85.

Schnall, A.M. & Genuth, S.M. (1976). Multiple endocrine adenomas in a patient with the Maffucci syndrome. *Am. J. Med.*, **61**, 952–6.

Schnur, R.E., Sellinger, B.T., Holmes, S.A. et al. (1996). Type 1 oculocutaneous albinism associated with a full-length deletion of the tyrosinase gene. *J. Invest. Dermatol.*, **106**, 1137–40.

Schorge, J.O., Muto, M.G., Welch, W.R., Bandera, C.A., Rubin, S.C., Bell, D.A., Berkowitz, R.S. & Mok, S.C. (1998). Molecular evidence for multifocal papillary serous carcinoma of the peritoneum in patients with germline BRCA1 mutations [see comments]. *J. Natl. Cancer Inst.*, **90**, 841–5.

Schorge, J.O., Muto, M.G., Lee, S.J., Huang, L.W., Welch, W.R., Bell, D.A., Keung, E.Z., Berkowitz, R.S. & Mok, S.C. (2000). BRCA1-related papillary serous carcinoma of the peritoneum has a unique molecular pathogenesis. *Cancer Res.*, **60**, 1361–4.

Schottenfeld, D.S. & Fraumeni, J.F. (1982). *Cancer Epidemiology and Prevention*. W.B. Saunders, Philadelphia.

Schrager, C.A., Schneider, D., Gruener, A.C., Tsou, H.C. & Peacocke, M. (1997). Clinical and pathological features of breast disease in Cowden's syndrome: an underrecognised syndrome with an increased risk of breast cancer. *Hum. Pathol.*, **29**, 47–53.

Schuffenecker, I., Ginet, N., Goldgar, D. et al. (1997). Prevalence and parental origin of *de novo RET* mutations in MEN 2A and FMTC. *Am. J. Hum. Genet.*, **60**, 233–7.

Schuffenecker, I., Virally-Monod, M., Brohet, R. et al. (1998). Risk and penetrance of primary hyperparathyroidism in MEN 2A families with codon 634 mutations of the *RET* proto-oncogene. *J. Clin. Endocrinol. Metab.*, **83**, 487–91.

Schulze, K.E., Rapini, R.P. & Duvic, M. (1989). Malignant melanoma in oculocutaneous albinism. *Arch. Dermatol.*, **125**, 1583–6.

Schwartz, A.G., King, M.C., Belle, S.H. et al. (1985). Risk of breast cancer to relatives of young breast cancer patients. *J. Natl. Cancer Inst.*, **75**, 665–8.

Schwartz, A.G., Yang, P. & Swanson, G.M. (1996). Familial risk of lung cancer among nonsmokers and their relatives. *Am. J. Epidemiol.*, **144**, 554–62.

Schwartz, C.E., Haber, D.A., Stanton, V.P. et al. (1991). Familial predisposition to Wilms' tumor does not segregate with the WT1 gene. *Genomics*, **10**, 927–30.

Schwartz, H.S., Zimmerman, N.B., Simon, M.A., Wroble, R.R., Millar, E.A. & Bonfiglio, M. (1987). The malignant potential of enchondromatosis. *J. Bone Joint Surg.*, **69A**, 269–74.

Schwartz, R.A. (1978). Basal cell naevus syndrome and upper gastrointestinal polyposis. *New Engl. J. Med.*, **299**, 49.

Schwartz, R.A., Goldberg, D.J., Mahmood, F. et al. (1989). The Muir–Torre syndrome: a disease of sebaceous and colonic neoplasms. *Dermatologica*, **178**, 23–8.

Schwartz, S., Flannery, D.B. & Cohen, M.M. (1985). Tests appropriate for the prenatal diagnosis of ataxia telangiectasia. *Prenat. Diagn.*, **5**, 9–14.

Scott, N., Lansdown, M., Diament, R. et al. (1990). *Helicobacter gastritis* intestinal metaplasia in a gastric cancer family. *Lancet*, **335**, 8691–728.

Scott, R.H. (2006). Syndromes and constitutional chromosomal abnormalities associated with Wilms tumour. *J. Med. Genet.*, [Epub ahead of print]

Scott, S.P., Bendix, R., Chen, P., Clark, R., Dork, T. & Lavin, M.F. (2002). Missense mutations but not allelic variants alter the function of ATM by dominant interference in patients with breast cancer. *Proc. Natl. Acad. Sci. USA*, **99**, 925–30.

Scully, R., Chen, J., Plug, A., Xiao, Y., Weaver, D., Feunteun, J., Ashley, T. & Livingston, D.M. (1997). Association of BRCA1 with Rad51 in mitotic and meiotic cells. *Cell*, **88**, 265–75.

Scully, R.E. (2000). Influence of origin of ovarian cancer on efficacy of screening [see comments]. *Lancet*, **355**, 1028–9.

Seizinger, B., Smith, D., Filling-Katz, M.R. et al. (1991). Genetic flanking markers refine the diagnostic criteria and provide new insights into the genetics of von Hippel–Lindau disease. *Proc. Natl. Acad. Sci. USA*, **88**, 2864–8.

Seizinger, B.R., Rouleau, G.A., Ozelius, L.J. et al. (1987). Genetic linkage of von Recklinghausen neurofibromatosis to the nerve growth receptor gene. *Cell*, **49**, 589–94.

Sellers, T.A., Bailey-Wilson, J.E., Elston, R.C. et al. (1990). Evidence for Mendelian inheritance in the pathogenesis of lung cancer. *J. Natl. Cancer Inst.*, **82**(15), 1272–9.

Sellers, T.A., Chen, P.L., Potter, J.D., Bailey-Wilson, J.E., Rothschild, H. & Elston, R. (1994). Segregation analysis of smoking-associated malignancies: evidence for Mendelian inheritance. *Am. J. Med. Genet.*, **52**, 308–14.

Sepp, T., Yates, J.R. & Green, A.J. (1996). Loss of heterozygosity in tuberous sclerosis hamartomas. *J. Med. Genet.*, **33**(11), 962–4.

Shannon, K.E., Gimm, O., Hinze, R., Dralle, H. & Eng, C. (1999). Germline V804M in the *RET* proto-oncogene in two apparently sporadic cases of MTC presenting in the seventh decade of life. *J. Endo. Genet.*, **1**, 39–46.

Shannon, R.S., Mann, J.R., Harper, E., Harnden, D.G., Morten, J.E.N. & Herbert, A. (1982). Wilms' tumour and aniridia: clinical and cytogenetic features. *Arch. Dis. Child.*, **57**, 685–90.

Sharan, S.K., Morimatsu, M., Albrecht, U., Lim, D.S., Regel, E., Dinh, C., Sands, A., Eichele, G., Hasty, P. & Bradley, A. (1997). Embryonic lethality and radiation hypersensitivity mediated by Rad51 in mice lacking Brca2 [see comments]. *Nature*, **386**, 804–10.

Sharer, N., Schwarz, M., Malone, G., Howarth, A., Painter, J., Super, M. & Braganza, J. (1998). Mutations of the cystic fibrosis gene in patients with chronic pancreatitis. *New Engl. J. Med.*, **339**, 645–52.

Shattuck, T.M., Valimaki, S., Obara, T. et al. (2003). Somatic and germ-line mutations of the HRPT2 gene in sporadic parathyroid carcinoma. *New Engl. J. Med.*, **349**, 1722–9.

Shattuck-Eidens, D., McClure, M., Simard, J., Labrie, F., Narod, S., Couch, F., Hoskins, K., Weber, B., Castilla, L., Erdos, M. et al. (1995). A collaborative survey of 80 mutations in the BRCA1 breast and ovarian cancer susceptibility gene. Implications for presymptomatic testing and screening. *J. Am. Med. Assoc.*, **273**, 535–41.

Shattuck-Eidens, D., Oliphant, A., McClure, M., Mcbride, C., Gupte, J., Rubano, T., Pruss, D., Tavtigian, S.V., Teng, D.H.F., Adey, N., Staebell, M., Gumpper, K., Lundstrom, R.,

Hulick, M., Kelly, M., Holmen, J., Lingenfelter, B., Manley, S., Fujimura, F., Luce, M., Ward, B., Cannonalbright, L., Steele, L., Offit, K., Gilewski, T., Thomas, A. et al. (1997). BRCA 1 sequence analysis in women at high risk for susceptibility mutations-risk factor analysis and implications for genetic testing. *J. Am. Med. Assoc.*, **278**, 1242–50.

Shaw, D., Blair, V., Framp, A. et al. (2005). Chromoendoscopic surveillance in hereditary diffuse gastric cancer: an alternative to prophylactic gastrectomy? *Gut.*, **54**, 461–8.

Shaw, J.M. (1968). Genetic aspects of urticaria pigmentosa. *Arch. Dermatol.*, **97**, 137–8.

Shay, J.W. & Wright, W.E. (2004). Telomeres in Dyskeratosis Congenita. *Nat. Genet.*, **36**, 437–8.

Shen, J.J., William, B.J., Zipursky, A. et al. (1995). Cytogenetic and molecular studies of Down's syndrome individuals with leukemia. *Am. J. Hum. Genet.*, **56**, 915–25.

Shia, J., Klimstra, D.S., Nafa, K., Offit, K., Guillem, J.G., Markowitz, A.J., Gerald, W.L. & Ellis, N.A. (2005). Value of immunohistochemical detection of DNA mismatch repair proteins in predicting germline mutation in hereditary colorectal neoplasms. *Am. J. Surg. Pathol.*, **29**(1), 96–104.

Shiflett, S.L., Kaplan, J. & Ward, D.M. (2002). Chediak–higashi syndrome: a rare disorder of lysosomes and L related organelles. *Pigm. Cell Res.*, **5**, 451–67.

Shine, I. & Allison, P.R. (1966). Carcinoma of the oesophagus with tylosis. *Lancet*, **i**, 951–3.

Shirer, J.A. & Ray, M.C. (1987). Familial occurrence of lichen sclerosis et atrophicus: case reports of a mother and daughter. *Arch. Dermatol.*, **123**, 485–8.

Shugart, Y.Y., Hemminki, K., Vaittinen, P., Kingman, A. & Dong, C. (2000). A genetic study of Hodgkin's lymphoma: an estimate of heritability and anticipation based on the familial cancer database in Sweden. *Hum. Genet.*, **106**(5), 553–6.

Shugart, Y.Y., Hemminki, K., Vaittinen, P. & Kingman, A. (2001). Apparent anticipation and heterogeneous transmission patterns in familial Hodgkin's and non-Hodgkin's lymphoma: report from a study based on Swedish cancer database. *Leuk. Lymphoma*, **42**(3), 407–15.

Sidransky, D. (1996). Is human PATCHED the gatekeeper of common skin cancers? *Nat. Genet.*, **14**, 7–8.

Sidransky, D. (1997). Nucleic acid-based methods for the detection of cancer. *Science*, **278**, 1054–8.

Sidransky, D., Tokino, T., Helzlsouer, K., Zehnbauer, B., Rausch, G., Shelton, B., Prestigiacomo, L., Vogelstein, B. & Davidson, N. (1992). Inherited p53 gene mutations in breast cancer. *Cancer Res.*, **52**, 2984–6.

Sieber, O.M., Heinimann, K. & Tomlinson, I.P. (2003). Genomic instability – the engine of tumorigenesis? *Nat. Rev. Cancer*, **3**(9), 701–8.

Silver, S.A., Wiley, J.M. & Perlman, E.J. (1994). DNA ploidy analysis of pediatrie germ cell tumours. *Mod. Pathol.*, **7**, 951–6.

Simon, A., Ohel, G., Neri, A. et al. (1985). Familial occurrence of mature ovarian teratomas. *Obstet. Gynecol.*, **66**, 278–9.

Singh, A.D., Shields, C.L., Shields, J.A., Eagle, R.C. & De Potter, P. (1995). Uveal melanoma and familial atypical mole and melanoma (FAM-M) syndrome. *Ophthalmic Genet.*, **16**, 53–61.

Singh, A.D., Wang, M.X., Donoso, L.A., Shields, C.L., De Potter, P. & Shields, J.A. (1996). Genetic aspects of uveal melanoma: a brief review. *Semin. Oncol.*, **23**, 768–72.

Sirinavin, C. & Trowbridge, A.A. (1975). Dyskeratosis congenita: clinical features and genetic aspects. *J. Med. Genet.*, **12**, 339–53.

Skogseid, B., Larsson, C., Lindgren, P.G. et al. (1992). Clinical and genetic features of adreno-cortical lesions in multiple endocrine neoplasia type 1. *J. Clin. Endocrinol. Metab.*, **75**, 76–81.

Skogseid, B., Rastad, J. & Öberg, K. (1994). Multiple endocrine neoplasia type 1. Clinical features and screening. *Endocrinol. Metab. Clin. N. Am.*, **23**, 1–18.

Smith, F. (2003). The molecular genetics of keratin disorders. *Am. J. Clin. Dermatol.*, **4**, 347–64.

Smith, D.P., Houghton, C. & Ponder, B.A.J. (1997). Germline mutation of *RET* codon 883 in two cases of *de novo* MEN 2B. *Oncogene*, **15**, 1213–17.

Smith, F.J., Corden, L.D., Rugg, E.L. et al. (1997). Missense mutations in keratin 17 cause either pachonychia congenita type 2 or a phenotype resembling steatocystoma mutiplex. *J. Invest. Dermatol.*, **108**, 220–3.

Smith, J.M., Kirk, E.P.E., Theodosopoulos, G. et al. (2002). Germline mutation of the tumour suppressor *PTEN* in Proteus syndrome. *J. Med. Genet.*, **39**, 937–40.

Smith, M.L., Cavenagh, J.D., Lister, T.A. & Fitzgibbon, J. (2004). Mutation of CEBPA in familial acute myeloid leukemia. *New Engl. J. Med.*, **351**, 2403–7.

Smith, O.P., Hann, I.M., Chessells, J.M., Reeves, B.R. & Milla, P. (1996). Haematological abnormalities in Shwachman–Diamond syndrome. *Br. J. Haemat.*, **94**, 279–84.

Smith, T.E., Lee, D., Turner, B.C., Carter, D. & Haffty, B.G. (2000). True recurrence vs. new primary ipsilateral breast tumor relapse: an analysis of clinical and pathologic differences and their implications in natural history, prognoses, and therapeutic management. *Int. J. Radiat. Oncol. Biol. Phys.*, **48**, 1281–9.

Smyrk, T.C., Watson, P., Kaul, K. et al. (2001). Tumour-infiltrating lymphocytes are a marker for microsatellite instability in colorectal cancer. *Cancer*, **91**, 2417–22.

Soares, P., Trovisco, V., Rocha, A.S. et al. (2003). BRAF mutations and RET/PTC rearrangements are alternative events in the etiopathogenesis of PTC. *Oncogene*, **22**, 4578–80.

Sonneveld, D.J., Sleijfer, D.T., Schrafford Koops, H., Sijmons, R.H., van der Graaf, W.T., Sluiter, W.J. & Hoekstra, H.J. (1999). Familial testicular cancer in a single-centre population. *Eur. J. Cancer*, **35**, 1368–73.

Sorensen, S.A., Mulvihill, J.J. & Nielsen, A. (1986). Long-term follow-up of von Recklinghausen neurofibromatosis. *New Engl. J. Med.*, **314**, 1010–15.

Sorlie, T., Tibshirani, R., Parker, J., Hastie, T., Marron, J.S., Nobel, A., Deng, S., Johnsen, H., Pesich, R., Geisler, S., Demeter, J., Perou, C.M., Lonning, P.E., Brown, P.O., Borresen-Dale, A.L. & Botstein, D. (2003). Repeated observation of breast tumor subtypes in independent gene expression data sets. *Proc. Natl. Acad. Sci. USA*, **100**, 8418–23.

Soufir, N., Avril, M., Chompret, A. et al. (1998). Prevalence of p16 and CDK4 germline mutations in 48 melanoma-prone families in France. *Hum. Mol. Genet.*, **7**, 209–16.

Soufir, N., Bressac-de Paillerets, B., Desjardins, L. et al. (2000). Individuals with presumably hereditary uveal melanoma do not harbour germline mutations in the coding regions of either the P16INK4A, P14ARF or cdk4 genes. *Br. J. Cancer*, **82**(4), 818–22.

Sozzi, G., Bongarzone, I., Miozzo, M. et al. (1992). A t(10;17) translocation creates the RET/PTC2 chimeric transforming sequence in papillary thyroid carcinoma. *Gene. Chromo. Cancer*, **9**, 244–50.

Spector, B.D., Filipovich, A.H., Perry, G.S. & Kersey, J.H. (1982). Epidemiology of cancer in ataxia telangiectasia. In *Ataxia Telangiectasis: A Cellular and Molecular Link between Cancer, Neuropathology and Immune Deficiency*, eds. Bridges, B.A. & Harnden, D.G. John Wiley & Sons, Chichester, pp. 103–38.

Spigelman, A.D. & Phillips, R.K.S. (1991). Screening for cancer and pre-cancer in the oesophagus, stomach and duodenum. *Hosp. Update*, **17**, 220–8.

Spigelman, A.D., Arese, P. & Phillips, R.K.S. (1995). Polyposis: the Peutz–Jeghers syndrome. *Br. J. Surg.*, **82**, 1311–14.

Spirio, L., Olschwang, S., Groden, J. et al. (1993). Alleles of the APC gene: an attenuated form of familial polyposis. *Cell*, **75**, 951–7.

Spirio, L.N., Samowitz, W., Robertson, J. et al. (1998). Alleles of APC modulate the frequency and classes of mutations that lead to colon polyps. *Nat. Genetics.*, **20**, 385–8.

Spitz, M.R., Hoque, A., Trizna, Z. et al. (1994). Mutagen sensitivity as a risk factor for second malignant tumors following malignancies of the upper aerodigestive tract. *J. Natl. Cancer Inst.*, **86**, 1681–4.

Spitz, M.R., Wei, Q., Deng, Q. et al. (2003). Genetic susceptibility to lung cancer and the role of DNA damage and repair. *Cancer Epidemiol. Biomark. Prev.*, **12**, 689–98.

Spitz, R.A., Strunk, K.M., Giebel, L.B. et al. (1990). Detection of mutations in the tyrosinase gene in a patient with type 1a oculocutaneous albinism. *New Engl. J. Med.*, **322**, 1724–7.

Srivastava, S., Zou, Z., Pirollo, K., Blattner, W. & Chang, E.H. (1990). Germ-line transmission of a mutated *p53* gene in a cancer-prone family with Li–Fraumeni syndrome. *Nature*, **348**, 747–9.

St John, D.V.B., McDennett, F.T., Hopper, V.L. et al. (1993). Cancer risks in relatives with common colorectal cancer. *Ann. Int. Med.*, **118**, 785–90.

Stankovic, T., Kidd, A.M., Sutcliffe, A., McGuire, G.M., Robinson, P., Weber, P., Bedenham, T., Bradwell, A.R., Easton, D.F., Lennox, G.G., Haites, N., Byrd, P.J. & Taylor, A.M. (1998). ATM mutations and phenotypes in ataxia-telangiectasia families in the British Isles: expression of mutant ATM and the risk of leukemia, lymphoma, and breast cancer. *Am. J. Hum. Genet.*, **62**, 334–45.

Starink, T.M., van der Veen, J.P.W., Arwert, F. et al. (1986). The cowden syndrome: a clinical and genetic study in 21 patients. *Clin. Genet.*, **29**, 222–33.

Starr, D.G., McClure, J.P. & Connor, J.M. (1985). Non-dermatological complications and genetic aspects of the Rothmund–Thomson syndrome. *Clin. Genet.*, **27**, 102–4.

Stefanini, M., Fawcett, H., Botta, E., Nardo, T. & Lehmann, A.R. (1996). Genetic analysis of twenty-two patients with Cockayne syndrome. *Hum. Genet.*, **97**, 418–23.

Steichen-Gersdorf, E., Trawoger, R., Duba, H.C., Mayr, U., Felber, S. & Utermann, G. (1993). Hypomelanosis of Ito in a girl with plexus papilloma and translocation (X;17). *Hum. Genet.*, **90**, 611–13.

Steinbach, F., Novick, A.C., Zincke, H. et al. (1995). Treatment of renal cell carcinoma in Vol Hippel—Lindau disease: a multicenter study. *J. Urol.*, **153**, 1812–16.

Steinbach, G., Lynch, P.M., Phillips, R.K. et al. (2000). The effect of celecoxib, a cyclooxygenase-2 inhibitor, in familial adenomatous polyposis. *New Engl. J. Med.*, **342**(26), 1946–52.

Steinberg, G.S., Carter, B.S., Beaty, T.H., Childs, B. & Walsh, P.C. (1990). Family history and the risk of prostate cancer. *Prostate*, **17**, 337–47.

Steiner, G., Schoenberg, M.P., Linn, J.F., Mao, L. & Sidransky, D. (1997). Detection of bladder cancer recurrence by microsatellite analysis of urine. *Nat. Med.*, **3**, 621–4.

Steiner, M.S., Goldman, S.M., Fishman, E.K. & Marshall, F.F. (1993). The natural history of renal angiomyolipoma. *J. Urol.*, **150**, 1782–6.

Stephenson, B.M., Finan, P.J., Gascoyne, J. et al. (1991). Frequency of familial colorectal cancer. *Br. J. Surg.*, **78**, 1162–6.

Stettner, A.R., Hartenbach, E.M., Schink, J.C., Huddart, R., Becker, J., Pauli, R., Long, R. & Laxova, R. (1999). Familial ovarian germ cell cancer: report and review. *Am. J. Med. Genet.*, **84**, 43–6.

Stevens, G., van Beukering, J., Jenkins, T. & Ramsay, M. (1995). An intragenic deletion of the P gene is the common mutation causing tyrosinine positive oculocutaneous albinism in Southern African negroids. *Am. J. Hum. Genet.*, **56**, 586–91.

Stewart, G.S., Maser, R.S., Stancovic, T. et al. (1999). The DNA strand double break repair gene hMRE11 is mutated in individuals with an ataxia-telangectasia-like disorder. *Cell*, **99**, 577–87.

Stickens, D., Clines, G., Burbee, D. et al. (1996). The EXT2 multiple exostoses gene defines a family of putative tumour suppressor genes. *Nat. Genet.*, **14**, 25–32.

Stieglitz, J.B. & Centerwall, W.R. (1983). Pachonychia congenita (Jadassohn–Lewandowsky syndrome) a seventeen member four generation pedigree with unusual respiratory and dental involvement. *Am. J. Med. Genet.*, **14**, 21–8.

Stiller, C.A., Chessells, J.M. & Fitchett, M. (1994). Neurofibromatosis and childhood leukaemia/lymphoma: a population based UKCCSG study. *Br. J. Cancer*, **70**, 969–72.

Stoll, C., Alembik, Y. & Truttman, M. (1996). Multiple familial lipomatosis with polyneuropathy, an inherited dominant condition. *Ann. Genet.*, **39**, 193–6.

Stoppa-Lyonnet, D., Laurent-Puig, P., Essioux, L., Pages, S., Ithier, G., Ligot, L., Fourquet, A., Salmon, R.J., Clough, K.B., Pouillart, P., Bonaiti-Pellie, C. & Thomas, G. (1997). BRCA1 sequence variations in 160 individuals referred to a breast/ovarian family cancer clinic. Institute Curie Breast Cancer Group [see comments]. *Am. J. Hum. Genet.*, **60**, 1021–30.

Stratakis, C.A. et al. (1996). Carney complex, a familial multiple neoplasia and lentigenosis syndrome: analysis of 11 kindreds and linkage to the short arm of chromosome 2. *J. Clin. Invest.*, **97**, 699–705.

Stratakis, C.A., Sarlis, N., Kirschner, L.S. et al. (1999). Paradoxical response to dexamethasone in the diagnosis of primary pigmented nodular adrenocortical disease. *Ann. Int. Med.*, **131**, 585–91.

Stratakis, C.A., Papageorgiou, T., Premkumar, A., Pack, S., Kirschner, L.S., Taymans, S.E., Zhuang, Z.P., Oelkers, W.H. & Carney, J.A. (2000). Ovarian lesions in Carney complex: clinical genetics and possible predisposition to malignancy. *J. Clin. Endocrinol. Metab.*, **85**, 4359–66.

Stratakis, C.A., Kirschner, L.S. & Carney, J.A. (2001). Clinical and molecular features of the Carney complex diagnostic criteria and recommendations for patient evaluation. *J. Clin. Endocrinol. Metab.*, **86**, 4041–6.

Stratton, J.F., Gayther, S.A., Russell, P. et al. (1997). Contribution of BRCA1 mutations to ovarian cancer. *New Engl. J. Med.*, **336**, 1125–30.

Stratton, J.F., Buckley, C.H., Lowe, D. & Ponder, B.A. (1999a). Comparison of prophylactic oophorectomy specimens from carriers and noncarriers of a BRCA1 or BRCA2 gene mutation. United Kingdom Coordinating Committee on Cancer Research (UKCCCR) Familial Ovarian Cancer Study Group. *J. Natl. Cancer Inst.*, **91**, 626–8.

Stratton, J.F., Thompson, D., Bobrow, L., Dalal, N., Gore, M., Bishop, D.T., Scott, I., Evans, G., Daly, P., Easton, D.F. & Ponder, B.A. (1999b). The genetic epidemiology of early-onset epithelial ovarian cancer: a population-based study. *Am. J. Hum. Genet.*, **65**, 1725–32.

Streubel, B. et al. (2003). T(14;18)(q32;q21) involving IGH and MALT1 is a frequent chromosomal aberration in MALT lymphoma. *Blood*, **101**(6), 2335–9.

Struewing, J.P., Abeliovich, D., Peretz, T., Avishai, N., Kaback, M.M., Collins, F.S. & Brody, L.C. (1995a). The carrier frequency of the BRCA1 185delAG mutation is approximately 1 percent in Ashkenazi Jewish individuals. *Nat. Genet.*, **11**, 198–200.

Struewing, J.P., Brody, L.C., Erdos, M.R. et al. (1995b). Detection of 8 BRCA1 mutations in 10 breast/ovarian cancer families, including one family with male breast cancer. *Am. J. Hum. Genet.*, **51**, 1–7.

Struewing, J.P., Hartege, P., Wacholder, S. et al. (1997). The risk of cancer associated with specific mutations of BRCA1 and BRCA2 among Ashkenazi Jews. *New Engl. J. Med.*, **336**, 1401–8.

Sty, J.R., Ruiz, M.E. & Carmody, T.J. (1996). Congenital generalised fibromatosis. Extraosseus accumulation of bone seeking radiopharmaceutical. *Clin. Nucl. Med.*, **21**, 413–14.

Su, H., Hu, N., Shih, J., Hu, Y., Wang, Q.H., Chuang, E.Y., Roth, M.J., Wang, C., Goldstein, A.M., Ding, T., Dawsey, S.M., Giffen, C., Emmert-Buck, M.R. & Taylor, P.R. (2003). Gene expression analysis of esophageal squamous cell carcinoma reveals consistent molecular profiles related to a family history of upper gastrointestinal cancer. *Cancer Res.*, **63**, 3872–6.

Su, W.P.D., Chun, S.I., Hammond, D.E. et al. (1990). Pachonychia congenita: a clinical study of 12 cases and review of the literature. *Pediatr. Dermatol.*, **7**, 33–8.

Sumegi, J., Huang, D., Lanyi, A., Davis, J.D., Seemayer, T.A., Maeda, A., Klein, G., Seri, M., Wakiguchi, H., Purtilo, D.T. & Gross, T.G. (2000). Correlation of mutations of the SH2D1A gene and Epstein–Barr virus infection with clinical phenotype and outcome in X-linked lymphoproliferative disease. *Blood*, **9**(6), 3118–25.

Summers, C.G., Getting, W.S. & King, R.A. (1996). Diagnosis of oculocutaneous albinism with molecular analysis. *Am. J. Ophthalmol.*, **121**, 724–6.

Sun, C.C., Lenoir, G., Lynch, H. & Narod, S.A. (1996). In-situ breast cancer and BRCA1. *Lancet*, **348**, 408.

Sun, T.C., Swee, R.G., Shives, T.C. & Unni, K.K. (1985). Chondrosarcoma in Mafrucci's syndrome. *J. Bone Joint Surg.*, **67A**, 1214–19.

Sun, X., Becker-Catania, S.G., Chun, H.H. et al. (2002). Early diagnosis of ataxia telangiectasia using radiosensitivity testing. *J. Paed.*, **140**, 724–31.

Sutcliffe, S., Pharoah, P.D.P., Easton, D.F. & Ponder, B.A.J. (2000). Ovarian and breast cancer risks to women in families with two or more cases of ovarian cancer. *Int. J. Cancer*, **87**, 110–17.

Suter, C.M., Martin, D.I. & Ward, R.L. (2004). Germline epimutation of MLH1 in individuals with multiple cancers. *Nat. Genet.*, **36**, 497–501.

Sutter, C., Dallenbach-Hellweg, G. & Schmidt, D. (2004). Molecular analysis of endometrial hyperplasia in HNPCC-suspicious patients may predict progression to endometrial carcinoma. *Int. J. Gynecol. Pathol.*, **23**(1), 18–25.

Swanson, G.P., Dobin, S.M., Arber, J.M. et al. (1997). Chromosome 11 abnormalities in Bowendisease of the vulva. *Cancer Genet. Cytogenet.*, **93**, 109–14.

Sweet, K. et al. (2002). *J. Clin. Oncol.*, **20**, 528–37.

Swenssen, O. (1999). Pachonychia congenita. Keratin gene mutations with pleiotropic effect. *Hantarzt*, **50**, 483–90.

Swerdlow, A.J., English, J.S.C. & Qiao, Z. (1995). The risk of melanoma in patients with congenital nevi: a cohort study. *J. Am. Acad. Dermatol.*, **32**, 595–9.

Swift, M. & Chase, C. (1979). Cancer in families with xeroderma pigmentosum. *J. Natl. Cancer Inst.*, **62**, 1415–21.

Swift, M., Caldwell, R.J. & Chase, C. (1980). Reassessment of cancer predisposition of Fanconi anemia heterozygotes. *J. Natl. Cancer Inst.*, **65**, 863–7.

Swift, M., Reifnauer, R.J., Morrell, D. et al. (1987). Breast and other cancers in families with ataxia-telangiectasia. *New Engl. J. Med.*, **316**, 1289–94.

Swift, M., Morrell, D., Massey, R.D. et al. (1991). Incidence of cancer in 161 families affected by ataxia-telangiectasia. *New Engl. J. Med.*, **325**, 1831–4.

Swinburn, P.A., Yeong, M.L., Lane, M.R., Nicholson, G.I. & Holdaway, I.M. (1988). Neurofibromatosis associated with somatostionoma: report of two patients. *Clin. Endocrinol.*, **28**, 353–9.

Syngal, S., Fox, E.A., Eng, C., Kolodner, R.D. & Garber, J.E. (2000). Sensitivity and specificity of clinical criteria for hereditary non-polyposis colorectal cancer associated mutations in MSH2 and MLH1. *J. Med. Genet.*, **37**(9), 641–5.

Szabo, C.I., Schutte, M., Broeks, A., Houwing-Duistermaat, J.J., Thorstenson, Y.R., Durocher, F., Oldenburg, R.A., Wasielewski, M., Odefrey, F., Thompson, D., Floore, A.N., Kraan, J., Klijn, J.G., van den Ouweland, A.M., Wagner, T.M., Devilee, P., Simard, J., Van't Veer, L.J., Goldgar, D.E. and Meijers-Heijboer, H. (2004). Are ATM mutations 7271T-->G and IVS10-6T-->G really high-risk breast cancer-susceptibility alleles? *Cancer Res.*, **64**(3), 840–3.

Szekely, G., Remenar, E., Kasler, M. & Gundy, S. (2003). Does the bleomycin sensitivity assay express cancer phenotype? *Mutagenesis*, **18**, 59–63.

Szepietowski, J.C., Wasik, F., Szybejko-Machaj, G. et al. (2001). Brook–Spiegler syndrome. *J. Eur. Acad. Dermatol. Venereol.*, **15**, 346–9.

Taalman, R.D.F.M., Hustinx, T.W.J., Weemaes, C.M.R. et al. (1989). Further delineation of the Nijmegen breakage syndrome. *Am. J. Med. Genet.*, **32**, 425–31.

Tabata, Y., Villanueva, J., Lee, S.M., Zhang, K., Kanegane, H., Miyawaki, T., Sumegi, J. & Filipovich, A.H. (2005). Rapid detection of intracellular SH2D1A protein in cytotoxic lymphocytes from patients with X-linked lymphoproliferative disease and their family members. *Blood*, **105**, 3066–71.

Tachibana, I., Smith, J.S., Sato, K., Hosek, S.M., Kimmel, D.W. & Jenkins, R.B. (2000). Investigation of germline PTEN, p53, p16(INK4A)/p14(ARF), and CDK4 alterations in familial glioma. *Am. J. Med. Genet.*, **92**, 136–41.

Taconis, W.K. (1988). Osteosarcoma in fibrous dysplasia. *Skeletal Radiol.*, **17**, 163–70.

Tai, D.I., Chen, C.H., Chang, T.T. et al. (2002). Eight-year nationwide survival analysis in relatives of patients with hepatocellular carcinoma: role of vital infection. *J. Gastroenterol. Hepatol.*, **17**, 682–9.

Takahashi, H., Behbakht, K., McGovern, P.E., Chiu, H.C., Couch, F.J., Weber, B.L., Friedman, L.S., King, M.C., Furusato, M., LiVolsi, V.A. et al. (1995). Mutation analysis of the BRCA1 gene in ovarian cancers. *Cancer Res.*, **55**, 2998–3002.

Takahashi, H., Chiu, H.C., Bandera, C.A., Behbakht, K., Liu, P.C., Couch, F.J., Weber, B.L., LiVolsi, V.A., Furusato, M., Rebane, B.A., Cardonick, A., Benjamin, I., Morgan, M.A., King, S.A., Mikuta, J.J., Rubin, S.C. & Boyd, J. (1996). Mutations of the BRCA2 gene in ovarian carcinomas. *Cancer Res.*, **56**, 2738–41.

Tamimi, H.K. & Bolen, J.W. (1984). Enchondramatosis (Ollier's disease) and ovarian juvenile granulosa cell tumour. *Cancer*, **53**, 1605–8.

Tamura, Y., Ishibashi, S., Gotoda, T. *et al.* (2002). A Kindred of familial acromegaly without evidence for linkage to MEN 1 locus. *Endocr. J.*, **49**, 425–31.

Tassone, P., Tagliaferri, P., Perricelli, A., Blotta, S., Quaresima, B., Martelli, M.L., Goel, A., Barbieri, V., Costanzo, F., Boland, C.R. & Venuta, S. (2003). BRCA1 expression modulates chemosensitivity of BRCA1-defective HCC1937 human breast cancer cells. *Br. J. Cancer*, **88**, 1285–91.

Tate, G., Suzuki, T., Kishimoto, K. et al. (2004). Novel mutations of EVER1/TMC6 gene in a Japanese patient with Epidermodysplasia verruciformis. *J. Hum. Genet.*, **49**, 223–5.

Taylor, G.M., Gokhale, D.A., Crowther, D. et al. (1996). Increased frequency of HLA-DPB1*0301 in Hodgkin's disease suggests that susceptibility is HVR-sequence and subtype-associated. *Leukemia*, **10**, 854–9.

Taylor, G.M., Gokhale, D.A., Crowther, D., Woll, P.J., Harris, M., Ryder, D., Ayres, M. & Radford, J.A. (1999). Further investigation of the role of HLA-DPB1 in adult Hodgkin's disease (HD) suggests an influence on susceptibility to different HD subtypes. *Br. J. Cancer*, **80**(9), 1405–11.

Taylor, M.D., Gokgoz, N., Andrulis, I.L., Mainprize, T.G., Drake, J.M. & Rutka, J.T. (2000). Familial posterior fossa brain tumors of infancy secondary to germline mutation of the hSNF5 gene. *Am. J. Hum. Genet.*, **66**, 1403–6.

Taylor, M.D., Liu, L., Raffel, C., Hui, C.C., Mainprize, T.G., Zhang, X., Agatep, R., Chiappa, S., Gao, L., Lowrance, A., Hao, A., Goldstein, A.M., Stavrou, T., Scherer, S.W., Dura, W.T., Wainwright, B., Squire, J.A., Rutka, J.T. & Hogg, D. (2002). Mutations in SUFU predispose to medulloblastoma. *Nat. Genet.*, **31**(3), 306–10.

Teh, B.T., Farnebo, F., Kristoffersson, U. et al. (1996). Autosomal dominant primary hyperparathyroidism and jaw tumor syndrome associated with renal hamartomas and cystic kidney disease: linkage to 1q21–q32 and loss of the wildtype allele in renal hamartomas. *J. Clin. Endocrinol. Metab.*, **81**, 4204–11.

Teh, B.T., McArdle, J., Chan, S.P. et al. (1997). Clinicopathologic studies of thymic carcinoids in multiple endocrine neoplasia type 1. *Medicine*, **76**, 21–9.

Teh, B.T., Farnebo, F., Twigg, S. et al. (1998). Familial isolated hyperparathyroidism maps to the hyperparathyroidism-jaw tumor locus in a subset of families. *J. Clin. Endocrinol. Metab.*, **83**, 2114–20.

Teich, N., Schulz, H.U., Witt, H., Bohmig, M. & Keim, V. (2003). N34S, a pancreatitis associated SPINK1 mutation, is not associated with sporadic pancreatic cancer. *Pancreatology*, **3**, 67–8.

Telatar, M., Wang, Z., Udar, N. et al. (1996). Ataxia-telangiectasia: mutations in *ATM* cDNA detected by protein truncation screening. *Am. J. Hum. Genet.*, **59**, 40–4.

Tello, R., Blickman, J.G., Buonomo, C. & Herrin, J. (1998). Meta analysis of the relationship between tuberous sclerosis complex and renal cell carcinoma. *Eur. J. Radiol.*, **27**, 131–8.

ten Bensel, R.W., Stadlan, E.M. & Krivit, W. (1964). The development of malignancy in the course of the Aldrich syndrome. *J. Pediatr.*, **68**, 761–7.

Thakker, R.V. (2000). Multiple endocranial neoplasia type I. *Endocrine Metab. Clin. North Amer.*, **29**, 541–67.

The European Chromosome 16 Tuberous Sclerosis Consortium (1993). Identification and characterisation of the tuberous sclerosis gene on chromosome 16. *Cell*, **75**, 1305–15.

Thompson, D. & Easton, D. (2001). Variation in cancer risks, by mutation position, in BRCA2 mutation carriers. *Am. J. Hum. Genet.*, **68**, 410–19.

Thompson, D. & Easton, D.F. (2002). Cancer incidence in BRCA1 mutation carriers. *J. Natl. Cancer Inst.*, **94**, 1358–65.

Thomson, D., Duedal, S., Kirner, J. et al. (2005). Cancer risks and mortality in heterozygous ATM mutation carriers. *J. Natl. Cancer Inst.*, **97**(11), 813–22.

Thoralacius, S., Sigurdsson, S., Bjarnadottir, H. et al. (1997). Study of a single BRCA2 mutation with high carrier frequency in a small population. *Am. J. Hum. Genet.*, **60**, 1079–84.

Thorensten, Y.R., Roxas, A., Kroiss, R. et al. (2003). Contributions of ATM mutations to familial breast and ovarian cancer. *Cancer Res.*, **63**, 3325–33.

Thunberg, U., Tobin, G., Johnson, A., Soderberg, O., Padyukov, L., Hultdin, M., Klareskog, L., Enblad, G., Sundstrom, C., Roos, G. & Rosenquist, R. (2002). Polymorphism in the P2X7 receptor gene and survival in chronic lymphocytic leukaemia. *Lancet*, **360**(9349), 1935–9.

Thuwe, I., Lundstrom, B. & Walinder, J. (1979). Familial brain tumour. *Lancet*, **i**, 504.

Tian, X.L. (2003). Identification of an angiogenic factor that when mutated causes susceptibility to klippel Trenaunay syndrome. *Nature*, **427**, 640–5.

Tidman, M.J. (1990). Skin malignancy in epidermolysis bullosa. In *Epidermolysis Bullosa*, eds. Priestly, G.C., Tidman, M.J., Weiss, J.B. & Eady, R.A.J. Dystrophic Epidermolysis Bullosa Research Association, Crowthorne, pp. 156–60.

Tiffet, O., Nicholson, A.G., Ladas, G., Sheppard, M.N. & Goldstraw, P. (2003). A clinico-pathologic study of 12 neuroendocrine tumors arising in the thymus. *Chest*, **124**, 141–6.

Tilanus-Linthorst, M., Verhoog, L., Obdeijn, I.M., Bartels, K., Menke-Pluymers, M., Eggermont, A., Klijn, J., Meijers-Heijboer, H., van der, K.T. & Brekelmans, C. (2002). A BRCA1/2 mutation, high breast density and prominent pushing margins of a tumor independently contribute to a frequent false-negative mammography. *Int. J. Cancer*, **102**, 91–5.

Till, M.M., Jones, L.H., Penticess, C.R. et al. (1975). Leukaemia in children and their grandparents: studies of immune function in six families. *Br. J. Haematol.*, **29**, 575–86.

Tinari, A., Pace, S., Fambrini, M. et al. (2002). Vulvar Pagets disease: review of the literature, considerations about histogenetic hypothesis and surgical approaches. *Eur. J. Gynae. Oncol.*, **23**, 551–2.

Tirkkonen, M., Johannsson, O., Agnarsson, B.A., Olsson, H., Ingvarsson, S., Karhu, R., Tanner, M., Isola, J., Barkardottir, R.B., Borg, A. & Kallioniemi, O.P. (1997). Distinct somatic genetic changes associated with tumor progression in carriers of BRCA1 and BRCA2 germ-line mutations. *Cancer Res.*, **57**, 1222–7.

Tischkowitz, M.D. & Hodgson, S.V. (2003). Fanconi anaemia. *J. Med. Genet.*, **40**, 1–10.

Tobachman, J.K., Greene, M.H., Tucker, M.A. et al. (1982). Intra-abdominal carcinomatosis after prophylactic oophorectomy in ovarian cancer-prone families. *Lancet*, **ii**, 795–7.

Toguchida, J., Ishizaki, K., Sasaki, M.S. et al. (1989). Preferential mutation of the paternally derived RB gene as the initial event in sporadic osteosarcoma. *Nature*, **338**, 156–8.

Toguchida, J., Yamaguchi, T., Dayton, S.H. et al. (1992). Prevalence and spectrum of germline mutations of the p53 gene among patients with sarcoma. *New Engl. J. Med.*, **326**, 1301–9.

Tokuhata, G.K. & Lilienfeld, A.M. (1963). Familial aggregation of lung cancer in humans. *J. Natl. Cancer Inst.*, **30**, 289–92.

Tolmie, J.L., Boyd, E., Batstone, P., Ferguson-Smith, M.E., al Roomi, L. & Connor, J.M. (1988). Siblings with chromosome mosaicism, microcephaly, and growth retardation: the phenotypic expression of a human mitotic mutant? *Hum. Genet.*, **80**(2), 197–200.

Tomanin, R., Sarto, F., Mazotti, D. et al. (1989). Louis–Barr syndrome: spontaneous and induced chromosomal aberrations in lymphocytes and micronuclei in lymphocytes, oral mucosa and hair root cells. *Hum. Genet.*, **85**, 31–8.

Tomita, Y., Sato-Matsumura, K.C., Sawanmura, D. et al. (2003). Simultaneous occurrence of 3 squamous cell carcinomas in a recessive dystrophic epidermolysis bullosa patient. *Acta. Dermatol. Venereol.*, **83**, 225–6.

Tomlinson, I.P., Alam, N.A., Rowan, A.J. et al. (2002). Germline mutations in FH predispose to dominantly inherited uterine fibroids, skin leiomyomata and papillary renal cell carcinoma. *Nat. Genet.*, **30**, 406–10.

Tonin, P., Weber, B., Offit, K., Couch, F., Rebbeck, T.R., Neuhasen, S., Godwin, A.K., Daly, M., Wagner-Costalas, J., Berman, D., Grana, G., Fox, E., Kane, M.F., Kolodner, R.D., Krainer, M., Haber, D.A., Struewing, J.P., Warner, E., Rosen, B., Lerman, C., Peshkin, B., Norton, L., Serova, O., Foulkes, W.D., Lynch, H.T., Lenoir, G.M., Narod, S.A. & Garber, J.E. (1996). Frequency of recurrent BRCA1 and BRCA2 mutations in Ashkenazi Jewish breast cancer families. *Nat. Med.*, **2**, 1183–96.

Tonin, P.N., Mes-Masson, A.M., Narod, S.A., Ghadirian, P. & Provencher, D. (1999). Founder BRCA1 and BRCA2 mutations in French Canadian ovarian cancer cases unselected for family history. *Clin. Genet.*, **55**, 318–24.

Tonin, P.N., Mes-Masson, A.-M., Futreal, P.A., Morgan, K., Mahon, M., Foulkes, W.D., Cole, D.E.C., Provencher, D., Ghadirian, P. & Narod, S.A. (1998). Founder *BRCA1* and *BRCA2* mutations in French Canadian breast and ovarian cancer families. *Am. J. Hum. Genet.*, **63**, 1341–51.

Tops, C.M.J., Vasen, H.F.A., van Berge Henegouwen, G. et al. (1992). Genetic evidence that Turcot syndrome is not allelic to familial adenamatous polyposis. *Am. Med. Genet.*, **43**, 888–93.

Toro, J.R., Glenn, G., Duray, P., Darling, T., Weirich, G., Zbar, B., Linehan, M. & Turner, M.L. (1999). Birt–Hogg–Dube syndrome: a novel marker of kidney neoplasia. *Arch. Dermatol.*, **135**(10), 1195–202.

Torres, C.F., Korones, D.N. & Pilcher, W. (1997). Multiple ependymomas in a patient with Turcot's syndrome. *Med. Pediatr. Oncol.*, **28**, 59–61.

Tos, M. & Thomsen, J. (1984). Epidemiology of acoustic neuromas. *J. Laryngol. Otol.*, **98**, 685–92.

Traverso, G., Shuber, A., Levin, B., Johnson, C., Olsson, L., Schoetz Jr, D.J., Hamilton, S.R., Boynton, K., Kinzler, K.W. & Vogelstein, B. (2002). Detection of APC mutations in fecal DNA from patients with colorectal tumors. *New Engl. J. Med.*, **346**, 311–20.

Traverso, G., Bettegowda, C., Kraus, J., Speicher, M.R., Kinzler, K.W., Vogelstein, B. & Lengauer, C. (2003). Hyper-recombination and genetic instability in BLM-deficient epithelial cells. *Cancer Res.*, **63**(24), 8578–81.

Treem, W.R. (2004). Emerging concepts in celiac disease. *Curr. Opin. Pediatr.*, **16**, 552–9.

Triantafillidis, J.K., Kosmidis, P. & Kottaridis, S. (1993). Familial stomach cancer. *Am. J. Gastroenterol.*, **88**, 1789–90.

Trimbath, J.D., Peterson, G.M., Erdman, S. et al. (2001). Café – au-lait spots and early-onset colorectal neoplasia: a variant of HNPCC? *Fam. Cancer*, **1**, 101–5.

Trizna, Z., Clayman, G.L., Spitz, M.R., Briggs, K.L. & Goepfert, H. (1995). Glutathione stransferase genotypes as risk factors for head and neck cancer. *Am. J. Surg.*, **170**, 499–501.

Trump, D., Farren, B., Wooding, C. et al. (1996). Clinical studies of multiple endocrine neoplasia type 1 (MEN 1). *Q. J. Med.*, **89**, 653–69.

Tsai, K.Y. & Tsao, H. (2004). The genetics of skin cancer. *Am. J. Med. Genet.*, **131C**, 82–92.

Tsuchiya, K., Reijo, R., Page, D.C. & Disteche, C.M. (1995). Gonadoblastoma: molecular definition of the susceptibility region on the Y chromosome. *Am. J. Hum. Genet.*, **57**, 1400–7.

Tuo, J., Jaruga, P., Rodriguez, H. et al. (2003). Primary fibroblasts of Cockayne syndrome patients are defective in cellular repair of 8-hydroxyguanine and 8-hydroxyadenine resulting from oxidative stress. *FASEB J.*, **17**, 668–74.

Turcot, J., Despres, J.P. & St Pierre, F. (1959). Malignant tumours of the central nervous system associated with familial polyposis of the colon. *Dis. Colon Rectum*, **2**, 465–8.

Turner, J.T., Cohen Jr, M.M., Bieseker, L.G. et al. (2001). Reassessment of the Proteus syndrome with application of diagnostic criteria to published cases. *Am. J. Med. Genet.*, **130A**, 111–22.

Tzonou, A., Day, N.E., Trichopoulos, D., Walker, A., Saliaraki, M., Papapostolou, M. & Polychronopoulou, A. (1984). The epidemiology of ovarian cancer in Greece: a case–control study. *Eur. J. Cancer clin. Oncol.*, **20**, 1045–52.

Uchino, S., Noguchi, S., Nagatomo, M. et al. (2000). Screening of the Men1 gene and discovery of germ-line and somatic mutations in apparently sporadic parathyroid tumors. *Cancer Res.*, **60**, 5553–7.

Uitto, J., Pulkkinent, L. & Ringpfeil, F. (2002). Progress in molecular genetics of heritable skin diseases: the paradigms of epidemoysis bullosa and pseudoxanthoma elasticum. *J. Invest. Dermotol. Symp. Proc.*, **7**(1), 6–16.

Ullmann, R., Petzmann, S., Klemen, H. et al. (2002). The position of pulmonary carcinoids within the spectrum of neuroendocrine tumours of the lung and other tissues. *Gene. Chromosome. Cancer*, **34**, 78–85.

Umar, A., Boland, C.R., Terdiman, J.P., Syngal, S., de La, C.A., Ruschoff, J., Fishel, R., Lindor, N.M., Burgart, L.J., Hamelin, R., Hamilton, S.R., Hiatt, R.A., Jass, J., Lindblom, A., Lynch, H.T., Peltomaki, P., Ramsey, S.D., Rodriguez-Bigas, M.A., Vasen, H.F., Hawk, E.T., Barrett, J.C., Freedman, A.N. & Srivastava, S. (2004a). Revised Bethesda guidelines for hereditary nonpolyposis colorectal cancer (Lynch syndrome) and microsatellite instability. *J. Natl. Cancer Inst.*, **96**, 261–8.

Umar, A., Risinger, J.I., Hawk, E.T. & Barrett, J.C. (2004b). Testing guidelines for hereditary non-polyposis colorectal cancer. *Nat. Rev. Cancer*, **4**(2), 153–8.

Urrita, R. & DiMagno, E.P. (1996). Genetic markers: the key to early diagnosis and improved survival in pancreatic cancer? Editorial. *Gastroenterology*, **110**, 306–10.

Ushio, K., Sasagawa, M., Doi, H. et al. (1976). Lesions associated with familial polyposis coli. Studies of lesions of the stomach, duodenum, bones and teeth. *Gastrointest. Radiol.*, **1**, 67.

Vabres, P., Lancombe, D., Rabinowitz, L.G. et al. (1995). The gene for Bazex–Dupre–Christol syndrome maps to chromosome Xq. *J. Invest. Dermatol.*, **105**, 87–9.

Valverde, P., Healy, E., Sikkink, S. et al. (1996). The Asp84Glu variant of the melanocortin 1 receptor (MC1R) is associated with melanoma. *Hum. Mol. Genet.*, **5**(10), 1663–6.

van, O.I. et al. (2003). Long-term psychological impact of carrying a BRCA1/2 mutation and prophylactic surgery: a 5-year follow-up study. *J. Clin. Oncol.*, **21**(20), 3867–74.

Van den Bos, M., Van den Hoven, M., Jongejan, E. et al. (2004). More differences between HNPCC-related and sporadic carcinomas from the endometrium as compared to the colon. *Am. J. Surg. Path.*, **28**, 706.

van der Horst, G.T. et al. (2002). UVB radiation-induced cancer predisposition in Cockayne syndrome group A (Csa) mutant mice. *DNA Repair (Amsterdam)*, **1**(2), 143–57.

Van der Looij, M., Szabo, C., Besznyak, I., Liszka, G., Csokay, B., Pulay, T., Toth, J., Devilee, P., King, M.C. & Olah, E. (2000). Prevalence of founder BRCA1 and BRCA2 mutations among breast and ovarian cancer patients in Hungary. *Int. J. Cancer*, **86**, 737–40.

van der Mey, A.G., Maaswinkel-Mooy, P.D., Cornelisse, C.J., Schmidt, P.H. & van de Kamp, J.J. (1989). Genomic imprinting in hereditary glomus tumours: evidence for new genetic theory. *Lancet*, **II**, 1291–4.

van der Velden, P.A., Sandkuijl, L.A., Bergman, W., Pavel, S., van Mourik, L., Frants, R.R. & Gruis, N.A. (2001). Melanocortin-1 receptor variant R151C modifies melanoma risk in Dutch families with melanoma. *Am. J. Hum. Genet.*, **69**(4), 774–9.

van Dijken, P.J., Woldendorp, K.H. & van Wouwe, J.P. (1996). Familial thrombocytosis in infancy presenting with a leukaemoid reaction. *Acta Pediatr.*, **85**, 1132–4.

van Haeringen, A., Bergman, W., Nelen, M.R. et al. (1989). Exclusion of the dysplastic nevus syndrome (DNS) locus from the short arm of chromosome 1 by linkage studies in Dutch families. *Genomics*, **5**, 61–4.

van Kessell, A.G. et al. (1999). Renal cell cancer: chromosome 3 translocations as risk factors. *J. Natl. Cancer. Inst.*, **91**(13), 1159–60.

van Meyel, D.J., Ramsay, D.A., Chambers, A.F., Macdonald, D.R. & Cairncross, J.G. (1994). Absence of hereditary mutations in exons 5 through 9 of the p53 gene and exon 24 of the neurofibromin gene in families with glioma. *Ann. Neurol.*, **35**, 120.

van Nagell, J., DePriest, P.D., Reedy, M.B., Gallion, H.H., Ueland, F.R., Pavlik, E.J. & Kryscio, R.J. (2000). The efficacy of transvaginal sonographic screening in asymptomatic women at risk for ovarian cancer. *Gynecol. Oncol.*, **77**, 350–6.

van Slegtenhorst, M., de Hoogt, R., Hermans, C. et al. (1997). Identification of the tuberous sclerosis gene TSC1 on chromosome 9q34. *Science*, **277**, 805–8.

Van Steensel, M.A., Jaspers, N.G. & Steijlen, P.M. (2001). A case of Rombo syndrome. *Br. J. Dermatol.*, **144**, 1215–8.

Van't Veer, L.J., Dai, H.Y., van de Vijver, M.J., He, Y.D.D., Hart, A.A.M., Mao, M., Peterse, H.L., van der Kooy, K., Marton, M.J., Witteveen, A.T., Schreiber, G.J., Kerkhoven, R.M., Roberts, C., Linsley, P.S., Bernards, R. & Friend, S.H. (2002). Gene expression profiling predicts clinical outcome of breast cancer. *Nature*, **415**, 530–6.

Vang, R., Taubenberger, J.K., Mannion, C.M. et al. (2000). Primary vulvar and vaginal extraosseous Ewing's sarcoma/peripheral neuroectodermal tumour: diagnostic confirmation with CD99 immunostaining and reverse transcriptase-polymerase chain reaction. *Int. J. Gynaecol. Pathol.*, **19**, 103–9.

Vanin, K., Scurry, J., Thorne, H. et al. (2002). Overexpression of wild-type p53 in lichen sclerosus adjacent human papillomavirus-negative vulvar cancer. *J. Invest. Dermatol.*, **119**, 1027–33.

Varley, J.M. (2003). Germline TP53 mutations and Li–Fraumeni syndrome. *Hum. Mutat.*, **21**, 313–20.

Varley, J.M., McGown, G., Thorncroft, M. et al. (1995). An extended Li–Fraumeni kindred with gastric carcinoma and a codon 175 mutation in TP53. *J. Med. Genet.*, **32**, 942–5.

Varley, J.M., McGown, G., Thorncroft, M. et al. (1997). Germ-line mutations of TP53 in Li–Fraumeni families: an extended study of 39 families. *Cancer Res.*, **57**, 3245–52.

Varon, R., Vissinga, C., Platzer, M., Cerosaletti, K.M., Chrzanowska, K.H., Saar, K., Beckmann, G., Seemanova, E., Cooper, P.R., Nowak, N.J., Stumm, M., Weemaes, C.M.R., Gatti, R.A., Wilson, R.K., Digweed, M., Rosenthal, A., Sperling, K., Concannon, P. & Reis, A. (1998). Nibrin, a novel DNA double-strand break repair protein, is mutated in Nijmegen breakage syndrome. *Cell*, **93**, 467–76.

Vasen, H.F., den Hartog Jager, F.C., Menko, F.H. et al. (1989). Screening for hereditary non-polyposis colorectal cancer: a study of 22 kindreds in the Netherlands. *Am. J. Med.*, **86**, 278–81.

Vasen, H.F., Wijnen, J.T., Menko, F.H. et al. (1996). Cancer risk in families with hereditary nonpolyposis colorectal cancer diagnosed by mutation analysis. *Gastroenterology*, **110**, 1020–7.

Vasen, H.F., Watson, P., Mecklin, J.P. & Lynch, H.T. (1999). New clinical criteria for hereditary nonpolyposis colorectal cancer (HNPCC, Lynch syndrome) proposed by the International Collaborative Group on HNPCC. *Gastroenterology*, **116**, 1453–6.

Vasen, H.F., Stormorken, A., Menko, F.H., Nagengast, F.M., Kleibeuker, J.H., Griffioen, G., Taal, B.G., Moller, P. & Wijnen, J.T. (2001). Msh2 mutation carriers are at higher risk of cancer than Mlh1 mutation carriers: a study of hereditary nonpolyposis colorectal cancer families. *J. Clin. Oncol.*, **19**(20), 4074–80.

Vasen, H.F.A., Mecklin, J.-P., Meera-Khan, P. & Lynch, H.T. (1991). The International Collaboration Group on Hereditary Nonpolyposis Colorectal Cancer (ICG-HNPCC). *Dis. Colon Rectum*, **34**, 424–5.

Vasen, H.F.A., Mecklin, J.P., Watson, P. et al. (1993). Surveillance in hereditary colorectal cancer: an international co-operative study of 165 families. *Dis. Colon Rectum*, **36**, 1–4.

Vasen, H.F.A., Taal, F.M., Nagengast, G. et al. (1995). Hereditary nonpolyposis colorectal cancer: results of long-term surveillance in 50 families. *Eur. J. Cancer*, **31A**, 1145–8.

Vaz, R.M. & Turner, C. (1986). Oilier disease (enchondromatosis) associated with ovarian juvenile granulosa cell tumour and precocious pseudopuberty. *J. Pediatr.*, **108**, 945–7.

Venkitaraman, A.R. (2002). Cancer susceptibility and the functions of BRCA1 and BRCA2. *Cell*, **108**, 171–82.

Venkitaraman, A.R. (2004). Tracing the network connecting BRCA and Fanconi anaemia proteins. *Nat. Rev. Cancer*, **4**, 266–76.

Vernia, S. (2003). Chelitis glandularis: a rare entity. *Br. J. Dermatol.*, **148**, 362.

Verp, M.S. & Simpson, J.L. (1987). Abnormal sexual differentiation and neoplasia. *Cancer Genet. Cytogenet.*, **25**, 191–218.

Veugelers, M., Wilke, D., Burton, K. et al. (2004). Comparative PRKAR1A genotype-phenotype analyses in humans with Carney complex and prkar1a haploinsufficient mice. *Proc. Natl. Acad. Sci.*, **101**, 14222–7.

Vieregge, P., Gerhard, L. & Nahser, H.C. (1987). Familial glioma: occurrence within the 'familial cancer syndrome' and systemic malformations. *J. Neurol.*, **234**, 220–32.

Viljeon, D., Pearn, J. & Beighton, P. (1984). Manifestations and natural history of idiopathic hemihypertrophy: a review of eleven cases. *Clin. Genet.*, **26**, 81–6.

Viljeon, D.L. (1988). Klippel–Trenaunay–Weber syndrome (angio-osteohypertrophy syndrome). *J. Med. Genet.*, **25**, 250–2.

Viniou, N., Terpos, E., Rombos, J. et al. (2001). Acute myeloid leukaemia in a patient with ataxia telangectasia: a case-report and review of the literature. *Leukaemia*, **15**, 1668–70.

Viskochil, D., Buchberg, A.M., Xu, G. et al. (1990). Deletions and a translocation interrupt a cloned gene at the neurofibromatosis type 1 locus. *Cell*, **62**, 187–92.

von Koch, C.S., Gulati, M., Aldape, K. & Berger, M.S. (2002). Familial medulloblastoma: case report of one family and review of the literature. *Neurosurgery*, **51**(1), 227–33.

Vousden, K.H. (1989). Human papillomaviruses and cervical carcinoma. *Cancer Cell.*, **1**, 43–50.

Voutsinas, S. & Wynne-Davies, R. (1983). The infrequency of malignant disease in dia-physial aclasis and neurofibromatosis. *J. Med. Genet.*, **20**, 345–9.

Vuilamy, T., Marrone, A., Szydlo, R. et al. (2004). Telomerase is a ribonucleoprotrein com-plex required for synthesis of DNA repeats at the ends of telomeres. The RNA com-ponent of this is mutated in dyskeratosis congenita. *Nat. Genet.*, **36**, 447–9.

Wachsmuth, R., Harland, M. & Newton Bishop, J. (1998). The atypical mole syndrome and predisposition to melanoma. *New Engl. J. Med.*, **339**, 348–9.

Wachsmuth, R.C.G., Rupert, M., Barrett, J.H., Saunders, C.L., Randerson-Moor, J.A., Eldridge, A., Martin, N.G., Bishop, D.T. & Newton-Bishop, J.A. (2001). Heritability and gene-environment interactions for melanocytic nevus density examined in a UK adoles-cent twin study. *J. Invest. Dermatol.*, **117**(2), 348–52.

Wagner, A., Barrows, A., Wijnen, J.T., van der, K.H., Franken, P.F., Verkuijlen, P., Nakagawa, H., Geugien, M., Jaghmohan-Changur, S., Breukel, C., Meijers-Heijboer, H., Morreau, H., van Puijenbroek, M., Burn, J., Coronel, S., Kinarski, Y., Okimoto, R., Watson, P., Lynch, J.F., de La, C.A., Lynch, H.T. & Fodde, R. (2003). Molecular analysis of hereditary nonpolyposis colorectal cancer in the United States: high mutation detec-tion rate among clinically selected families and characterization of an American founder genomic deletion of the MSH2 gene. *Am. J. Hum. Genet.*, **72**(5), 1088–1100.

Wagner, J.E., Tolar, J., Levran, O., Scholl, T., Deffenbaugh, A., Satagopan, J., Ben-Porat, L., Mah, K., Batish, S.D., Kutler, D.I., MacMillan, M.L., Hanenberg, H. & Auerbach, A.D. (2004). Germline mutations in BRCA2: shared genetic susceptibility to breast cancer, early onset leukemia and Fanconi anemia. *Blood*, **103**(7), 2554–9.

Wagner, T.M., Moslinger, R., Zielinski, C., Scheiner, O. and Breiteneder, H. (1996). New Austrian mutation in BRCA1 gene detected in three unrelated HBOC families [letter]. *Lancet*, **347**, 1263.

Wahlen, T. & Astedt, B. (1965). Familial occurrence of coexisting leiomyoma of vulva and oesophagus. *Acta Obstet. Gynecol. Scand.*, **44**, 197–203.

Waite, K.A. & Eng, C. (2003). From developmental disorder to heritable cancer: it's all in the BMP/TGF-B family. *Nat. Rev. Genet.*, **4**, 763–73.

Wallace, M.R., Marchuk, D.A., Andersen, L.B. et al. (1990). Type 1 neurofibromatosis gene: identification of a large transcript disrupted in three NF1 patients. *Science*, **249**, 181–6.

Walsh, N., Qizilbash, A., Banergee, R. & Waugh, G.A. (1987). Biliary neoplasia in Gardner's syndrome. *Arch. Pathol. Lab. Med.*, **111**, 76–7.

Walshe, J.M., Waldenstrom, E., Sams, V. et al. (2003). Abdominal malignancies in patients with Wilson's disease. *Quar. J. Med.*, **96**, 657–62.

Walther, M.M., Choyke, P.L., Glenn, G., Lyne, J.C., Rayford, W., Venzon, D. & Linehan, W.M. (1999a). Renal cancer in families with hereditary renal cancer: prospective analysis of a tumor size threshold for renal parenchymal sparing surgery. *J. Urol.*, **161**, 1475–9.

Walther, M.M., Herring, J., Enquist, E., Keiser, H.R. & Linehan, W.M. (1999b). von Recklinghausen's disease and pheochromocytomas. *J. Urol.*, **162**, 1582–6.

Wands, J. & Blum, H.E. (1991). Primary hepatocellular carcinoma. *New Engl. J. Med.*, **325**, 729–31.

Wang, J., German, J., Ashby, K. & French, S.W. (1999). Ulcerative colitis complicated by dysplasia–adenoma–carcinoma in a man with Bloom's syndrome. *J. Clin. Gastroenterol.*, **28**(4), 380–2.

Wang, L., Cunningham, J.M., Winters, J.L., Guenther, J.C., French, A.J., Boardman, L.A., Burgart, L.J., McDonnell, S.K., Schaid, D.J. & Thibodeau, S.N. (2003). BRAF mutations in colon cancer are not likely attributable to defective DNA mismatch repair. *Cancer Res.*, **63**, 5209–12.

Wang, L.L., Levy, M.L., Lewis, R.A. et al. (2001). Clinical manifestations in a cohort of 41 Rothmund–Thomson syndrome patients. *Am. J. Med. Genet.*, **102**, 11–17.

Wang, L.L., Gannavarapu, A., Kozinetz, C.A. et al. (2003). Association between osteosarcoma and deleterious mutations in the RECQL4 gene in Rothmund–Thomson syndrome. *J. Natl. Cancer Inst.*, **95**, 669–74.

Wang, Y., Cortez, D., Yazdi, P., Neff, N., Elledge, S.J. & Qin, J. (2000). BASC, a super complex of BRCA1-associated proteins involved in the recognition and repair of aberrant DNA structures. *Gene. Dev.*, **14**, 927–39.

Wank, R. & Thomssen, C. (1991). High risk of squamous cell carcinoma of the cervix for women with HLA-DQw3. *Nature*, **352**, 723–5.

Wanq, Q., Timmr, A.A., Szafranski, P. et al. (2001). Identification and molecular characterisation of de novo translocation t(8;14) (q22.3;q13) associated with a vascular and tissue overgrowth syndrome. *Cytogenet. Cell Genet.*, **95**, 183–8.

Wanschura, S., Belge, G., Stenman, G. et al. (1996). Mapping of the translocation breakpoints of primary peliomorphic adenomas and lipomas within a common region of chromosome 12. *Cancer Genet. Cytogenet.*, **86**, 39–45.

Warburton, D., Anyane-Yeboa, K., Taterka, P., Yu, C.Y. & Olsen, D. (1991). Mosaic variegated aneuploidy with microcephaly: a new human mitotic mutant? *Ann. Genet.*, **34**(3–4), 287–92.

Ward, D.M., Shiflett, S.L. & Kaplan, J. (2002). Chediak–Higashi syndrome: a clinical and molecular view of a rare lysosomal storage disease. *Curr. Mol. Med.*, **2**, 469–77.

Warner, E., Foulkes, W., Goodwin, P., Meschino, W., Blondal, J., Paterson, C., Ozcelik, H., Goss, P., Allingham-Hawkins, D., Hamel, N., Di Prospero, L., Contiga, V., Serruya, C., Klein, M., Moslehi, R., Honeyford, J., Liede, A., Glendon, C., Brunet, J.S. & Narod, S. (1999). Prevalence and penetrance of BRCA1 and BRCA2 gene mutations in unselected Ashkenazi Jewish women with breast cancer. *J. Natl. Cancer Inst.*, **91**, 1241–7.

Warner, E., Plewes, D.B., Hill, K.A., Causer, P.A., Zubovits, J.T., Jong, R.A., Cutrara, M.R., DeBoer, G., Yaffe, M.J., Messner, S.J., Meschino, W.S., Piron, C.A. and Narod, S.A. (2004). Surveillance of BRCA1 and BRCA2 mutation carriers with magnetic resonance imaging, ultrasound, mammography, and clinical breast examination. *J. Am. Med. Assoc.*, **292**(11), 1317–25.

Washecka, R. & Hanna, M. (1991). Malignant renal tumours in tuberous sclerosis. *Urology*, **37**, 340–3.

Watson, P. & Lynch, H.T. (2001). Cancer risk in mismatch repair gene mutation carriers. *Fam. Cancer*, **1**, 57–60.

Watson, P., Lin, K.M., Rodruigez-Bigas, M.A. et al. (1998). Colorectal carcinoma survival among hereditary nonpolyposis colorectal cancer family members. *Cancer*, **83**, 259–66.

Wautot, V., Vercherat, C., Lespinasse, J. et al. (2002). Germline mutation profile of MEN1 in multiple endocrine neoplasia type 1: search for correlation between phenotype and the functional domains of the MEN1 protein. *Hum. Mutat.*, **20**, 35–47.

Webb, D.W., Fryer, A.E. & Osborne, J.P. (1996). Morbidity associated with tuberous sclerosis: a population study. *Dev. Med. Child Neurol.*, **38**, 146–55.

Webster, A. et al. (1998). An analysis of phenotypic variation in the familial cancer syndrome von Hippel-Lindau disease: evidence for modifier effects. *Am. J. Hum. Genet.*, **63**, 1025–35.

Webster, A.R., Maher, E.R. & Moore, A.T. (1999). Clinical characteristics of ocular angiomatosis in von Hippel–Lindau disease and correlation with germline mutation. *Arch. Ophthalmol.*, **117**, 371–8.

Webster, A.R., Maher, E.R., Bird, A.C. & Moore, A.T. (2000). Risk of multisystem disease in isolated ocular angioma (haemangioblastoma). *J. Med. Genet.*, **37**, 62–3.

Wechter, M.E., Gruber, S.B., Haefner, H.K. et al. (2004). Vulvar melanoma: a report of 20 cases and review of the literature. *J. Am. Acad. Dermatol.*, **50**, 554–62.

Weinblatt, M. & Kochen, J. (1991). An unusual family cancer syndrome manifested in young siblings. *Cancer*, **68**, 1068–70.

Weinstein, L.S., Shenker, A., Geiman, V., Merino, M.J., Friedman, E. & Spiegel, A.M. (1991). Activating mutations of the stimulatory G protein in the McCune–Albright syndrome. *New Engl. J. Med.*, **325**, 1688–95.

Weinstein, L.S., Chen, M. & Liu, J. (2002). Gs(alpha) mutations and imprinting defects in human disease. *Ann. NY Acad. Sci.*, **968**, 173–97.

Weirich, G., Glenn, G., Junker, K. et al. (1998). Familial renal oncocytoma: clinicopathological study of 5 families. *J. Urol.*, **160**, 335–40.

Weksberg, R., Nishikawa, J., Caluseriu, O., Fei, Y.L., Shuman, C., Wei, C., Steele, L., Cameron, J., Smith, A., Ambus, I., Li, M., Ray, P.N., Sadowski, P. & Squire, J. (2001). Tumor development in the Beckwith–Wiedemann syndrome is associated with a variety of constitutional molecular 11p15 alterations including imprinting defects of KCNQ1OT1. *Hum. Mol. Genet.*, **10**, 2989–3000.

Weksberg, R., Smith, A.C., Squire, J. & Sadowski, P. (2003). Beckwith–Wiedemann syndrome demonstrates a role for epigenetic control of normal development. *Hum. Mol. Genet.*, 12 Spec No 1, R61–8.

Welch, J.P., Wells, R.S. & Kerr, C.B. (1968). Ancell-Spiegler cylindromas (turban tumours) and Brook-Fordyce trichoepitheliomas: evidence for a single genetic entity. *J. Med. Genet.*, **5**, 29–35.

Wells, R.S., Higgs, J.M., Macdonald, A. et al. (1972). Familial chronic mucocutaneous candidiasis. *J. Med. Genet.*, **9**, 302–10.

Wells, S.A., Baylin, S.B., Linehan, W.M., Farrell, R.E., Cox, E.B. & Cooper, C.W. (1978). Provocative agents and the diagnosis of medullary carcinoma of the thyroid gland. *Ann. Surg.*, **188**, 139–41.

Wells, S.A., Chi, D.D., Toshima, D. et al. (1994). Predictive DNA testing and prophylactic thyroidectomy in patients at risk for multiple endocrine neoplasia type 2A. *Ann. Surg.*, **200**, 237–50.

Werness, B.A., Afify, A.M., Bielat, K.L., Eltabbakh, G.H., Piver, M.S. & Paterson, J.M. (1999). Altered surface and cyst epithelium of ovaries removed prophylactically from women with a family history of ovarian cancer. *Hum. Pathol.*, **30**, 151–7.

Werness, B.A., Parvatiyar, P., Ramus, S.J., Whittemore, A.S., Garlinghouse-Jones, K., Oakley-Girvan, I., DiCioccio, R.A., Wiest, J., Tsukada, Y., Ponder, B.A.J. & Piver, M.S. (2000). Ovarian carcinoma in situ with germline BRCA1 mutation and loss of heterozygosity at BRCA1 and TP53. *J. Natl. Cancer Inst.*, **92**, 1088–91.

Wertelecki, W., Rouleau, G.A., Superneau, D.W. et al. (1988). Neurofibromatosis 2: clinical and DNA linkage studies of a large kindred. *New Engl. J. Med.*, **319**, 278–83.

Wessels, L.F.A., van Welsem, T., Hart, A.A.M., Van't Veer, L.J., Reinders, M.J.T. & Nederlof, P.M. (2002). Molecular classification of breast carcinomas by comparative genomic hybridization: a specific somatic genetic profile for BRCA1 tumors. *Cancer Res.*, **62**, 7110–17.

Westergaard, H. (1996). Colorectal cancer: the role of screening and surveillance. *J. Invest. Med.*, **44**, 216–27.

Westman, J., Hampel, H. & Bradley, T. (2000). Efficacy of a touch screen computer based familiy cancer history questionaire and subsequent cancer risk assessment. *J. Med. Genet.*, **37**, 354–60.

Wetzels, R.H., Kuijpers, H.J., Lane, E.B., Leigh, I.M., Troyanovsky, S.M., Holland, R., van Haelst, U.J. & Ramaekers, F.C. (1991). Basal cell-specific and hyperproliferation-related keratins in human breast cancer. *Am. J. Pathol.*, **138**, 751–63.

Wetzels, R.H.W., Holland, R., Vanhaelst, U.J.G.M., Lane, E.B., Leigh, I.M. & Ramaekers, F.C.S. (1989). Detection of basement-membrane components and basal-cell keratin-14 in noninvasive and invasive carcinomas of the breast. *Am. J. Pathol.*, **134**, 571–9.

Whitcomb, D.C., Gorry, M.C., Preston, R.A. et al. (1996). Hereditary pancreatitis is caused by a mutation in the cationic trypsinogen gene. *Nat. Genet.*, **14**, 141–5.

Whitelaw, S.C., Murday, V.A., Tomlinson, I.P.M. et al. (1997). Clinical and molecular features of the hereditary mixed polyposis syndrome. *Gastroenterology*, **112**, 327–34.

Whiteside, D., McLeod, R., Graham, G., Steckley, J.L., Booth, K., Somerville, M.J. & Andrew, S.E. (2002). A homozygous germ-line mutation in the human MSH2 gene predisposes to hematological malignancy and multiple cafe-au-lait spots. *Cancer Res.*, **62**(2), 359–62.

Whittemore, A.S., Gong, G. & Itnyre, J. (1997). Prevalence and contribution of BRCA1 mutations in breast cancer and ovarian cancer: results from three U.S. population-based case-control studies of ovarian cancer. *Am. J. Hum. Genet.*, **60**, 496–504.

Whittemore, A.S., Balise, R.R., Pharoah, P.D., DiCioccio, R.A., Oakley-Girvan, I., Ramus, S.J., Daly, M., Usinowicz, M.B., Garlinghouse-Jones, K., Ponder, B.A., Buys, S., Senie, R., Andrulis, I., John, E., Hopper, J.L. & Piver, M.S. (2004a). Oral contraceptive use and ovarian cancer risk among carriers of BRCA1 or BRCA2 mutations. *Br. J. Cancer*, **91**, 1911–15.

Whittemore, A.S., Gongm G., John, E.M., McGuire, V., Li, F.P., Ostrow, K.L., Dicioccio, R., Felberg, A. & West, D.W. (2004b). Prevalence of BRCA1 mutation carriers among US non-hispanic Whites. *Cancer Epidemiol. Biomark. Prev.*, **13**, 2078–83.

Wick, M.R., Scheithauer, B.W., Dines, D.E. et al. (1982). Thymic neoplasia in 2 male siblings. *Mayo Clin. Proc.*, **57**, 653–6.

Wicking, C., Shanlay, S., Smyth, I., Gillies, S., Negus, K., Graham, S., Suthers, G., Haites, N., Edwards, M., Wainwright, B. & Chenevix-Trench, G. (1997). Most germ-line mutations in the nevoid basal cell carcinoma syndrome lead to a premature termination of the PATCHED protein, and no genotype-phenotype correlations are evident. *Am. J. Hum. Genet.*, **60**(1), 21–6.

Wiedemann, H.-R. (1983). Tumours and hemihypertrophy associated with Wiedemann–Beckwith syndrome. *Eur. J. Pediatr.*, **141**, 129.

Wiench, M., Wygoda, Z., Gubala, E. et al. (2001). Estimation of risk of inherited medullary thyroid carcinoma in apparent sporadic patients. *J. Clin. Oncol.*, **19**, 1374–80.

Wienecke, R., Konig, A. & De Clue, J.E. (1995). Identification of tuberin, the tuberose sclerosis-2 product. Tuberin possesses specific Rap/GAP activity. *J. Biol. Chem.*, **270**, 16409–14.

Wiernik, P.H., Wang, S.Q., Hu, X.-P., Marino, P. & Paietta, E. (2000). Age of onset evidence for anticipation in familial non-Hodgkin's lymphoma. *Br. J. Haemat.*, **108**, 72–9.

Wiggs, J., Nordenskjold, M. & Yandell, D. (1988). Prediction of the risk of hereditary retinoblastoma, using DNA polymorphisms within the retinoblastoma gene. *New Engl. J. Med.*, **318**, 151–7.

Wijnen, J., Khan, P.M., Vasen, H. et al. (1997). Hereditary nonpolyposis colorectal cancer families not complying with the Amsterdam criteria show extremely low frequency of mismatch-repairgene mutations. *Am. J. Hum. Genet.*, **61**, 329–35.

Wijnen, J. et al. (1998). Clinical findings with implications for genetic testing in families with clustering of colorectal cancer. *New Engl. J. Med.*, **339**, 511–18.

Wijnen, J., de Leew, W., Nvasen, H. et al. (1999). Familial endometrial cancer in female carriers of MSH6 germline mutations. *Nat. Genet.*, **23**, 142–4.

Wiley, J.S. et al. (2002). A loss-of-function polymorphic mutation in the cytolytic P2X7 receptor gene and chronic lymphocytic leukaemia: a molecular study. *Lancet.*, **359**(9312), 1114–9.

Williams, C.B. & Fairclough, P.D. (1991). Colonoscopy. *Curr. Opin. Gastroenterol.*, **7**, 55–65.

Williams, C.B., Goldblatt, M. & Delaney, P.V. (1982). Top and tail endoscopy and follow-up in Peutz–Jeghers syndrome. *Endoscopy*, **14**, 22–34.

Williams, W.R. & Strong, L.C. (1985). Genetic epidemiology of soft tissue sarcomas in children. In *Familial Cancer*, eds. Müller, H.J. & Weber, W. *First International Research Conference on Familial Cancer*, Basel. Karger, Basel, pp. 151–3.

Wilson, D. & Boland, J. (1994). Sporadic multiple lipomatosis: a case report and review of the literature. *W. Va Med. J.*, **90**, 145–6.

Wilson, G.N., Squires Jr, R.H. & Weinberg, A.G. (1991). Keratitis, hepatitis, icthyosis and deafness: report and review of KID syndrome. *Am. J. Med. Genet.*, **40**, 255–60.

Winawer, S.J., Zauber, A.G., O'Brien, M.J. et al. (1993). Randomised comparison of surveillance intervals after colonoscopic removal of newly diagnosed adenomas. The National Polyp Study Workgroup. *New Engl. J. Med.*, **328**, 901–6.

Winawer, S., Fletcher, R., Rex, D. et al. (2003). Colorectal cancer screening and surveillance; clinical guidelines and rationale—Update based on new evidence. *Gastroenterology*, **124**, 554–60.

Witt, H., Luck, W., Becker, M., Bohmig, M., Kage, A., Truninger, K., Ammann, R.W., O'Reilly, D., Kingsnorth, A., Schulz, H.U., Halangk, W., Kielstein, V., Knoefel, W.T., Teich, N. & Keim, V. (2001). Mutation in the SPINK1 trypsin inhibitor gene, alcohol use, and chronic pancreatitis. *J. Am. Med. Assoc.*, **285**, 2716–17.

Wohlik, N., Cote, G.J., Bugalho, M.M.J. et al. (1996). Relevance of RET proto-oncogene mutations in sporadic medullary thyroid carcinoma. *J. Clin. Endocrinol. Metab.*, **81**, 3740–5.

Wong, A.K., Pero, R., Ormonde, P.A., Tavtigian, S.V. & Bartel, P.L. (1997). RAD51 interacts with the evolutionarily conserved BRC motifs in the human breast cancer susceptibility gene brca2. *J. Biol. Chem.*, **272**, 31941–4.

Wood, N.J. & Duffy, S.R. (2003). The outcome of endometrial carcinoma surveillance by ultrasound scan in women at risk of hereditary nonpolyposis colorectal carcinoma and familial colorectal carcinoma. *Am. Cancer Soc.*, **1772**, 3.

Woods, W.G., Roloff, J.S., Lukens, J.N. & Krivit, W. (1981). The occurrence of leukemia in patients with the Shwachman syndrome. *J. Pediatr.*, **90**, 425–9.

Woods, W.G., Tuchman, M., Robison, L.L. et al. (1996). A population-based study of the usefulness of screening for neuroblastoma. *Lancet*, **348**, 1682–7.

Woods, W.G., Gao, R.N., Shuster, J.J., Robison, L.L., Bernstein, M., Weitzman, S., Bunin, G., Levy, I., Brossard, J., Dougherty, G., Tuchman, M. & Lemieux, B. (2002). Screening of infants and mortality due to neuroblastoma. *New Engl. J. Med.*, **346**, 1041–6.

Woodward, E.R., Eng, C., McMahon, R., Voutilainen, R., Affara, N.A., Ponder, B.A.J. & Maher, E.R. (1997). Genetic predisposition to pheochromocytoma: analysis of candidate genes GDNF, RET and VHL. *Hum. Mol. Genet.*, **6**, 1051–6.

Woodward, E.R. et al. (2000). Familial clear cell renal cell carcinoma (FCRC): clinical features and mutation analysis of the VHL, MET, and CUL2 candidate genes. *J. Med. Genet.*, **37**(5), 348–53.

Wooster, R., Ford, D., Mangion, J. et al. (1993). Absence of linkage to the ataxia telangiectasia locus in familial breast cancer. *Hum. Genet.*, **92**, 91–4.

Wooster, R., Neuhausen, S., Mangion, J. et al. (1994). Localisation of a breast cancer susceptibility gene (BRCA2) to chromosome 13q by genetic linkage analysis. *Science*, **265**, 2088–90.

Wooster, R., Bignell, G., Lancaster, J. et al. (1995). Identification of the breast cancer susceptibility gene BRCA2. *Nature*, **378**, 789–92.

Wu, A.U., Trumble, T.E. & Ruwe, P.A. (1991). Familial incidence of Paget's disease and secondary osteogenic sarcoma. A report of three cases in a single family. *Clin. Orthop.*, **265**, 306–9.

Wu, L.C., Wang, Z.W., Tsan, J.T., Spillman, M.A., Phung, A., Xu, X.L., Yang, M.C., Hwang, L.Y., Bowcock, A.M. & Baer, R. (1996). Identification of a RING protein that can interact in vivo with the BRCA1 gene product. *Nat. Genet.*, **14**, 430–40.

Wu, X., Lippman, S.M., Lee, J.J., Zhu, Y., Wei, Q.V., Thomas, M., Hong, W.K. & Spitz, M.R. (2002). Chromosome instability in lymphocytes: a potential indicator of predisposition to oral premalignant lesions. *Cancer Res.*, **62**, 2813–18.

Wu, X., Zhao, H., Do, K.A., Johnson, M.M., Dong, Q., Hong, W.K. & Spitz, M.R. (2004). Serum levels of insulin growth factor (IGF-I) and IGF-binding protein predict risk of second primary tumors in patients with head and neck cancer. *Clin. Cancer Res.*, **10**, 3988–95.

Wu, Y., Berends, M.J., Post, J.G. et al. (2001). Germline mutations in EXO1 gene in patients with hereditary non-polyposis colorectal cancer (HNPCC) and atypical HNPCC forms. *Gastroenterology*, **120**, 1580–7.

Wuyts, W., Van Hul, W., Wauters, J. et al. (1996). Positional cloning of a gene involved in hereditary multiple exostoses. *Hum. Mol. Genet.*, **5**, 1547–57.

Wynder, E.L., Dodo, H. & Barber, H.R. (1969). Epidemiology of cancer of the ovary. *Cancer*, **23**, 352–70.

Xiong, W., Zeng, Z.Y., Xia, J.H. et al. (2004). A susceptibility locus at chromosome 3p21 linked to familial nasopharyngeal carcinoma. *Cancer Res.*, **64**, 1972–4.

Yamashita, Y., Sagawa, T., Fujimoto, T., Sugawara, T., Yamada, H., Hoshi, N., Sakuragi, N., Ishioka, C. & Fujimoto, S. (1999). BRCA1 mutation testing for Japanese patients with ovarian cancer in breast cancer screening. *Breast Cancer Res. Treat.*, **58**, 11–17.

Yang, P., Grufferman, M.J., Houry, A.G. et al. (1995). Association of childhood rhabdomyosarcoma with neurofibromatosis type 1 and birth defects. *Genet. Epidemiol.*, **12**, 467–74.

Yarden, R.I. & Brody, L.C. (1999). BRCA1 interacts with components of the histone deacetylase complex. *Proc. Natl. Acad. Sci. USA*, **96**, 4983–8.

Yates, V.D., Wilroy, R.S., Whittington, G.L. & Simmons, J.C.H. (1983). Anterior sacral defects; an autosomal dominantly inherited condition. *J. Pediatr.*, **102**, 239–42.

Ye, Z., Song, H. & Guo, Y. (2004). Glutathione S-transferase M1, T1 status and the risk of head and neck cancer: a meta-analysis. *J. Med. Genet.*, **41**, 360–5.

Yokota, T., Tachizawa, T., Fukino, K., Teramoto, A., Kouno, J., Matsumoto, K. & Emi, M. (2003). A family with spinal anaplastic ependymoma: evidence of loss of chromosome 22q in tumor. *J. Hum. Genet.*, **48**(11), 598–602.

Yonemoto, R.H. et al. (1969). Familial polyposis of the entire gastrointestinal tract. *Arch. Surg.*, **99**, 427–34.

Yong, D., Lim, J.G., Choi, J.R. et al. (2000). A case of Klinefelter syndrome with retroperitoneal teratoma. *Yonsei. Med. J.*, **41**, 136–9.

Yotsumoto, S., Hashignchi, T. & Chen, X. (2003). Novel mutations in GJBZ encoding connexin 26 in Japanese patients with keratitis–ichthyosis–deafness syndrome. *Br. J. Dermatol.*, **148**, 649–53.

Youinou, P., Le Goff, P., Saleun, J.P. et al. (1978). Familial occurrence of monoclonal gammopathies. *Biomedicine*, **28**, 226–32.

Yu, C.E., Oshima, J., Fu, Y.H. et al. (1996). Positional cloning of the Werner's syndrome gene. *Science*, **272**, 258–62.

Yuan, S.S.F., Lee, S.Y., Chen, G., Song, M.H., Tomlinson, G.E. & Lee, E.Y.H.P. (1999). BRCA2 is required for ionizing radiation-induced assembly of rad51 complex in vivo. *Cancer Res.*, **59**, 3547–51.

Yuasa, H., Tokito, S. & Tokunaga, M. (1993). Primary carcinoma of the choroid plexus in Li–Fraumeni syndrome: case report. *Neurosurgery*, **32**, 131–3.

Zbar, B., Tory, K., Merino, M. et al. (1994). Hereditary papillary renal carcinoma. *J. Urol.*, **151**, 561–6.

Zbar, B., Glenn, G., Lubensky, I. et al. (1995). Hereditary papillary renal cell carcinoma: clinical studies in 10 families. *J. Urol.*, **153**, 907–12.

Zbar, B., Alvord, W.G., Glenn, G., Turner, M., Pavlovich, C.P., Schmidt, L., Walther, M., Choyke, P., Weirich, G., Hewitt, S.M., Duray, P., Gabril, F., Greenberg, C., Merino, M.J., Toro, J. & Linehan, W.M. (2002). Risk of renal and colonic neoplasms and spontaneous pneumothorax in the Birt–Hogg–Dube syndrome. *Cancer Epidemiol. Biomark. Prev.*, **11**(4), 393–400.

Zha, S., Yegnasubramin, V., Nelson, W.G. et al. (2004). Cyclooxygenases in cancer: progress and perspective. *Cancer Lett.*, **215**, 1–20.

Zhang, W., Bailey-Wilson, J.E., Li, W., Wang, X., Zhang, C., Mao, X., Liu, Z., Zhou, C. & Wu, M. (2000). Segregation analysis of esophageal cancer in a moderately high-incidence area of northern China. *Am. J. Hum. Genet.*, **67**(1), 110–19.

Zhanq, Q., Zhao, B., Li, W. et al. (2002). Ru 2 & Ru encode some of the genes mutated in human Hermansky–Pudlak syndrome. *Nat. Genet.*, **33**, 145–53.

Zhong, Q. et al. (1999). Association of BRCA1 with the hRad50–hMre11–p95 complex and the DNA damage response. *Science*, **285**(5428), 747–50.

Zhou, X.P., Marsh, D.J., Hampel, H., Mulliken, J.B., Gimm, O. & Eng, C. (2000). Germline and germline mosaic mutations associated with a Proteus-like syndrome of hemihypertrophy, lower limb asymmetry, arterio-venous malformations and lipomatosis. *Hum. Mol. Genet.*, **9**, 765–8.

Zhou, X.P., Hampel, H., Thiele, H. et al. (2001a). Association of germline mutation in the *PTEN* tumour suppressor gene and a subset of Proteus sand Proteus-like syndromes. *Lancet*, **358**, 210–1.

Zhou, X.P., Woodford-Richens, K., Lehtonen, R. et al. (2001b). Germline mutations in *BMPR1A/ALK3* cause a subset of juvenile polyposis syndrome and of Cowden and Bannayan–Riley–Ruvalcaba syndromes. *Am. J. Hum. Genet.*, **69**, 704–11.

Zhou, X.P., Kuismanen, S., Nyström-Lahti, M., Peltomaki, P. & Eng, C. (2002). Distinct *PTEN* mutational spectra in endometrial carcinomas from hereditary non-polyposis colorectal cancer cases compared to sporadic microsatellite unstable tumors. *Hum. Mol. Genet.*, **11**, 445–50.

Zhou, X.P., Marsh, D.J., Morrison, C.D., Maxwell, M., Reifenberger, G. & Eng, C. (2003a). Germline and somatic PTEN mutations and decreased expression of PTEN protein and dysfunction of the PI3K/Akt pathway in Lhermitte-Duclos disease. *Am. J. Hum. Genet.*, **73**, 1191–8.

Zhou, X.P., Waite, K.A., Pilarski, R. et al. (2003b). Germline *PTEN* promoter mutations and deletions in Cowden/Bannayan–Riley–Ruvalcaba syndrome result in aberrant PTEN protein and dysregulation of the phosphoinositol-3-kinase/Akt pathway. *Am. J. Hum. Genet.*, **73**, 404–11.

Zhu, G., Duffy, D., Eldridge, A. et al. (1999). A major quantitative-trait locus for mole density is linked to the familial melanoma gene CDKN2A: a maximum-likelihood combined linkage and association analysis in twins and their sibs. *Am. J. Hum. Genet.*, **65**, 483–92.

Zhu, X., Dunn, J.M., Phillips, R.A. et al. (1989). Preferential germline mutation of the paternal allele in retinoblastoma. *Nature*, **340**, 312–14.

Zhuang, Z., Vortmeyer, A.O., Pack, S. et al. (1997). Somatic mutations of the *MEN1* tumor suppressor gene in sporadic gastrinomas and insulinomas. *Cancer Res.*, **57**, 4682–6.

Zipursky, A., Poon, A. & Doyle, J. (1992). Leukemia in Down syndrome. *Pediatr. Hematol. Oncol.*, **9**, 139–49.

Zuccurello, D., Salpietro, D.C., Gangemi, S. et al. (2002). Familial chronic nail candidiasis with ICAM-1 deficiency: a new form of chronic mucocutaneous candidiasis. *J. Med. Genet.*, **39**, 671–5.

Zugel, N.P., Hehl, J.A., Jechart, G. et al. (2001). Colorectal carcinoma in Cronkhite–Canada syndrome. *Z. Gastroenterol.*, **39**, 365–7.

Zuo, L., Weger, J., Yang, Q. et al. (1996). Germline mutations in the p16INK4a binding domain of CDK4 in familial melanoma. *Nat. Genet.*, **12**, 97–9.

Zuppan, P., Hall, J.M., Lee, M.K. et al. (1991). Possible linkage of estrogen receptor gene to breast cancer in a family with late-onset disease. *Am. J. Hum. Genet.*, **48**, 1065–8.

Zwetsloot, C.P., Kros, J.M. & Paz y Geuze, H.D. (1991). Familial occurrence of tumours of the choroid plexus. *J. Med. Genet.*, **28**, 492–4.

Index

Note: page numbers in *italics* refer to figures and tables